Critical Acclaim
for *Betrayed as Boys*

"This volume provides important tools not only for clinicians working with individuals, families and groups, but also for educators and others interested in psychodynamic perspectives on trauma, gender, and sexuality." —*Digest of Neurology and Psychiatry*

"[A] comprehensive, insightful book. . . . Should be of great interest to all therapists working in this burgeoning area of clinical practice." —*American Journal of Psychotherapy*

"The author provides in-depth analysis of the effect of sexual abuse on boys/men and provides a sophisticated tying together of the cultural, developmental, and personality factors influencing the patients' adjustment. . . . This book adds to the literature of an underexplored area. . . . Upper-division undergraduates through professionals." —*Choice*

"A welcome addition to the emerging literature on healing and recovery for men who were sexually abused as children. [Gartner's] clear and articulate style of writing makes this book interesting to read and easy to digest. Although this material is written primarily for clinicians, it is clearly understandable for a wide range of readers, and therefore accessible to those sexually abused men who seek to know more about the intricacies of their own therapy process. The book is comprehensive in its scope and builds on a thorough review of existing research and literature. The author maintains a careful blend of research citations and clinical vignettes. By integrating existing research with his own clinical observations and practical experiences, Gartner powerfully nudges the reader toward application rather than theoretical pondering. . . . Clinicians who read this book will be invigorated to apply what they have learned to their work with male clients who have histories of sexual abuse." —*Journal of Contemporary Psychotherapy*

BETRAYED
AS
BOYS

Psychodynamic Treatment of Sexually Abused Men

RICHARD B. GARTNER

THE GUILFORD PRESS
New York   London

Published by The Guilford Press
A Division of Guilford Publications, Inc.
72 Spring Street, New York, NY 10012
http://www.guilford.com

Printed in the United States of America

This book is printed on acid-free paper.

Last digit is print number: 9 8 7 6 5 4

Library of Congress Cataloging-in-Publication Data

Gartner, Richard B.
  Betrayed as boys : psychodynamic treatment of sexually
    abused men / Richard B. Gartner.
      p.   cm.
    Includes bibliographical references and index.
    ISBN 1-57230-467-7 (hc.)   ISBN 1-57230-644-0 (pbk.)
    1. Adult child sexual abuse victims.   2. Male sexual abuse
  victims.   3. Psychodynamic psychotherapy.   I. Title.
    [DNLM: 1. Psychotherapy—in adulthood.   2. Child Abuse,
  Sexual—therapy.   3. Men—psychology.   WM 420 G244b 1999]
  RC569.5.A28G37   1999
  616.85′83690651—dc21
  DNLM/DLC
  for Library of Congress   98-55694
                                                                     CIP

*Dedicated to the memory of
Benjamin Wolstein
(1922–1998),
whose capacity for
emotional presence,
interpersonal engagement,
and intellectual persistence
astounded me,
infused me,
and helped me become the
psychoanalyst and person I am.*

About the Author

Richard B. Gartner, PhD, trained as both a family therapist and an inter-personal psychoanalyst. A graduate of the William Alanson White Insti-tute in New York City, he is now the Director of the Institute's Center for the Study of Psychological Trauma as well as founder and Director of the Sexual Abuse Program that operates under the Center's auspices. He has written and spoken extensively on the treatment of men sexually abused as boys, and is the editor of *Memories of Sexual Betrayal: Truth, Fantasy, Repression, and Dissociation* (Jason Aronson, 1997). Dr. Gart-ner is a Supervisor of Psychotherapy and on the teaching faculty at the White Institute; is a consultant and supervisor at the Center for Abuse and Incest at the Manhattan Institute for Psychoanalysis; is on the edito-rial boards of *Contemporary Psychoanalysis* and the *American Journal of Psychoanalysis*; and serves on the Board of Directors of the National Organization on Male Sexual Victimization. He practices in Manhattan and Brooklyn.

Acknowledgments

This book was first conceived in Philadelphia in 1992. I was attending a meeting of the Division of Psychoanalysis of the American Psychological Association to present the first paper I had written about male sexual victimization. While in Philadelphia, I met Sue Shapiro, Mary Gail Frawley (now Frawley-O'Dea), and Jody Messler Davies, who were all presenting papers related to the sexual abuse of girls. Jody and Mary Gail had together recently published an important article on dissociation and were in the midst of writing their book on treating sexually abused women. Over a long dinner, during which we shared much about our professional and personal lives, Jody and Sue commented on the paucity of literature about sexually abused men and their treatment. They encouraged me to write a book about my work, and, basking in the warmth of new friendship, collegiality, and a very good bottle of wine, I agreed.

Thus began a long journey. These three colleagues have been wonderfully encouraging in diverse ways throughout this process, and Dr. Shapiro has written a thoughtful and evocative contribution that appears as part of Chapter 10. Among others who treat sexually abused adults, Michelle Price, Ernesto Mujica, David Lisak, and Elizabeth Hegeman have also been especially generous with their thoughts, ideas, and support.

For the past few years, I have had the great fortune to have two professional homes. First, I was given the opportunity to allow my ideas to gestate in the receptive milieu of the William Alanson White Institute's

Sexual Abuse Program. I thank Marylou Lionells, the Institute's director, for developing its tradition of pragmatic psychoanalysis into the Center for the Study of Psychological Trauma, and for naming me director of the Center as well as of the Sexual Abuse Program that flourishes within it. The ongoing presence of the psychoanalysts from the Sexual Abuse Program in our monthly clinical seminars has helped me shape my thoughts and gain the courage to do very difficult work; I wish to thank my colleagues Arlene McKay, Olga Cheselka, Julie Marcuse, Helene Kafka, Jill Bellinson, Sarah Stemp, Margit Winckler, Karen Marisak, Tina Harrell, Elizabeth Halsted, Berryl Fox, Carol Albert, Anton Hart, Daniel Gensler, Elena Skolnick, Chris Russo, Evelyn Hartman, Eric Dammann, Meryl Weinman, Dodi Goldman, Bert Schaffner, Judd Bortner, and Rebecca Curtis, in addition to Drs. Mujica and Hegeman.

My second professional home is in the National Organization on Male Sexual Victimization (NOMSV), which has given me a rare and cherished national and international network of friends and colleagues. Their intense commitment, their emotional warmth and accessibility, and their willingness to share their considerable expertise and wisdom in a nonhierarchical manner have offered me a safe venue in which to develop new ideas and thrive. Michael Castellana, Randy Fitzgerald, Howard Fradkin, Andrew Mai, Tom Rini, Karl Trappe, Mary Froning, Ken Singer, Larry Morris, Jim Struve, Mic Hunter, Peter Dimock, Neal King, Eugene Porter, Chris Carracher, Don Wright, Mikele Rauch, John Jones, Bill Maloney, Shawn Sullivan, Matthew Gilbert, Fred Tolson, Dave McCall, and Neil Cabe have all become very dear to me.

Over the years, I have presented aspects of my work in many locales. As my ideas have evolved, they have been sharpened, enriched, and strengthened by responsive audiences who heard me speak under the auspices of the William Alanson White Institute; the National Organization on Male Sexual Victimization; Divisions 39 (Psychoanalysis) and 51 (Men and Masculinity) of the American Psychological Association; the Manhattan Institute for Psychoanalysis; the Postgraduate Center for Mental Health; the Institute for Contemporary Psychotherapy; New York University; Adelphi University; Columbia University; Vassar College; Oberlin College; Manhattan Psychiatric Center; the Psychoanalytic Connection; the International Society for Traumatic Stress Studies; the hospital-based rape intervention programs in New York City; the National Organization for Men against Sexism; the Harm Reduction Coalition; the Learning Alliance of New York; the Sandor Ferenczi Society of Budapest; and the Eastern Group Psychotherapy Society. I thank them all.

Since 1982, I have met weekly with a small group of extraordinary colleagues who became close friends. The Viceroys, as we informally call ourselves, have been unshakable and loving in their affirmation of my work. John O'Leary was the first to insist that I write about my clinical ideas. Mark Blechner and Sandra Buechler have been careful, encouraging, and astute readers of virtually every professional paper I have written since we met. Allison Stern Rosen and Robert Watson have likewise been steadfast in their support.

I thank Jane Gartner, Karen Saakvitne, Karen Hopenwasser, and Sue Bronson, in addition to Drs. Frawley-O'Dea, Buechler, Lisak, Blechner, Shapiro, and Hegeman, for their willingness to read and comment perceptively on parts or all of my manuscript.

I also wish to thank Jim Hopper, Steven Knoblauch, Sue Grand, James Cassese, Emily McNally, Ron Winchel, Jack Drescher, Michelle Sidrane, Muriel Dimen, Adrienne Harris, Tony Sidoti, Kathleen White, Sondra Wilk, and Brian Donoghue for their help and support at various points in the development of *Betrayed as Boys*.

Kitty Moore at The Guilford Press has been a wonderful editor who knew when to be sympathetic and when to tell me to just do it. Both attitudes were truly supportive.

The men I write about in this book were my collaborators in a very direct way. I thank them all: Abe, Andreas, Beau, Bruno, Chet, Cory, David, Devin, Ed, Ezra, Felix, Frank, Gene, Greg, Harris, Hugo, Ira, Isaac, Jared, Julian, Keith, Kyle, Lewis, Lorenzo, Max, Neal, Owen, Patrick, Quinn, Ramon, Seth, Teo, Uri, Victor, Willem, Xavier, Yale, and Zak.

During the countless hours that I devoted to *Betrayed as Boys,* Jane, Josh, and Elana each maintained a capacity for humor and communicated an immense pride in my efforts. Certainly they behaved with more grace and generosity than I think I could have summoned up under similar circumstances. They helped me focus my thinking, solved MacIntosh mysteries for me, and gave me a nurturing space in which my ideas could germinate and bloom. To merely say thank you to them is to demonstrate the inadequacy of language to convey emotional meaning. I am so grateful for their presence in my life!

Contents

Introduction

In 1988, I started treating the first man I specifically conceptualized as having been sexually abused in boyhood. I had been in practice for more than fifteen years, as a dynamically oriented psychotherapist, as a systems-oriented family therapist, and finally as an interpersonal psychoanalyst. In retrospect, I realize that patient, whom I call Patrick in my clinical descriptions later in this book, was certainly not the first man I treated who had a history of childhood sexual betrayal. He was not even the first to tell me about inappropriate or unwanted premature sexual experiences with older friends, relatives, or caretakers. I was, however, a product of my own training and a prevailing conventional wisdom among clinicians that such stories should be treated cautiously because of the likelihood that they emerged from patients' fantasy lives and wish fulfillments. So, while I had not doubted my patients' stories, I also had not encoded them as descriptions of sexual abuse. Nor had I thought about patterns of behavior common in men with histories of childhood sexual betrayal.

My work with Patrick proved to be a watershed for me. As he slowly began to recall horrifying stories of sexual abuse in early childhood, I was forced to rethink how to understand them. If they were entirely fantasies, then Patrick was floridly psychotic, which I did not believe. But if his stories were even partly true, then he had been the victim of grievous crimes perpetrated by his father and brother. As time went on, the picture became fuller as his sister confirmed that she too had been sexually abused by their father. My doubts about Patrick's stories dissipated. Instead, I began to think about how his adult symptoms of recurrent depression, night terrors about a stranger breaking into his room, obsessive but impersonal sexual fantasies, long-term isolation, and difficulties in interpersonal relationships all made sense in the context of chronic sexual abuse in early childhood.

In time, I educated myself about the literature on childhood sexual abuse, which focuses mainly on women. As I sought help from colleagues, my interest in sexually abused men[1] grew, and I began to get referrals of other men (and women) with similar histories. More referrals came when I started a group for these men after I could not find one in New York City for Patrick.

Once I began to work with men who defined themselves as having been sexually abused, I started to think about other patients differently. I was more likely to inquire into their early sexual histories. Interestingly, more patients told me about inappropriately sexual childhood histories without my ever asking. My receptivity about the subject had in some way been communicated to them.

When a patient I had treated for several years during and after my psychoanalytic training returned to see me after an absence of some five years, I was especially struck by how much my thinking had been transformed. He reminded me that just before he stopped treatment he had asked whether I thought he might have had a history of boyhood sexual abuse, even though he had no actual memories of it. Confused about how to explore this possibility in the absence of memories, I had given an equivocal response. He now told me that shortly thereafter he stopped the treatment "in despair."

Yet I now realized how limited my thinking had been. This man's symptom picture, which included obsessive and compulsive sexuality, masochism, cross-dressing, and severe interpersonal isolation and distrust, was certainly consonant with a history of childhood sexual abuse. Nevertheless, I had never thought in such terms during his earlier treatment. Nor had it ever been brought up by any of the four excellent teachers and supervisors to whom I had presented my work with him while in training.

My work with this man in his second treatment sequence did not reveal overt childhood sexual abuse. Nevertheless, the incestuous sexuality and abusiveness he witnessed in his extended family came to the forefront as inappropriately stimulating. From this, I came to see him as having suffered a covert sexual betrayal as a boy.

---

[1] I have chosen wherever possible to use the term "sexually abused man" rather than the words "victim" or "survivor" as I discuss this population. I consider both of these to be overused and limiting terms that diminish the uniqueness of the individual with a sexual abuse history. See Hunter and Gerber (1990) for a discussion of them.

This is the kind of pattern I was now able to recognize and work with in my male patients. Sexual abuse is certainly not a universal experience for boys, nor is it the explanation in every case for complex symptomatic pictures like those I describe in this book. It is, however, far more often present in boys' histories than any of us would like to believe.

Incest and the sexual abuse of children have long been taboo and misunderstood subjects in the popular culture and in the clinical literature. Sexual victimization of all children has chronically been denied in our society. The sexual victimization of boys, however, is even more universally minimized, underestimated, and ridiculed than the abuse of girls, for reasons I will discuss throughout this book, but especially in Chapters 2 and 3.[2]

Perhaps these social views of male sexual victimization have started to change as stories about boys' sexual victimization gain greater currency in the popular press. I will discuss in Chapter 2 the well-publicized cases of two women brought up on child rape charges for their sexual involvement with boys. Scandals have also been widely reported about extrafamilial victimization of boys by men in church, scouting, Internet, child care, and sports venues. I refer here to such stories as:

- The sexual abuse of young boys by Catholic priests and seminarians in such diverse locations as Maryland, California, and Texas, leading to numerous guilty pleas and successful civil suits (*New York Times,* December 2, 1993, p. A18; *New York Times,* October 21, 1995, p. I10; *New York Times,* July 25, 1997, pp. A1, A23);
- The multiple successful suits against the Boy Scouts of America brought by former scouts and their families because of sexual abuse by scoutmasters (Boyle, 1994);
- The criminal convictions and financial settlements in Newfoundland and Ontario during the 1980s and early 1990s following the revelation of sexual, emotional, and physical abuse by Christian Brothers of hundreds of boys confined to training schools (Henton and McCann, 1995);
- The male nanny who pled guilty to abusing a twelve-year-old boy in Armonk, New York, while already on probation for abusing a nine-year-old boy in Greenwich, Connecticut (*New York Times,* September 26, 1996, p. B6);

---

[2] The sexual victimization of adult men is also a compelling issue that is often minimized. However, it is beyond the scope of this book. For an extended discussion of the rape of adult men, see Scarce's *Male on Male Rape* (1997; see also Mezey and King, 1992).

- The guilty plea of a Canadian hockey coach accused of molesting several young hockey players, followed by the further accusation by National Hockey League player Sheldon Kennedy that he too had been abused by this coach as a teenager (*New York Times*, January 4, 1997, p. I34, and January 16, 1997, p. A10), in turn followed by the arrest and subsequent conviction of Toronto Maple Leaf Garden employees who lured at least twenty-four boys into exchanging sex for hockey tickets, hockey sticks, and player autographs (*New York Times*, February 20, 1997, p. B19); and

- The controversy when a teenage boy accused of sexually assaulting and murdering an eleven-year-old boy was revealed to have been himself abused by an adult man he met in an America On-Line chat room (*New York Times*, October 3, 1997, p. B6).

Interestingly, in each of these stories the victimizer came from outside the family. This does reflect some research findings that most abused boys suffer from extrafamilial victimization. Incestuous abuse of boys is virtually never reported in the press, however, even though its prevalence is also well documented, as we will see in Chapter 1. Indeed, denial of the extent of childhood incest has been almost universal in our society. There is a deep cultural taboo against accepting how common it is. To believe in the widespread incidence of incest is to question the sanctity of the family, where children are thought to be protected from harm.

The pervasiveness of the denial of childhood sexual betrayal, especially the sexual abuse of boys, was illuminated for me several years ago. I was invited to an international conference to give a paper about the treatment of sexually abused men. Just as I was leaving for the foreign city that was hosting the meeting, the conference program arrived. My paper was not listed in it. Surprised, I called the program chair when I arrived. He did not remember me or my paper. At that moment, I felt the sense of unreality that patients have told me they experience in the face of their family's denial of ongoing sexual abuse. Flustered and confused after a day-long flight, I momentarily wondered if I was mistaken about the initial request to read my paper. I grounded myself when I realized that the conference chair's letter of invitation was in my hand as I spoke to him. He apologized and found a place for me on a panel at the meeting, albeit one on which none of the other papers related to mine. The addition of my paper to the program was announced once at the conference opening, but was not listed on any of the notices posted around the meeting rooms until I insisted. At the panel itself, the moderator, an American scholar and psychoanalyst, permitted the speaker before me to continue for fifteen minutes beyond his allotted twenty-five. Seven minutes after I began to talk about the experiences of sexually abused men, however, this moderator handed me a note that read "Can you wrap this up? We're supposed to be having a coffee break now." Luckily, several colleagues in the audience protested that they wanted to hear my paper.

These events were not directed at me personally. At first, I thought my experience arose from the overall disorganization of the conference itself. Now, however, I realize that hearing about boyhood sexual abuse is intolerable to many of us. Our unconscious reactions affect how we feel, how we act, and how we enact.

Stories of childhood sexual abuse have been central to acrimonious debates as long as psychological treatment itself has existed. This started when Freud's early work on hysteria (Breuer and Freud, 1893–1895; Freud, 1896) was followed by his retreat from the so-called seduction theory. Later, there was a notorious dispute between him and his closest and most gifted student, Sandor Ferenczi, after Ferenczi (1933) wrote a paper, "Confusion of Tongues between Adults and the Child," that cogently described how sexual trauma affects a child in later life. In the decades that followed, childhood incest and other childhood sexual betrayals were relegated to the realm of fantasy throughout the psychoanalytic, psychiatric, and psychological literatures. As recently as 1976, a leading psychiatric textbook claimed that actual incest between father and daughter occurred only once in a million cases (Freedman, Kaplan, and Sadock, 1976).

Since 1980, however, the pendulum has been swinging away from the fantasy theory about sexual betrayal, and a rich literature has emerged in both the psychoanalytic and trauma-based arenas of sexual abuse work. This literature, in turn, has stimulated new controversy. In particular, criticism has been made by those who felt too easy credence was given to patients' vague memories or to therapists' feelings that abuse took place.

It is indeed possible both for memories of abuse that have been long forgotten to be remembered and for adults to construct pseudomemories for events that never occurred (Alpert et al., 1994; see also Lindsay and Read, 1994). I have elsewhere edited a book that considers this complex controversy about memories of sexual betrayal (Gartner, 1997c). In this book, unless otherwise noted, I accept the patient's memory as basically true, though not necessarily representing a point-to-point, literal, videotape-like recollection. Such recall is rare when any adult remembers what happened at a developmentally early stage of life. Instead, I believe the essence of my patients' stories, which usually means that severe boundary violations took place, some of a specifically and explicitly sexual nature, and that frequently the abusers were trusted parents and caretakers (see Hedges, 1994).

This is a book about what happens to boys who grow up in pernicious circumstances, often in a family where incestuous boundary violations repeatedly recur. It is also about the psychotherapeutic treatment of these boys when they become men who at last must face their abusive histories. Finally, it is about the inner experience of therapists who try to draw on their skill and inner resources as they evolve in very complex treatment situations.

In my discussion, I will draw on the existing body of literature about sexually abused men and illustrate from my own clinical practice how these themes recur in psychodynamic psychotherapy and psychoanalysis with them.[3] Many of the stories of abuse recounted in this book are difficult to read. They were difficult for me to hear and believe when my patients told them. I have tried to convey the horror of these men's boyhood abuse, giving details of the sexual activity involved without sensationalizing it. Readers themselves may experience some measure of the trauma involved as they reflect on what these men endured as boys.

Soon after I started writing this book, I attended a conference about male sexual victimization. I had been floundering to find my voice as I wrote, unsure of who my audience really was. At the conference, I met three men and one woman who allowed me to find my focus. I wrote this book trying to speak to these individuals and others like them.

The first was a graduate student in science at a university in a western state, a young man who had only recently begun to realize the extent of his boyhood sexual betrayal. He had found an understanding therapist, but had not told anyone else about his abuse. Nor did he know any other men with sexual abuse histories. He came to the conference with trepidation, and there he was amazed to find a community of (mostly) men who seemed to understand the issues he had struggled with in virtual solitude. He was exhilarated when we met, saying he was happy and feeling more freely connected to others than he ever had before.

The second man was a therapist from a small city in the Midwest. He was experienced in treating a wide range of individuals, and was clearly earnest and serious about his work. A growing number of men with sexual abuse histories were coming into his practice, and he found that the principles of therapy he had learned during his training did not always seem to apply to his work with them. The professional books he had consulted helped some, but they concentrated mainly on sexually

---

[3] The case descriptions in this book have been disguised to preserve the men's anonymity. Identifying features have been changed if I felt such changes would not betray the integrity of the story being told. In all cases, pseudonyms are used.

abused women, and their framework only partially fit the work he was doing with men. He tried networking with other professionals in the conservative community he lived in. Many seemed not to understand that men could be sexually abused and felt he was on some private, quixotic mission, possibly for dark countertransferential reasons. Some therapists who worked with female rape victims were more helpful, but others seemed to believe that men were rarely if ever abused, and that any man coming for treatment about abuse was himself an abuser. Feeling professionally isolated and overburdened, he turned to the Internet for information. There, he found several useful web sites, and also saw a notice for the conference where we met. It was scheduled to begin two weeks later. Quickly changing his vacation schedule, he traveled across the country to this meeting. It was a revelation for him to talk there to other therapists who for years had been grappling with issues related to male sexual victimization. In workshop after workshop, he learned more and more about work with this population, discovered he had a lot to offer other practitioners about treatment, and found a clinician in a city about three hours away from him who was experienced in working with sexually abused men and was willing to serve as a consultant and supervisor when they returned home.

The third man was an experienced psychoanalytically trained therapist from a southeastern community. Of retirement age, he said he came to the conference for help in writing an article about treating patients with trauma histories. At first, his comments at presentations focused on the intellectual and didactic components of what was being addressed. He seemed to be trying to minimize or deflect others from the wells of feeling that were being tapped by the material. After listening to both therapists and nonclinicians express their emotional responses to what they were hearing, he rigidified his intellectualized approach until he was confronted about this by another member of a workshop he took. He grew silent, then, astonishingly, began to weep. He poured out the story of his own childhood sexual abuse. In the fifty or more years since these experiences, he had never hinted about them to another soul except his analyst, and even then he apparently had minimized their impact. By the end of the conference, he found several kindred spirits, seemed looser and far more open, and also achieved his initial goal of learning more about the psychological impact of trauma.

The fourth person I met at the conference was a woman who worked at a rape intervention program in a big inner-city hospital. Her agency, originally dedicated to working with women sexually mistreated as adults or children, was treating increasing numbers of men with sexual abuse histories. She saw many of these men for brief therapy, and also ran short-term groups for them, sometimes with a male colleague and sometimes alone. The men resembled in important ways the women she was used to treating. She had grown increasingly aware, however, of differences between the two groups, and had come to this conference to crystallize her thinking in order to work better with a male population.

As I address a readership of individuals like these four, my writing, like my clinical work, is informed by my background in interpersonal psychoanalysis,[4] family systems theory, and work with trauma. I expect readers to have had diverse professional and theoretical experiences, and I therefore discuss theory and research that will be new to some but familiar to others. In particular, I have emphasized the theoretical underpinnings that influence my understanding of such important issues as masculine gender identity, sexual orientation, family systems, dissociative processes, and transference/countertransference phenomena. These theoretical discussions are interlaced with the clinical examples that appear throughout the book.

This book is structured as follows: In the first chapter, terms are explained, research is summarized, and the population of men described in the book is defined. The second, third, and fourth chapters develop ideas about how boys are likely to encode premature sexual situations with women as well as with men, and how these processes interact with internalized ideas about masculinity and homosexuality. The fifth and sixth chapters analyze the familial and interpersonal contexts of abuse and their influence on a boy's responses to sexual trauma. The seventh chapter describes the dissociative process that often helps a child survive an initial abuse experience, but then is problematic if it becomes his characteristic way of dealing with stress. The eighth chapter demonstrates how early sexual trauma, chronic boundary violation, and dissociation all influence an adult man's interpersonal relatedness. The ninth and tenth chapters focus on the vicissitudes of therapeutic relationships with sexually abused men. The eleventh chapter concentrates on working with sexually abused men in group therapy.

My writing is deeply influenced by my belief that, for most sexually abused men in psychotherapy and psychoanalysis, symptom removal is not nearly sufficient as a goal. Instead, these men want and need to develop a more nearly consolidated sense of self, a greater attunement to their emotional lives, and an increased ability to develop and maintain a

---

[4] Interpersonal psychoanalytic theory, emphasizing the influence of actual interpersonal experiences on personality and the therapeutic relationship, is based on the work of Harry Stack Sullivan and Erich Fromm, among others. It is closely identified with relational psychoanalytic theory, which adds to it aspects of object relations theory, stemming from Melanie Klein's work. The terms are often used interchangeably, as I do at times in this book.

tie with an intimate other. And, I believe, this is most likely to happen in a therapeutic experience that carefully examines the relational aspects of all actions and internal psychological events.

I do not intend to dictate to clinicians about how men sexually abused as boys should be treated. To try to write such a book would do a deep disservice to the uniqueness, complexity, and ambiguities of each man's life trajectory and individuality. It would compartmentalize the diverse experiences my patients had as boys who were sexually betrayed and, later, as men who dealt with their sexual betrayals in singular ways. It would also falsely imply that I work the same way with men with similar histories.

Instead, my intention is to raise, delineate, and develop the themes that often face the man with such a history and the clinician working with him. I expect that each therapist treating this population will develop distinct styles of working, based partly on the subpopulation he or she treats; partly on his or her own personality as well as theoretical and professional interests; and partly on the life situation of the man in therapy.

When I'm in my consulting room with a sexually abused man, the themes I outline in this book usually recede into the background as the intricacies of his specific situation, history, and character become the foreground of our work. No one is fully defined by an abuse history. In my clinical illustrations, therefore, I do not limit myself to issues directly related to sexual betrayal. Instead, I try to describe individuals as they revealed themselves to me, communicating the diversity, fullness, and uniqueness of each treatment situation. (Readers wishing to integrate multiple descriptions of these men may want to consult the Appendix: Cross-References to Personal Histories, pp. 325–326.) Inevitably, however, my portrayals lose some of the distinctiveness and complexity of each man and of our work together as I use them to highlight a particular theme or technique. For this, I apologize both to the reader and to the men I discuss.

Most of all, I give my heartfelt thanks to those who gave me permission to describe our work. My relationships with the thirty-eight men I have written about in this book have moved me and changed how I look at human interaction. These men have courageously faced terrifying pasts. As I once wrote, "Their stories have stirred me, their resolution in the face of their histories has astonished me. I have learned from them more than I can say" (Gartner, 1997c, p. xiv).

CHAPTER 1

———◆———

The Sexual Betrayal of Boys

He sat in the chair opposite me, a college-educated professional in his late thirties, intelligent and responsible. He sounded like a man who had achieved every goal he had set for himself: a successful career, an enduring marriage, two young children he loved. In many ways, he seemed to have followed a direct path toward the good life. Yet, as he emotionlessly told me the story of his childhood and adolescence, he revealed that underneath this splendid facade lay a hidden abscess filled with as-yet-unfelt anguish.

Gene[1] grew up in a working-class home, the son of hard-working parents. He and his sisters never wanted for material things. On the surface, their parents' relationship looked no different from that of many couples of their class and ethnic background. There was little affection between the two, but that was not unusual, as Gene understood things. He never thought about the emotional deadness between them. On the contrary, he had been glad his home was not the scene of the domestic violence characteristic of others in his neighborhood. But at least three times a week from the time he was eight until Gene finally put a stop to it at age nineteen, he and his father silently engaged in mutual oral sexual activity.

It was not necessary for Gene's father to use physical force to abuse

---

[1] For a comprehensive listing of the multiple descriptions of the men in this book, the reader is directed to the Appendix: Cross-References to Personal Histories following the Afterword.

his son. Instead, he trained Gene from an early age to accept molestations as part of his daily routine, and even to look forward to the mixture of closeness and arousal in their encounters. Gene's father told him
this was something between the two of them, something not to be discussed with anyone else, and Gene obeyed. Gene said that, as time went
on, he assumed most boys had similar relationships with their fathers,
and believed they all knew not to talk about it to outsiders, including
one another.

Gene did not remember how he felt during the incest. Indeed, he
could not say how he felt through most of his childhood or adulthood.
He grew up isolated socially from both boys and girls, and never had a
date till he was well into his twenties. He did not attempt sexual intercourse with a woman until his wedding night, when he was past thirty.
Looking back, he said he had never let himself think about the abuse. He
had never forgotten what happened, but he had not allowed his memories to become part of his conscious sense of who he was. The price he
had unknowingly paid was a general constriction of behavior, thought,
and emotion.

When his son was born, Gene began to experience disturbing feelings, and found he could not let himself touch the baby except in awk-
ward, stilted ways. He refused to change his son's diapers or to bathe
him, although he had done these things for his older child, a daughter.
He began to feel flashes of anxiety, and images of sex with his father
came unbidden to his mind at odd times. He could hardly talk to his
father when he visited his parents, and suddenly he realized that he was
afraid to leave his son at his parents' home.

The implications of his history unnerved Gene, and he began to feel
he was disintegrating. The next months were tumultuous. He asked himself terrible questions. Why had he allowed the abuse? What kind of
man was he to have permitted such a thing? Should he tell his wife and
his sisters not to leave their children with his father? Should he tell his
ailing mother what had happened? Should he confront his father? What
was the meaning of the images of bondage and homosexual sex that now
flooded his fantasy life? Had his shame about incest and his determination not to let it turn him gay blinded him to his very real sexual and
emotional desire for men? Or were his fantasies some kind of replication
of his abuse experiences? How could he manage the overpowering feelings of rage and despair that possessed him when he allowed himself any
feelings at all? Could he ever go back to the comfortable life he'd led
before these appalling motifs leaped out of his unconscious?

Gene moved in several directions as he struggled. He told his wife, and
then his sisters, about the abuse, and then felt guilty about the abyss this
inevitably created in his extended family's interrelationships. Emotional

agitation and sexual acting out ruptured his relationship with his wife, perhaps permanently. He stopped talking to his father. The father pressed him for a reason, and Gene finally told him. His father professed amazement: "That was such a big deal to you?" The father then became deeply depressed. At first, Gene was glad to have hurt his father. Soon, however, he felt guilty about his father's depression. Indeed, he began to feel responsible for cheering him up. For the moment, he became his father's caretaker and no longer allowed himself to feel angry at him.

Gene's past sexual betrayal had caught up to him and threatened to inundate him completely. His story contained elements common to many sexually abused men's stories: dissociation, isolation, flashbacks, sexual dysfunction, secrecy, shame, emotional and behavioral constriction, fierce rage, fear of being unmanly, and horror of being turned into a homosexual. He had a family whose surface harmony hid dark secrets, and he felt emotionally responsible for a molester who professed to have no idea he had been abusive.

This book is about Gene and the many other men who in manhood are forced to face their sexual betrayal as boys.

BETRAYAL, ABUSE, INCEST, AND TRAUMA

Gene was sexually betrayed by his father. Other equally valid ways to describe his experience are that he was sexually abused, he was a victim of paternal incest, and he was traumatized by premature childhood sexual experiences with his father. Each of these phrases focuses on a different aspect of what happened to Gene. Although in the rest of this book it may at times seem as though I use these terms interchangeably, I will now delineate the differences among them.

"Sexual betrayal" encompasses a greater range of human experience than the more common expressions "sexual abuse," "incest," and "sexual trauma." Put simply, *betrayal* is the violation of implicit or explicit trust. It is by definition an interpersonal experience. The closer and more necessary the relationship in which it appears, the greater the degree of betrayal in the violation (Freyd, 1996). In betrayal, seemingly unbreakable bonds are broken (Cheselka, 1996), and treachery is introduced into the most private, personal, and trusting relationships. The betrayed individual feels jagged, awry, fractured, recklessly hurt. As Cheselka (1996) describes its relational consequences, betrayal is "a violation not only of trust and of the other, but of the sanctity of intimate relationships. . . . *An implicit covenant has been broken or denied.* . . . It changes something fundamental; a belief or a frame of reference from which to view the world of interpersonal relationships" (pp. 3–4). This break in the interpersonal frame of reference is the heart of any betrayal, sexual or otherwise. The effects of personal betrayal on an individual's worldview are profound, and its consequences for future intimate relationships can be disastrous.

Abuse is a potent form of betrayal, and includes an added component of exploitation. When one individual abuses another, the abuser is using a power relationship in order to satisfy his or her own needs without regard to the needs of the person being abused. Abuse comes in many forms. Physical, emotional, and economic abuse often accompany sexual abuse, and they can be equally drastic and heinous in their results. It is sexual abuse, however, that is the primary focus of this book, namely, the childhood sexual abuse of boys and its effects as they grow into men.

Sexual abuse consists of sexual behavior by which the abuser takes advantage of a power differential with a dependent or vulnerable victim in order to satisfy the abuser's own needs. It involves "the misuse of the immature child by the adult for the solving of problems and satisfying adult needs, while disregarding the appropriate needs and developmental state of the child" (B. Steele, 1981, p. 233). These needs take a sexual form, but sexuality is often not the primary underlying motivation. The abuser's motives may include insecurity and a consequent need for power; or an inability to self-soothe in ways not involving sexual aggression; or an inner urgency to have interpersonal contact, even in a distorted, punishing form (see Groth and Oliveri, 1989; Salter, 1995; and Holmes and Slap, 1998, for fuller discussions of the motivations and characteristics of abusers).

When sexual abuse occurs between two adults, there is usually clear physical or psychological coercion. When a child is involved, however, the sexual activity may sometimes appear consensual. At the core of this interaction, however, *assent is not possible*. Children do not have the capacity to give informed consent to sexual activities with adults. Yet children are easily swayed by grown-ups, and abusers, who may or may not be chronological adults, take advantage of this tendency in order to exploit them. A child is not developmentally capable of considering or comprehending the emotional implications of sexual behavior with an adult, especially one who in some way, real or symbolic, has control over the child's fate. As we will see in numerous examples throughout this book, however, many children are incapable of understanding that they could not consent to their abuse. Unfortunately, this leads to an adult conviction that they were responsible for what happened to them.

Thus, all sexual acts between children and people who have power over them are sexually abusive. This is true if the power derives from the actual structure of the relationship (as in the case, for example, of a child abused by a babysitter, teacher, or parent). But it is equally true if the power is inferred by the child because of the age difference between him and the abuser (as in the case, for example, of a young boy abused by a teenager in the neighborhood who is not his caretaker). It is also true no matter how willing the child appears to be to participate in the sexual activity (see Ehrenberg, 1992). "Willing" or not, the child is abused by having the natural developmental unfolding of his sexuality violated and hurried into awareness. His very *childhood* is violated. Occasionally, men have asserted—sometimes convincingly—that they were not hurt by premature sexual experiences with adults. Far more often, however, there are both subtle and obvious negative sequelae.

Incest is a psychologically catastrophic form of sexual abuse. It has even more far-reaching consequences than extrafamilial sexual abuse because it occurs, often chronically, in the context of a family system that somehow supports it. This is particularly true when the abuser is a parent, because the child grows up chronically trapped in at least one twisted primary relationship. Incest therefore constitutes betrayal at a most profound level.

However, although usually thought of as sexual activity between near blood relatives, incest can also be construed in a larger sense as any "violation of a position of power, trust, and protection" (Lew, 1988, p. 16). By this broad definition, *any* older caretaker who sexually betrays a child is committing a form of incest. For the child, the result may be nearly the same as betrayal by a parent: a shattering of the natural trust he has in the adults who care for him.

Betrayal, abuse, and incest are interpersonal concepts that comment on the nature of the relationship between abuser and victim. By contrast, *trauma*—and in general I am referring to psychological rather than physical trauma—refers to the effect of the betrayal on the victim. Trauma is a reaction to an overwhelming life experience. Traumatic events are unexpected, unusual, often coming without warning, exceeding a person's capacity to deal with them and seriously disrupting his or her psychological stability and frame of reference (McCann and Pearlman, 1990).

REACTIONS TO ABUSE AND TRAUMA

No specific clinical picture points incontrovertibly to childhood sexual trauma. Nevertheless, common symptoms of psychological trauma appear regularly in both women and men with sexual abuse histories. These effects have been widely documented. They include severe interpersonal isolation, complex relational difficulties, and posttraumatic stress disorder (PTSD).

PTSD is a syndrome with a well-known cluster of symptoms (see Figley, 1985, 1986; van der Kolk, 1987, 1995, 1996; van der Kolk and Greenberg, 1987; van der Kolk, McFarlane, and Weisaeth, 1996; Herman, 1992; Saigh, 1992). It may occur as an immediate response to a traumatic situation, or its onset may be delayed for months or even years. A prime characteristic of PTSD is hyperarousal, often accompanied by intrusive thoughts, that is, flashbacks in any sensory modality that come unbidden, often repetitively. These may take the form of nightmares or night terrors in which the trauma is relived either realistically or symbolically. Consider these examples of hyperarousal in PTSD symptoms from the cases I discuss in this book: Cory had a flashback during sex with his wife, suddenly seeing his mother's face on her after she touched him in a particular way. He leaped up and pushed his wife away, shouting, "Don't touch me!" Patrick had night terrors about a stranger breaking into his room. He installed multiple locks on his door at home and took special padlocks with him to use in hotel rooms when he traveled, but always slept uneasily. Andreas felt bodily paralysis if his boss praised his work because he felt like their relationship had instantly become frighteningly intimate. He turned down special gifts his boss tried to give him for a job well done.

Simultaneous with hyperarousal, an individual may feel numb, removed from the world, and interpersonally detached. He is likely to have a sense of foreboding about the future and to be very constricted in his emotional responsiveness to others. Devin married a woman to whom he had very little sense of connection. In a short time, he could not perform sexually with her, and could only feel arousal with strangers or prostitutes. Andreas maintained that he experienced no emotions at all except for anxiety, fear, and anger. Although able to perform sexually with his wife, he experienced no pleasurable sensations during sexual activities. He insisted he had no feelings about anyone except his children.

Some of the symptoms usually associated with PTSD can be conceived as helpful adaptations, leading to habituation and counterconditioning if they unfold in safety. In such situations, flashbacks occur while the individual is relaxed, and the trauma thereby becomes paired with relaxation. When this happens, PTSD usually lasts for a relatively short time (Briere, 1995). For example, take the case of a person in a car accident who follows the advice often given in this situation: drive again as soon as possible. This allows any traumatic reactions that have become linked to the driving situation to get habituated, and for newer, nontraumatic reactions to get paired with driving. By contrast, an individual who waits months before attempting to drive again may develop the more severe symptoms of chronic PTSD and be unable to drive.

In other cases, such as the examples of Cory, Patrick, and Andreas noted above, the individual cannot tolerate his painful emotional state. He does not habituate the trauma because he cannot relax during flashbacks. He lives in a chronically hyperaroused state characterized by jumpiness, irritability, and somatization. Unable to desensitize his experience, he learns to avoid his painful emotional state through cognitive, behavioral, or dissociative means (Briere, 1995). In *cognitive* avoidance, he pushes upsetting thoughts out of his mind. This can be a conscious defense, and to a degree it is helpful and adaptive. *Behavioral* avoidance involves refraining from activity that might disturb him, such as sex or intimate relationships. *Dissociative* avoidance is a defensive severing of conscious connections between thoughts, feelings, memories, or behavior. Through dissociation, the individual decreases the impact of a traumatic event by only partly experiencing it (see Chapter 7).

Bessel van der Kolk and his colleagues (van der Kolk, 1987, 1995, 1996; van der Kolk and Greenberg, 1987; van der Kolk et al., 1996) have worked extensively on specifying the psychophysiological counterparts of PTSD. In general, they say, response to trauma is bimodal, with overreactivity concurrent with seeming insensibility as "hypermnesia, hyperreactivity to stimuli, and traumatic reexperiencing coexist with psychic numbing, avoidance, amnesia, and anhedonia" (van der Kolk, 1995, p. 31). Prolonged traumatic stress results in brain changes and a deregulated autonomic nervous system. This may either mediate or exacerbate cognitive and behavioral symptoms. Noting that people shut down in response to chronic hyperarousal, van der Kolk finds that the magnitude of exposure, degree of previous trauma, and the existence or nonexistence of a social support system are the strongest influences on whether chronic PTSD develops.

Extreme helplessness increases the traumatic impact of an event. But there is wide variation in different individuals' reactions to similar events. A circumstance that is traumatic to one person may be managed more easily by another. What is crucial is not an external judgment about how severely disturbing an experience is, but rather the way the individual subjectively registers it (Steele and Colrain, 1990). Some boys may be exposed to enormous over- or understimulation without the traumatic response that might be expected, while others are painfully reactive to circumstances that might seem less catastrophic to an "objective" outsider (Sugarman, 1994). As Crowder (1995) notes, "A client's perception of the intrusiveness of any specific sexual activity is subjective. . . . It is the client's *experience* that needs to be addressed in therapy rather than whether the behavior is objectively considered intrusive" (p. 3, emphasis added; see also Cassese, in press).

Behavior that is abusive and betraying may therefore *in some cases* not be traumatic to the victim. In these *rare* situations, a boy who has been sexually abused may not feel traumatized, particularly if he is past puberty, if the abuser is the same gender as the boy's sexual object choice (whether same or opposite sex), and if the abuse was not violent or otherwise obviously coercive. *However, the nontraumatic impact on the victim does not make the behavior itself less abusive.*

We have to be very careful when considering this issue, as boys are likely to think of premature sex as "sexual initiation" under these circumstances, for reasons I discuss in Chapters 2 and 3. This often happens on a conscious level for a boy even if the behavior has been exploitative and even if he has negative unconscious reactions to the abuse (see, for example, the case of Ed, pp. 48–51).

A man's understanding and experience of what happened to him may change over the course of treatment as he considers its ramifications and aftereffects in a different perspective. Sexual betrayal may have been positively framed, disguised as education, love, mutuality, hygiene, medicine ("It's what the doctor ordered"), recreation ("This is a game"), making a child into a surrogate spouse, payment of a debt owed the adult, or a fair trade for something the adult did for the child. When abuse is orchestrated as a loving, caring, or playful act, the child is betrayed not only by the behavior itself, but by the lies, mystification, and confusion surrounding it. He may learn to equate abuse with love, or care, or play, with potentially disastrous consequences, as we will see throughout this book (see especially Chapter 8). It is in the unraveling of his mystification that a man may develop a new perspective on what happened. Therapists may also be confused by this initial positive framing of betrayals, and therefore fail to recognize abusive experiences (Maltz, 1991).

Nevertheless, if a man claims that premature sex that took place in an abusive situation was not traumatic, or even claims that it was desired by him, we must accept this as a possibility. At the same time, we must continue to listen for other, less conscious reactions. For instance, we must evaluate whether he has an exaggerated capacity for denial and a consequent inability to appraise realistically the effects of abusive behavior. Likewise, the therapist and the abused man need to look at how the man's life is going, assessing, for example, whether on some level there are repetitions of the abuse in his current relationships, and judging whether there is a general emotional sparseness and constriction in his life arising from deprivations that accompanied the betrayal. Even if we accept the man's positive or neutral feelings about the experience and his belief that the outcome was benign or positive, we may need to help him come to terms with the fact that he was exploited (Fitzgerald, in Morris, Hunter, Struve, and Fitzgerald, 1997).

MYTHS ABOUT BOYHOOD
SEXUAL VICTIMIZATION

Preconceptions abound about the sexual abuse of boys and men. Some of the most common of these myths include:

- Men cannot be sexually abused.
- Women do not abuse sexually.
- Sexual abuse is always overt.
- Sexual abuse turns a boy gay.
- Sexually abused boys almost inevitably become sexually abusive men.
- Victimizers are always conscious of the abuse they are committing.
- Male victimizers who molest boys consider themselves homosexual and are sexually interested in other men.
- If you have allowed abuse, then you are a sissy or a weakling.
- Children can always say no to abuse if violence is not used. If they don't, they must have wanted the abuse to occur.
- If a boy becomes sexually aroused, he is an equal participant in the abuse.

Each of these myths reverberates for sexually abused boys and men, raising painful questions and suffusing deep shame. Yet none of them is true. Along with other preconceptions, they have all been refuted by an expanding body of literature about boyhood sexual victimization.

A GROWING BODY OF KNOWLEDGE

In the outpouring of books and papers on childhood sexual abuse that have appeared since 1980, the emphasis has nearly always been on sexually abused girls and their reactions to the abuse as women. While nearly all writers acknowledge that boys are also subject to sexual abuse, the focus on women has misleadingly implied that the occurrence of sexual abuse among boys is rare. In addition, it is assumed that boys' experiences are basically similar to girls', and that their treatment therefore follows similar lines. As recently as 1996, one writer suggested that the dearth of published material about sexually abused boys reflects a low incidence rate (Siegel, 1996).

When David Finkelhor surveyed the existing literature on sexual abuse of boys in 1984, he concluded that this area headed the list of sexual abuse areas that were "in crying need of research. . . . Probably, the

most serious question in regard to boys is how their victimization differs
from that of girls and how clinicians can take this difference into
account. . . . [E]ven purely descriptive accounts would be an important
resource given the current state of ignorance on the subject" (p. 230). In
1990, Urquiza and Capra wrote with justification that "if the body of
literature concerning female victims is still in its infancy . . . , the parallel
body of literature concerning males may best be described as in an
embryonic stage" (p. 126). The psychoanalytic literature was even more
sparse.

We have progressed since the early 1980s. Sexually abused men
now have access to material that helps them make sense of their victimization experiences. A number of books intended for nonprofessionals
have been written concerning boyhood sexual betrayal. These include
men's first-person accounts of childhood sexual abuse as well as books
by professionals intended for a lay audience (Mura, 1987; Bear and
Dimock, 1988; Lew, 1988; Loving in Fear, 1989; Thomas, 1989;
Estrada, 1990; Grubman-Black, 1990; Hunter, 1990a; Adams, 1991;
Sanders, 1991; Berendzen and Palmer, 1993; Hopkins, 1993; King,
1995; Ryan, 1995; Wiehe, 1996).

In addition to these books intended for nonprofessionals, scholarly
knowledge about sexually abused men has been enhanced by the professional writings of clinicians and researchers like Nasjaleti (1980); Finkelhor (1981, 1984; Finkelhor and Associates, 1986); Johnson and
Shrier (1985, 1987); Pierce and Pierce (1985; Pierce, 1987); Blanchard
(1986); Freeman-Longo (1986); Friedrich and associates (Friedrich, Berliner, Urquiza, and Beilke, 1986; Friedrich, Urquiza, and Beilke, 1986;
Friedrich, Beilke, and Urquiza, 1987, 1988; Friedrich and Luecke, 1988;
Friedrich, 1995); Porter (1986); Briere (Briere and Runtz, 1987, 1988;
Briere, Evans, Runtz, and Wall, 1988); Bruckner and Johnson (1987);
Fromuth and Burkhart (1987, 1989); Risin and Koss (1987); Reinhart
(1987); Sebold (1987); Dimock (1988); Johanek (1988); Vander Mey
(1988); Bolton, Morris, and MacEachron (1989); Everstine and Everstine (1989); Myers (1989); Pescosolido (1989); K. Singer (1989);
Gilgun (1990, 1991; Gilgun and Reiser, 1990); Hunter (1990b, 1990c);
Kendall-Tackett and Simon (1992); Mezey and King (1992); Watkins
and Bentovin (1992); Black and DeBlassie (1993); Gonsiorek (1993,
cited in Mendel, 1995; Gonsiorek, Bera, and Le Tourneau, 1994); Lisak
(1993, 1994, 1995; Lisak and Luster, 1994; Lisak, Hopper, and Song,
1996); Levesque (1994); Collings (1995); Mendel (1995); Dhaliwal,
Gauzas, Antonowicz, and Ross (1996); Bauserman and Rind (1997);
Chandy, Blum, and Resnick (1997); Gill and Tutty (1997); and Holmes
and Slap (1998). Some psychoanalysts, including Kramer (1974, 1990),
Margolis (1977, 1984), Shengold (1989), B. Steele (1990, 1991),

Ehrenberg (1992), Knoblauch (1993), Gartner (1994, 1996a, 1996b, 1997a, 1997b), and Hegeman (1995a, 1995b), have also written detailed case histories and discussions of their treatment of sexually abused men.

This literature dispels many of the myths about male sexual victimization and also supports the idea that men sexually abused in boyhood form a distinct population. Sexual abuse has different meanings for boys and girls, and these different meanings have implications for how the child reacts to it, defines it, and deals with it later on as an adult.

PREVALENCE OF BOYHOOD
SEXUAL VICTIMIZATION

The results of surveys since the mid-1980s documenting the prevalence of childhood sexual abuse are shocking. The most convincing are studies of nonclinical populations, randomly selected from the general population, and therefore not necessarily in psychotherapeutic treatment for the aftermath of sexual trauma or any other reason. (See Finkelhor and Associates, 1986; Bolton et al., 1989; Urquiza and Keating, 1990; Herman, 1992; and Lindsay and Read, 1994, for more extensive discussions of the prevalence of sexual abuse.)

Let us first look briefly at the studies of women and girls. Diana Russell (1983, 1984, 1986) interviewed 900 randomly sampled women in depth and found that approximately one-third reported direct childhood sexual abuse. When noncontact abuse (see below) was included, the figure rose to over half. Similar findings are reported by other sophisticated epidemiologists, including David Finkelhor (1984) and Gail Wyatt (1985). Of those women reporting childhood sexual abuse, over 40 percent say that they were abused incestuously.

Prevalence studies of sexually abused men are not as consistent in their findings as studies of women. In the 166 studies published between 1985 and 1997 that were surveyed by Holmes and Slap (1998), the prevalence estimates of the sexual abuse of boys ranged from 4 percent to 76 percent. This lack of consistency seems to arise in part from problems defining abuse and abusive relationships. Framing questions about early childhood sexuality as abuse may skew results with men who believe their premature sexual experiences were benign. Also, many of the early studies were done on clinical groups rather than random samples of the general population of men. (See Hopper, 1997, for a discussion of methodology issues in studies of male sexual victimization.)

According to Bruckner and Johnson (1987), the 1984 Canadian Badgley report found that 33 percent of Canadian men are sexually victimized at some point in their lives. Of these, 75 percent of the victimizations occur to boys under the age of 17, and 25 percent of those are serious chargeable assaults under Canadian criminal law. In the United States, according to the American Humane Society as cited by Dimock (1988), reports of both male and female sexual abuse victims rose from 1980 till 1984. The figures reported for boys rose more sharply, however, from 15.7 percent in 1980 to 21.7 percent in 1984. In a study of high school boys in Oregon, Nelson, Higginson, and Grant-Worley (1994) found that 2 percent of them had been abused in the previous *week*.

The difficulty of evaluating prevalence studies for boys is explored in *The Male Survivor* (1995), Matthew Mendel's work on the impact of sexual abuse on boys and men.[2] Mendel reviews the literature on the prevalence of the sexual abuse of boys and on the descriptive characteristics of men with childhood sexual abuse histories (pp. 40–71). Mendel considers methodological and definitional issues, the proportion of male to female victims, and such descriptive characteristics as the age of the victim when abuse began, the type and severity of abuse, the sex of the abuser, the relationship between victim and abuser, and the number of abusers. I briefly review here his findings about prevalence studies.

Noting the wide variation in estimates of the prevalence of sexual abuse of boys (from 2.5 percent to 33 percent in the surveys he cites), Mendel cites the methodological discrepancies in the studies, particularly differences among the populations studied and varied definitions of abuse. Thus, studies of prison populations, for example, or sexual offenders, or runaway adolescents may have limited generalizability to other populations. Even random nonclinical undergraduate samples are likely to underrepresent minority groups and men of lower socioeconomic backgrounds. Similarly, studies that look only at abuse either by men or by women, or that define abuse in terms of whether the experience was considered emotionally upsetting by the man himself, will not match surveys that use other definitions.

In addition, the language used when asking about sexual abuse skews the results for men. Boys often hesitate to define premature sexual behavior as abusive or even disturbing, for reasons I will discuss in Chapters 2, 3, and 4. Fromuth and Burkhart (1987, 1989) therefore recommend using terms like "sexual interactions" rather than "sexual abuse" when conducting surveys about male sexual victimization. Even with the lowered probability of boys openly stating that they have been sexually abused, however, a 1998 Harris survey of 3,162 adolescent boys found that one in eight answered affirmatively to the direct question of whether he had ever been sexually abused (*New York Times,* June 26, 1998, p. A11).

---

[2] See also Urquiza and Keating (1990), Violato and Genuis (1993), and Hopper (1997).

In a sophisticated study of a nonclinical male population that is analogous to Russell's work with women, Lisak, Hopper, and Song (1996) surveyed nearly 600 college men. They administered questionnaires carefully phrased to ask about specific events (for example, being touched sexually) rather than to elicit judgments about those events (for example, being abused). Based on responses, they classified their population into men with histories of sexual abuse, men with histories of physical abuse, men with histories of both sexual and physical abuse, and men who had not been abused. Their findings are summarized as follows:

- Of the men in their sample, 18 percent reported direct sexual abuse by the age of sixteen. When noncontact abuse was included, the figure rose to 28 percent. By comparison, 34 percent of the men they surveyed reported physical abuse.
- For the men who were sexually abused, the average age of the first sexual abuse incident was 10.1 years, with a range from 2 to 15 years for the age of first victimization (D. Lisak, personal communication). By comparison, when there was physical abuse, the average age of the first incident was 7.3 years.
- The use of force, intimidation, or threats was reported by 36 percent of the sexually abused men, while 43 percent reported more covert "seduction" and 22 percent claimed that they had participated voluntarily.
- Sixty-one percent of the sexual abusers were male and 28 percent were female. Eleven percent of those who were sexually abused reporting having both male and female abusers. For boys who were physically abused, 58 percent had male abusers, 11 percent had female abusers, and 31 percent said they were physically abused by both male and female victimizers.
- Extrafamilial abuse was involved for 79 percent of the sexually abused men. By contrast, 70 percent of those who were physically abused reported victimizers from within their own families.

These last figures are similar to the extrafamilial sexual abuse reported by 83 percent of the sexually abused men studied by Finkelhor (1984). Note, however, the contrasting findings of the large 1998 Harris survey, where about one-third of sexually abused boys reported that their abuse occurred at home, and 45 percent said the sexual abuser was a family member (*New York Times*, June 26, 1998, p. A11). In my own clinical practice, as represented by the cases reported throughout this book, intrafamilial sexual abuse has accounted for a much larger proportion of the population than in the Lisak and Finkelhor studies, one closer to the results reported by Harris. My impression that intrafamilial abuse is more common than Lisak and Finkelhor found is supported by Wright (1997a), who believes the discrepancy is due to incest being more underreported for men than extrafamilial abuse. An alternate explanation is that in general incest has more damaging psychological ramifications than extrafamilial abuse because of its embeddedness in crucial early relationships. It therefore may be more frequently traumatic, and its victims would thus be more likely to seek psychological help. In Mendel's (1995) nonrandom sample of men in psychotherapy who identified themselves as sexually abused, *all* described intrafamilial sexual betrayal. I emphasize, however, that I am talking here about general trends, not in any way implying that for a specific boy extrafamilial abuse is less traumatic than incest.

In sum, I want to underline Lisak et al.'s prevalence figures (Urquiza and Keating, 1990, report similar results). *Approximately one in six men reported direct inappropriate sexual contact by age sixteen.* An additional one in ten reported inappropriate noncontact sexual activity by that age. This means that approximately one in four men has a sexual abuse history. These would be enormous numbers even if they were somewhat inflated. On the contrary, though, the figures for men are likely to be underreported (Dimock, 1989a; Peake, 1989; Mendel, 1995).

DEFINING SEXUAL ABUSE

The inconsistency of research findings about male sexual victimization is due not only to research design, but also to varied definitions of sexual abuse (Holmes and Slap, 1998). A clinician who listens to a man's experience of his own specific history is privy to many clues about whether a particular situation was or was not traumatic. Defining abuse in a more general sense, as researchers must do, is more complicated. What constitutes abuse? What specific behaviors are we talking about? What is the cutoff age below which a youth should be considered a victim of abuse? What relationship must he have with his victimizer? What is the age difference between them? Clinicians have leeway in answering these questions. Researchers, however, must make arbitrary decisions about these and other questions when surveying large populations for sexual abuse histories. These decisions inevitably skew their results in one direction or the other.

Thus, studies differ in the upper range of the age of the child who is considered to have been abused. Some consider puberty as the limit, as Kinsey, Pomeroy, and Martin (1948) did. Others have chosen various ages in adolescence, even up to age twenty-one. For my own purposes, I generally consider the legal age of consent (seventeen for boys in New

York State) as the upper marker for childhood (as opposed to adult) sexual abuse (see Urquiza and Keating, 1990).

It is also important to consider the age difference between the victim and his victimizer. This usually differentiates abusive situations from mutual childhood sexual exploration with playmates and peers. The age difference required to denote a sexually abusive situation varies considerably in different studies. While nearly every observer would consider sexual behavior between a prepubescent child and an adult to be abusive, there is not always agreement when the age difference is smaller or the victim is postpubescent. Some studies have required a three-, five-, or even ten-year difference between victim and victimizer.

As a clinician, I am able to investigate the man's experience of a situation more thoroughly than most researchers do when I consider whether he has been abused. This requires understanding the *relationship* with the abuser as well as the age difference. When the relationship is such that the victimizer (often a caretaker) is in a position of power and trust, this adds to the coercion implicit in the relationship. And, for young children, even a three-year age difference implies a considerable power differential.

Studies may also use different behavioral definitions of abuse. In the next section, I will discuss more specifically the range of sexually abusive behaviors described by men I have treated. For the moment, drawing chiefly on the work of Dimock (1988), Gilgun (1990), and Maloney (1995), I want to convey in a more general sense what we mean by sexual abuse.

Contact abuse is usually a chargeable crime. It may involve the penetration, attempted penetration, or stimulation of the boy's body by a penis, finger, tongue, or other part of the victimizer's body, or by an object used by the abuser. It may also be genital or anal touch of the victimizer by the child, including fellatio, masturbation, intercourse, or intromission of any kind. Touching of breasts is included, as are forced unnecessary enemas, coercing a child to be sexual with animals, or engaging a child in prostitution.

Noncontact sexual abuse includes a wide range of behaviors, some more easily documented than others: masturbating or otherwise being sexual in front of a child; exposing genitals to a child for sexual gratification; encouraging a child to be sexual with others; practicing voyeurism; photographing a child for sexual purposes; showing a child pornography or making it available to him; engaging in sexualized talk with a child or confiding to him about sexual issues; ridiculing a child's sexual development, preferences, or organs; forcing a child to dress in an overrevealing manner; stripping oneself and/or a child in order to hit or spank him, or getting sexual pleasure from spanking; employing sexually charged verbal or emotional abuse; having a child witness the sexual abuse of others; using sexual punishments; manifesting unusual interest in and asking questions about sexuality; taking too much interest in baths at an inappropriate age; applying medication on genitals or cleaning genitals when a child is old enough to do it himself (this does include contact, of course, but is usually too subtle to be considered contact abuse); and employing seductive looks or talk to a child that violate generational or personal boundaries.

Some of these forms of noncontact sexual abuse are obvious, but others are subtle and covert. It is unlikely that any prevalence study will include such *covert sexual abuse* in its definition of abuse, yet this category forms an important subgroup in the population of men sexually abused as boys. Brandt and Tisza (1977) call this "sexual misuse" (p. 80), while Bolton et al. (1989) term it "the abuse of sexuality" (p. 87). In its interpersonal essence, covert sexual betrayal is very similar to overt abuse, despite differences in the actions involved.

Covert incest is often defined relationally rather than behaviorally. According to Maloney (1995), it "occurs when a child becomes the object of a parent's affection, love, passion and preoccupation. The boundary between caring and incestuous love is crossed when the relationship with the child exists to meet the needs of the parent rather than the needs of the child" (p. 5). It includes excitatory and sexualized relationships, even when there is no clear-cut, explicit sexual activity between the individuals. We may think of these relationships as psychological incest, since they involve psychological rather than physical boundary violations of a child (see Chapter 6). Herman (1981) and Mendel (1995) both discuss the perniciousness of this dynamic, which Love (1990) calls "emotional incest." Abusers may be unconscious of the covert sexual betrayal involved in such psychological or emotional incest. In the relationship between Keith and his seductive mother, for example, she seems never to have considered the implications of the sexually tinged, psychologically merged relationship she established with her son.

If we use "abuse" as a legal term, that is, if we use it only to apply to chargeable behaviors that could be prosecuted as abusive, we leave out these covert relationships. They have strong erotic components, however, and would not occur without the power differential in the relationship. Although I often use the word "abuse" throughout this book when describing both overt and covert sexual betrayals, it might be more accurate to use another term, for example, "transgression," for covert abuse in order to convey the difference between relationships that would be legally defined as abusive and those betrayals that could not be prosecuted but nevertheless violate the psychosexual boundaries of a boy.

But legal definitions are not necessarily appropriate in human situations. As Brooke Hopkins (1993) says in writing about his own sexual betrayal by his mother,

> Whether or not one wishes to call her behavior seductive is beside the point. The point is that it involved the emotional and physical exploitation of her child; it involved *using* him to satisfy her own emotional and physical needs. This may not have been something for which she might have been found criminally guilty (the law is too crude an instrument to regulate this kind of behavior), but it was wrong nevertheless, behavior that no amount of passivity, no claims not to have been better informed can mask. (p. 52)

BEHAVIORAL DESCRIPTIONS OF SEXUAL BETRAYAL FOR BOYS

In the previous section I described how sexual abuse may generally be defined. In this section I will be more specific, and discuss the range of abuse situations that have been described in my own clinical practice with sexually abused men. I divide sexual abuse situations into three groups: those involving penetration, those involving inappropriate tactile contact or overtly sexual noncontact behavior, and those involving noncontact seduction and excitation. These are roughly equivalent to the categories of abuse devised for women by D. Russell (1986).

When actual penetration of the child or the adult is involved, whether orally, anally, or vaginally, we have no trouble characterizing the act as sexually abusive for boys or girls. In these clear-cut cases described by my patients, the abuser usually was male and used his penis, fingers, tongue, or an object to penetrate the child. Women, of course, are also capable of performing many of these acts, and in my work I have on occasion heard about women who penetrated boys, often by using fingers or giving enemas.

Inappropriate touching or rubbing of either the child's or the abuser's body, sometimes leading to orgasm for either or both, again clearly reflects a sexually abusive situation. Abuse of this type described by my patients has included a four-year-old boy being bounced on an uncle's lap while a story was being read until the uncle ejaculated; a father attempting to cup his fourteen-year-old son's genitalia in his hands in order to help him decide what size jock strap he should wear; and a teenage boy, with the family's knowledge, repeatedly being masturbated and sucked to orgasm by a brain-injured older brother. Some of my patients have also described childhood incidents in which they were encouraged to touch a woman's breasts, their penises were touched by women, or they were otherwise touched inappropriately by a woman, often in the guise of physical caretaking.

As noted above, inappropriately seductive behavior when there is no direct contact is more difficult to define clearly as abuse. These seductive patterns of behavior are especially damaging to the developing boy when they occur with a parent (see Adams, 1991). In the literature on women, Herman (1981) discusses the dynamics of families in which fathers are seductive but not overtly abusive with their daughters. In the clinical literature about men, the inappropriately seductive mother and her son have, of course, been frequently described, though usually their relationship has not been labeled as sexually abusive. Nevertheless, I believe women are at least as likely to be covert or seductive abusers as men are. This may reflect narcissistic sexuality on the part of the abuser as much as or more than the abuse of power often seen with overt molestation. As Keith put it when describing his enmeshed and merged relationship with his mother, "We didn't have sex but we sure had sexuality every day."

Extreme examples of seductive abuse reported by my patients have ranged from a father sleeping in a twin bed with his son from age six to age ten, supposedly to allay the boy's fears of the dark, to a mother inviting her nine-year-old son to urinate through her legs into her menstrual blood while his sister watched. *Subtle* seductive abuse is the hardest of all to characterize definitively. My patients have described more of this kind of abuse from women than from men. Their reports have included a mother who habitually sat naked on the toilet, stroking her body while talking on the phone with the bathroom door open; and a father giving his preadolescent son detailed descriptions of his mother's sexual inadequacies and the contrasting sexual delights the father found with his mistresses.

It is arguable whether any specific seductive relationship or incident can be called sexual abuse. Hopkins (1993) addresses this point when writing about his relationship with his mother:

> Does this constitute abuse? Clearly, not in any active sense. But given the physiological and psychological impact of such actions upon the developmental process, the damage they inflict upon the growing child, it constitutes *some* form of the use of a child to satisfy adult needs. Call it what you will, the result is the same: pain that lasts for a very long time. (p. 50)

In my discussion throughout this book, I only include cases of seductive abuse where the man either defined himself as a survivor of sexual abuse before seeing me or was so clear in his eventual perceptions of the experience that there was no question in either of our minds that a sexual betrayal had occurred. Many of these men also wondered whether there had not also been more direct sexual molestation in their histories, though such memories were not necessarily recalled in our work.

THE AFTERMATH
OF BOYHOOD SEXUAL BETRAYAL

As Holmes and Slap (1998) conclude, "the sexual abuse of boys is common, underreported, underrecognized, and undertreated" (p. 1860). The research and clinical findings reported in the literature about the aftereffects of boyhood sexual abuse are complex, and have been carefully reviewed elsewhere (Bruckner and Johnson, 1987; Dimock, 1988, 1989b; Lew, 1988; Bolton et al., 1989; Pescosolido, 1989; Hunter, 1990a; Olson, 1990; Urquiza and Capra, 1990; Watkins and Bentovin, 1992; Lisak, 1994; Collings, 1995; Mendel, 1995; Lisak et al., 1996; Hopper, 1997; Holmes and Slap, 1998; Cassese, in press; K. Singer, n. d.). Drawing on this work, I summarize the literature findings, referencing chapters in this book that deal specifically with the issues raised:

• There is a higher general prevalence of sexual abuse of girls than boys. Among sexually abused children, a greater proportion of boys than girls suffer extrafamilial abuse (see this chapter). However, intrafamilial abuse, especially incest within the immediate family, is a powerful predictor of greater disturbance in later life for boys.

• Boys at greatest risk for sexual abuse are those living with neither or only one parent; those whose parents are separated, divorced, and/or remarried; those whose parents abuse alcohol or are involved in criminal behavior; and those who are nonwhite, of lower socioeconomic status, under thirteen years of age, and/or disabled.

• Among sexually abused children, a smaller proportion of boys than girls report the abuse, partly because fewer boys and men consciously identify their experiences as abusive. Cognitively, they may feel less traumatized, despite having a wide range of symptoms related to abuse. This raises the question of whether they are less disturbed by their abuse than girls, on the one hand, or are better able to deny trauma, on the other (see Chapters 2 and 3).

• Male victims of sexual abuse are less likely than female victims to seek psychotherapeutic help at some point in their lives, although they are more likely than nonabused men to seek therapy for issues that *seem* unrelated to abuse (see Chapter 3).

- Boys (like girls) often hold themselves responsible for their abuse, feeling they should have prevented it (see Chapters 2 and 3), or that they deserved it because they are "bad" or "dirty." This is less frightening than experiencing that the world is unpredictable or that their families do not take care of them.

- Like sexually abused women, many sexually abused men exhibit guilt, anxiety, depression, shame, and low self-esteem. Frequently, they are actively self-destructive and self-mutilating. They make more suicide attempts than nonabused men, and may exhibit covert suicidal behavior by needlessly putting themselves in high-risk situations (see Chapters 3, 7, and 8). They are at greater risk than nonabused men for developing major depression, bulimia, antisocial personality disorder, behavior problems, PTSD, and borderline personality disorder.

- Boys who are sexually abused are more likely than sexually abused girls to act aggressively as they progress in their lives. As a group, they are more likely than nonabused boys to engage in criminal behavior, although there is great individual variability about this. It is not uncommon for sexually abused adolescent boys to become hustlers (see Chapters 3 and 8), just as sexually abused girls become prostitutes more often than nonabused girls do.

- Sexually abused men are more likely than sexually abused women to fantasize about or desire sexual activity with children, although most do not themselves become sexual abusers (see Chapters 3, 5, 8, and 11).

- Sexually abused men are prone to have dysfunctional psychological and physiological reactions to stress, as well as poor body imagery. Hypertension, chest pains, sleep disturbance, nightmares, shortness of breath, dizziness, and anorexia or bulimia are common somatic symptoms (see Chapter 7). Men who suffered anal trauma are especially susceptible to constipation and encopresis (loss of bowel control). Even as boys, they are more likely than their nonabused peers to develop drug and/or alcohol addictions.

- Sexual abuse often precipitates crises about sexual orientation and gender identity in boys and men. These are related to shameful feelings of being less manly because of victimization. Also, beliefs that sexual victimization influences later sexual orientation and/or is a sign of one's "true" orientation may lead to anxiety or homophobia. Some sexually abused men consider themselves heterosexual but engage in sexual behavior at times with other men, with varying degrees of pleasure and satisfaction. Others believe their homosexual orientation was caused by an abuse history, whether the abuser was male or female. Still others retreat from all sexual contact. Of this last group, some are clear about their orientation but are phobic about sexual intimacy. Others have little concept of sexual orientation at all, and, more to the point, have never developed psychosexually to a point where sexual relatedness and orientation are even issues for them (see Chapters 3 and 4).

• Men with sexual abuse histories often have severe problems relating intimately to both men and women (see Chapter 8). They are far more likely than nonabused men to report sexual problems, including sexual dysfunction. Many associate sexuality with pain and humiliation. They may repeat a victim–victimizer pattern in relationships, often alternating between being the abused and the abuser. They may not feel capable of turning down unwanted sexual overtures or of taking the steps necessary to protect themselves from sexually transmitted disease. For these and other related reasons, many men become phobic about interpersonal sexuality. For others, emotional needs can only be met symbolically, through sexual contact, which has come to mean love and nurturance. Because of fears of relatedness, however, they may not be able to be intimate, sexual, and emotional with the same person over time. Situational impotence is common, especially with partners to whom they have emotional attachments. They score lower than sexually abused women on sexual self-esteem measures, although both groups score lower than nonvictims.

• Sexually abused men tend to be hypervigilant about other men, especially if they had a male abuser (see Chapter 3). They may avoid all-male groups of any kind (see Chapter 11), and may be especially anxious in situations where they might be seen unclothed by other men, such as locker rooms or public lavatories. It may be easier for them to express emotional problems to women than to men.

• Believing they cannot protect their interpersonal boundaries (see Chapter 6), many sexually abused men develop problems with trust. They unrealistically expect others to see their failures and vulnerabilities, and consequently to take advantage of them. The lack of safety they feel in interpersonal situations often causes them to lead isolated, alienated lives in which their underlying loneliness is masked by a conscious attitude that they do not need other people (see Chapter 8).

• Sexually abused men often view life in dichotomous black-or-white terms. They are likely to have a high need for interpersonal control (see Chapter 8), and often engage in power struggles with others. They may seem stubborn and rigid, on the one hand, yet appear passive and conforming, on the other. Each of these character styles protects the man from feelings of vulnerability.

• Sexually abused men are often either emotionally numb and withdrawn or filled with uncontrolled and frightening rage and aggression. These tendencies may alternate in the same man. When dissociation and lack of affect fail to protect him from his inner emotional turmoil, retaliation fantasies are common, as is fantasized tortured internal replaying of the original trauma (see Chapters 7 and 8).

• It is common for sexually abused men to exhibit many self-soothing, compulsive behaviors, including alcoholism, drug addiction, workaholism, overeating, and compulsive spending, exercising, or gambling. Sexual compulsivity is also common, especially compulsive masturbation, viewing of pornography, and seeking of anonymous partners. In addition to its self-soothing aspects, sexual compulsivity represents for many men a repetitive attempt at mastery over their original sexual victimization. However, they may interpret it as a sign that they are out of control sexually and really wanted their abuse. For men who become Don Juans (recurrently seeking female partners), compulsive sexuality is a way of repeatedly proving to themselves that they are not gay or weak, or of giving themselves an emotional high to prove they are not totally deadened to feeling (see Chapters 2, 3, 7, and 8).

These descriptions highlight a number of dissimilarities between male and female victims. Yet I also want to emphasize that men and women who have been sexually abused are much more similar than different. Both are likely to exhibit symptoms of PTSD, including flashbacks, night terrors, interpersonal isolation, and cycling between emotional hyperarousal and psychic numbing. Both often have characterological problems involving trust, depression, masochism, shame, dissociation, boundary violations, and addictive and other compulsive behaviors. As Crowder (1995) notes, "Both male and female victims of sexual trauma feel isolated and marginalized. Both struggle with low self-esteem and a damaged sense of self. Ultimately, healing and recovery for both male and female victims involve embracing all aspects of one's humanity, a process that goes beyond gender" (p. 37). Thus, many of the points I make here and throughout this book about sexually abused men are also true in some measure of women who have been sexually abused, though the clinical picture often looks different.

With regard to the differences between men and women, Briere (1995) has argued that sexually abused men encounter more difficulties and are harder to treat than sexually abused women. He particularly notes the problems sexually abused men have in their abilities to manage interpersonal boundaries, handle feelings, and regulate affect. While emphasizing that the coping mechanisms men use to tolerate extreme stress should be thought of as adaptations rather than as symptoms, he notes their long-term effects in cognitive, affective, and interpersonal spheres. Cognitively, they commonly lead to low self-esteem, a feeling that the boy is bad, and the belief that he deserved his maltreatment. Affectively, they result in anxiety, depression, and anger (Briere et al.,

1988). Interpersonally, the problems are complex, as we will see throughout this book (see especially Chapter 8), with some avoiding all interpersonal relationships when possible.

ABUSE IN THE CONTEXT
OF A MAN'S PSYCHIC LIFE

It is tempting to believe that abuse is virtually the sole influence on a betrayed boy's later psychological distress. Adults with childhood sexual abuse histories commonly identify themselves as victims and blame abuse for all their difficulties, at least during parts of their recovery period. And, indeed, as Gillman (1986) observes, trauma may be "an organizer for development. Although all or part of trauma may be out of awareness, something is embedded in the personality, a focus that draws into it posttraumatic events, to be dealt with over and over again" (p. 75).

Yet abuse is never the lone cause of all of a man's problems. While character development may be influenced by trauma, it also influences reactions to trauma. In working with traumatized individuals, it is critical to consider questions like these: How is a child's character affected by early recurring trauma? How does earlier character development affect the way a child then deals with trauma? And what is the interplay between these two dynamics in an unfolding treatment?

When interpersonal betrayal is the ultimate source of trauma, as is inevitably the case in sexual abuse, then these questions must be asked again from a relational perspective. Trauma is likely to crystallize the existing relational patterns that predate it (Lionells, 1998), but these patterns may be helpful in softening traumatic impact. What was the child's relational matrix preceding the trauma? Did he previously have an interpersonal life sufficiently rich that the relational effect of trauma on him can be mediated? What crucial relationships have been shattered through traumatic interpersonal behavior? Are there any relationships that have been safeguarded for the child? How has trauma affected his ability to continue in those relationships not directly involved in his betrayal?

All forms of early trauma can powerfully affect later character development. Yet other factors also affect how a child experiences sexual abuse. Every abused child was, of course, already developing his personality when his abuse occurred. His reactions to abuse are influenced by his developing personality, his family and cultural context, his psychological resources, and the external events in his life. Previous character development is especially important if abuse occurs to an older boy whose personality is further evolved than a younger boy's. He has already tested his capacity to cope with stress and trauma. In fact, his already-existing character, as it emerges through these coping strategies, may have made him vulnerable to abuse. For example, early life experiences may have made it problematic for him to form attachments to others, and this may have caused him to be especially susceptible to victimization. Ramon, for example, found the focused attention and seemingly gentle protectiveness of a man in his neighborhood to be a balm for his raw sense of deprivation and fear. These feelings themselves developed from his reactions to his parents' physically abusive relationship, his father's desertion of the family, and his being left alone much of the time while his mother worked. Needing sustenance and safety, he soon felt he had found both in his relationship with the neighbor, a relationship that included anal intercourse.

For the clinician, as for the sexually abused man, there is a temptation to oversimplify. I have wished at times, for example, that I could point with certainty to events in a man's history that led inevitably to specific psychological effects in his later life. Such reductionistic thinking, however, leads to stereotyping individuals without regard for the wide range of reactions people actually have to traumatic events. Therefore it is important to remember that:

- Men who were abused incestuously are not always distinctly different from those who were abused by individuals outside their family;
- Those abused before puberty do not show unambiguous differences from those abused in adolescence;
- Those abused on one or two occasions are not necessarily distinguishable from those who suffered chronic abuse;
- Boys abused by men do not always develop different features from those abused by women;
- The use of force or coercion may not inevitably yield a different picture than abuse where the betrayal is framed as loving and affectionate; and
- There are no clear differences in the aftermaths of boys who have one or another specific age difference from their molesters.[3]

It should not be surprising that such clear-cut differentiations cannot be made with confidence. Many factors influence how abuse affects a boy's maturational process. Consider, for example, such factors as whether the

---

[3] See Urquiza and Capra (1990) and Mendel (1995) for attempts to sort through these issues.

boy had someone to confide in; his family's strengths and weaknesses in a variety of areas; whether he felt compelled to conceal the abuse; and his individual temperament, character, creativity, and unique psychological makeup. These and other aspects of his inner or outer world decisively influence the boy's psychic development and serve to ameliorate, accentuate, or refocus the effects of his abuse (see Fischer, 1991).

GOALS, PROCESS, AND THEMES IN TREATMENT

What can we hope will happen by the end of psychotherapy for an adult who was sexually abused in childhood? Price (1994) anticipates that "the patient will move from being an incest survivor to a person with a history of incest" (p. 228). Dimock (1988) looks forward to him becoming "an adult who can take care of himself in a better way than he was cared for as a child" (p. 217). For Crowder (1995),

> [H]ealing from sexual trauma is a process that leads the survivor from a position of making abuse-reactive life decisions, based on past learning, to a new position of making proactive life decisions and choices based on present needs. As the survivor makes his unconscious coping strategies conscious, his personal autonomy increases. Flashbacks of the abuse become reclaimed memories, inexplicable fears and anxieties become associations to present environmental triggers that echo abuse-related experiences, and some chronic somatic complaints become the signals for recognizing unmet physical and emotional needs. (p. 42)

My patient Ezra put it more succinctly: "I'm coming to therapy to allow the abuse *to have happened.*" He had always known that sexually abusive events had occurred, but he experienced no feeling attached to that knowledge. He wanted to let the abuse experience become part of him in toto so that the deadness he had created in his center to protect himself from his trauma would no longer be necessary. He wanted to *remember* the abuse rather than to reenact it (Galperin, 1998).

It is, of course, essential to be able to help a man heal from the directly disabling effects of trauma. However, although this is a necessary objective of treatment, it is an insufficient goal. In order to stop a sexual betrayal from being the engine that runs a man's life, therapy must also deal with the spreading effects of sexual abuse. In particular, such relational aftermaths as interpersonal isolation, distrust, and the inability to live intimately in relation to a loved one must be addressed. This takes a long time, and I believe that in the majority of cases long-term treatment is most effective for this task. At the same time, specific situations may require shorter-term interventions because of the constraints of time, finances, or the reluctance of a man to stay in treatment longer. Such shorter treatments can be very useful; indeed, for some men, they are all that is needed. Others may need a period of time out of therapy to see how they now fare in the world. Some of these may return for future treatment sequences when they feel ready to continue the therapeutic work.

A number of writers have addressed the steps and/or the process of therapy with sexually abused adults (Courtois, 1988; Briere, 1989, 1991, 1992; Kluft, 1989a; Sgroi, 1989; Sanderson, 1990; Dolan, 1991; Herman, 1992; Davies and Frawley, 1994; van der Kolk et al., 1996), and specifically with men (Lew, 1988; Bolton et al., 1989; Hunter, 1990a; Gonsiorek et al., 1994; Crowder, 1995; Dimock, 1996). In general, the recovery process described in these works involves:

1. Acknowledging that victimization occurred;
2. Seeing its historical and familial context;
3. Discharging the intense affect surrounding it (particularly grief, terror, and rage), having first buttressed the patient's capacity to endure intense feelings and thus having created a greater sense of safety;
4. Recognizing its impact and separating out the child's traumatic reaction from the adult's greater capacity to withstand over-whelming experience;
5. Perceiving its dysfunctional influences on the adult's current day-to-day functioning and relearning patterns of living; and
6. Consolidating learning and putting the abuse into perspective so it recedes in importance and no longer dominates how the patient lives.

In my experience, these stages of recovery are conceptually useful, but they certainly do not occur in the ordered way this description implies. (Nor, to be sure, do these writers suggest that actual therapy necessarily follows such a neat path.) Further, I believe therapeutic work is rarely over when abuse is accepted and integrated into a man's self-image. This may be true in some cases, but for most men this point marks the beginning of the hardest part of their treatment. This is the long period when they struggle with the many ramifications, both subtle and overt, of their abuse experience (see Piers, 1998). During this phase, my interpersonal psychoanalytic training most obviously affects how I work. It leads me to focus with the patient on his relational world, both outside the therapy room and, most powerfully, within the live context of our therapeutic relationship. This is how I believe long-lasting change comes about, and this is what I describe in this book.

Working relationally with a sexually abused patient can be difficult for the therapist to endure (see Chapters 9 and 10). Virtually every writer alludes to the intense interpersonal vicissitudes of working with this population, but few actually convey these in their writing (Davies and Frawley, 1994, are a notable exception). It can be nearly unbearable for the therapist to allow the patient to tell his story in the only way he can. His communication may involve both detailed verbal descriptions of horrible acts and excruciating nonverbal reenactments of dissociated traumatic experience (see Chapters 7, 9, and 10). In either case, it impacts on the therapist in ways that themselves can be traumatic (see Chapter 9).

In this book, I write about themes that have recurred in the therapy of the men I have treated. Rather than focus on technical considerations, I elaborate on this thematic discussion with illustrations from my practice indicating the complexities of the work and demonstrating how issues develop in a specific individual's treatment. These recurring themes can serve the therapist as a kind of compass in the treatment. Believing as I do that all therapists bring unique capacities to clinical encounters, as do all patients, I do not advocate that readers try to do as I do. Rather, I hope my descriptions will stimulate therapists to consider how they would work with the themes we universally encounter. In addition, I hope they will consider how to capitalize on their own distinctive blend of personality, skill, and life experience as these themes emerge in their own patients' treatments.

THE MEN IN THIS BOOK

I base this book on my work with sexually abused men for over ten years. I have had numerous consultations with these men, have treated them in individual and group therapy, and have supervised other therapists doing similar work. In most of my discussion, I group together two subpopulations: boys who have suffered from incestuous abuse and boys whose abusers came from outside their families—usually adults who violated positions of power and trust. While these two subgroups may exhibit some differences in terms of psychological sequelae of abuse, I believe they are more similar than different.

The hundred or so men I have worked with have generally been high-functioning and impressive despite clear areas of profound psychological scarring and dysfunction.[4] This is not to say that all boys who

---

[4] See van der Kolk (1987), Herman (1981), and Davies and Frawley (1992, 1994) for similar impressions of sexually abused women.

were sexually abused grow up to be high-functioning. The men I have seen have managed, after all, to lead lives that somehow brought them to a psychoanalyst's office, which may suggest that they are psychologically stronger, more evolved, and less damaged than others with similar histories. This point is also made by Shengold (1989), who feels as I do that "my case material will seem mild indeed to those dealing with battered and sexually assaulted children who turn up in police stations and hospital emergency rooms" (p. 3). Again like Shengold, however, I believe my observations apply to a wider spectrum of sexually abused men than I have treated.

Many of my patients defined themselves as survivors of sexual abuse before seeing me, because knowledge of my interest in working with this population has encouraged referrals from such sources as rape intervention programs and self-help groups. Thus, my patient population may be somewhat different from those of clinicians whose patients have usually recovered memories of abuse during treatment. On the other hand, while they usually remembered abuse before seeing me, most of my patients experienced amnesia regarding it during some part of their life. This is in keeping with recent research about the extent of amnesia for childhood sexual abuse (Briere and Conte, 1993; Williams, 1994). Most of my patients recalled premature sexual experiences while not in therapy, although a significant minority regained memories while in treatment with another therapist.

While memories of early trauma may sometimes reflect the distortions of a child's viewpoint, I generally accept that they represent the man's psychological experience as well as an approximation of what a neutral observer would confirm did happen. Many men dealing with concerns about sexual abuse express doubts about their memories, especially if these are vague. Usually they want fervently to "prove" one way or the other whether they were in fact abused. Most often their initial hope is that they will prove they were *not* abused, preferring to think of themselves as crazy than their families as abusive or neglectful. It paradoxically restores hope for a boy to do this, because it supports the fantasy that he is "bad" and caused his abuse while his caretakers are "good" and love him. If this is so, then he can perfect himself and become loveable, thereby changing his abusive situation (Schwartz, Galperin, and Masters, 1995a).

Hearing men deal with memories that are nonspecific or shadowy has led me to conceptualize my sexual abuse work as much in terms of boundary violations of the child as of sexual activity with him (see Chapter 6). Every sexually abused adult has suffered a severe invasion of physical, sexual, and psychological space. It is sometimes helpful to concentrate on this psychological invasion rather than always to focus on whether a specific abusive act "really" took place. Doing so gets me out of the role of psychoanalytic detective and back into the role of interpreter of psychological experience. After all, I can never say definitively that a patient was sexually abused, because I was not there (see Courtois, 1992). I can, however, address his feelings of profound and traumatic violation, and the way this sense of violation affects his current life.

As a group, sexually abused men who choose to enter therapy, however reluctantly, are likely to have developed internalizing defenses in reaction to their abuse, as well as to other aspects of their lives. Those who do not seek treatment, by contrast, are more likely to have developed externalizing defenses (see Chapter 3), which may lead them to act out abusively. While several of the men I have worked with were sexual abusers themselves as older children or teenagers, none reported being an adult offender. All came into treatment voluntarily. I am thus writing about only a segment of the larger group of sexually abused men. While some in that larger population do become abusive themselves, most do not (see the discussion of the work of Lisak et al., 1996, in Chapter 3). Some come to therapy voluntarily, while others are forced to come because of antisocial behavior, which may include being sexually abusive. (Both of these factors are complexly related to whether the man encodes his abuse experience as "abuse" or "sexual initiation" and whether he feels feminized by his victimization. I will address these issues in Chapters 2, 3, and 4.)

My patients' treatments have lasted from a minimum of three sessions to over seven years, at a rate of one to four times weekly. The men have ranged in age from sixteen to seventy-two. I have seen gay and straight men in about equal numbers, and both these groups have reported abuse by men and by women. Most of the men have been white, although there have been some men of African-American, Asian, Native American, and Latino backgrounds. The great majority have had at least some college education. Many have had backgrounds that included neglect and verbal or physical abuse in addition to sexual abuse. Approximately half of the men whose stories are described in this book were referred for psychotropic medication, usually antidepressants, but occasionally drugs for sleep or anxiety disorders.[5]

The subject of sexually abused adults confronting abusers as part of

---

[5] I will not be discussing psychotropic medication in any comprehensive way in this book, but I do feel that when indicated it can be a very helpful adjunct of psychotherapy, especially for men whose dissociated memories are suddenly emerging into full emotional awareness, who have been mired in long-term depression, or who are highly anxious.

the treatment has been discussed in the literature (for example, Courtois, 1988). The abusers of most of the men I have treated were dead at the time of treatment, which in itself raises the question of whether men are less likely than women to be able to face their abuse while the abuser lives. Even when the abuser is alive, in my experience, women have been more likely than men to want such adult confrontations with abusers. This may be due to shame issues, but also to the possibility that further physical abuse in such situations is especially strong when both partici-pants are men.[6]

The question of suing perpetrators of abuse has also occupied the attention of the media and some writers. None of the men I have treated has sought legal remedy for sexual abuse. My own belief is that seeking legal redress for childhood sexual abuse is rarely a healing process. On occasion, using the legal system in this way may satisfy a need for the truth to be revealed. However, court cases can drag on for years, forcing the abused individual to stay emotionally focused on his betrayal. In addition, the outcome is never assured, and even when an individual wins in court he may well not feel any better about what happened to him.[7] In terms of his psychotherapy, knowing that a therapist may be called upon to support a legal case vastly complicates the treatment. Different standards of proof are necessarily required for work with a troubled patient than for legal proof that a person is guilty of child molestation. And the relationship between patient and therapist, complicated enough when it does not involve a legal battle, can become hopelessly entangled in expectations on both sides that the therapist will advocate for the patient in court. (See my previous discussion of this issue; Gartner, 1997d.)

BETRAYAL BY A TRUSTED CARETAKER

The abusers of the men I have treated included fathers, mothers, broth-ers, sisters, female and male babysitters, grandfathers, teachers, neigh-bors, a family doctor, a godfather, a priest, a nun, and the director of a summer camp. No man I have treated was *only* abused by strangers. Nearly all of them were violated as boys by adults in positions of power and trust.

The betrayal of a trusted relationship is frequently more traumatic than the sexual acts themselves. This is a fundamental truth that must be

---

[6] For a harrowing first-person account of how an adult confrontation between a man and his abusive father turned violent, see Lew's (1988) case of "Philip" (pp. 78–90).

[7] See Shapiro (1997) for another viewpoint.

understood when working with sexually abused adults. Because of its importance, I end this opening chapter with an adult's perceptions as he looked back on his boyhood betrayal. Ross Cheit (quoted in Freyd, 1996), a professor at Brown University, recovered memories in adulthood of sexual abuse by a much-admired and beloved conductor of a children's music group. These memories were confirmed to have occurred. Here is Cheit's description of the heartbreaking grief he felt about his violation:

> "I thought about these actions in terms of what this man meant to me in my life, in terms of a relationship rather than in terms of just actions. . . . I thought he was a great guy. I really admired him. I read these letters [I wrote about him at the time]. And the whole thing shifted from just 'those acts' to complete betrayal. And I broke down that night and cried in a way I had never cried before. And I was sobbing, saying the whole time, he was such a great guy." (p. 9)

CHAPTER 2

Encoding Sexual Abuse
as Sexual Initiation

Boys are socialized to believe that men want sex whenever it is offered to them. The sexual behavior of adults with boys has often been misunderstood and underreported because it is not considered abusive or even unwelcome. If boys have premature sexual experiences, especially with girls and women, they are thought to be "sexually initiated," not molested. This results from the false belief that boys and men cannot be sexually victimized. They thus often come to think of themselves, at least consciously, as fortunate rather than as exploited in these sexual encounters. Popular literature is replete with examples of "coming-of-age" stories in which boys are introduced to sexuality in a positive way by older women, as we shall see in this chapter. Thus, boys may not have an acceptable way of understanding premature sexual experience with women as anything but enjoyable. If they do not welcome sexuality with women, they feel deviant, and may expect others to see them that way too. For all these reasons, the sexual betrayal of boys by women, both overt and covert, is especially underreported and underrecognized, even though, as Lisak et al. (1996) report, 39 percent of the men in their sample who acknowledged sexual abuse histories reported having female victimizers.

Sex with men usually has very different connotations, whether the boy is headed for a predominantly gay or for a predominantly straight

42

orientation. I will limit my discussion of sex between boys and men in this chapter to situations in which a boy developing a gay identity encodes the sexual activity as consonant with his own erotic desires. In Chapter 3, I will analyze the masculine gender ideals that influence how sexual abuse is encoded. In Chapter 4, I will discuss same-sex situations in which intertwined conflicts about sexual orientation and masculine gender identity confound how both predominantly straight and predominantly gay boys may encode same-sex abuse.

In this chapter, I will focus on how boys encode sexual situations with women, and then discuss how these issues play out in mother–son incestuous relationships. I will then consider the circumstance of a gay boy who considers himself a full partner in sexual activity with a man. Finally, I will highlight how the encoding of abuse interacts with sexual object choice, and the contrasting encoding problems of both straight and gay boys who are abused by men versus those abused by women.

ARE BOYS IN CHARGE OF SEX WITH WOMEN?

Consider a cartoon that appeared in *The New Yorker* on August 25, 1997: The scene is a young boy's bedroom. The window shade is down. The paraphernalia of young boyhood are strewn all over the room. On the wall are pennants and a poster. The bureau displays a model airplane, and the drawers are open with his clothes spilling out. A baseball bat leans against the wall. Scattered about the floor are a board game, a model car, and a football. Clothes are in disarray on the floor and chair. In the bed are a boy of perhaps ten or eleven and a young woman apparently in her late teens or early twenties. Both are sitting up, both are naked, and both are smoking in a postcoital scene straight out of a French film of the 1960s. The woman is a glassy-eyed blonde, exhaling clouds of smoke. The boy gestures grandly to her as he says in the caption, "I want you to know, Sheila, that you'll always be more than just another babysitter to me."

The joke is clear. The boy, prepubescent or perhaps in early puberty, is in charge of the sexual encounter with his much older babysitter. He is letting her know that their relationship will end but that she will be a wonderful memory as he goes on to other, perhaps better, conquests. If we see anything below the surface of this cartoon, it is that the woman is the victim of a cad who is trying to let her down gently. Meanwhile, we see him as a skilled and lucky seducer. Such is the collective societal view of premature sex between a young boy and an older woman. She has been generous to him, and is certainly not a sexual abuser. If anything, she has been used by a lecher who is responsible for what is happening and is to be admired for his success with her. It is assumed that he has no anxiety about their relationship.

If you are amused by this cartoon's image, imagine for a moment that the sexes are reversed, that a ten-year-old girl is naked in her bed with her twenty-year-old male baby-sitter, smoking a cigarette and telling him he'll always have a special place in her heart. For most of us, the joke is suddenly no longer funny. We understand that young girls should not be in bed with their baby-sitters, and we would consider the man the predator and the girl the victim, unlike the portrayal of the couple in the cartoon. This imaginary reversal of the sexes highlights our double standard about child sexual abuse.

CAN WOMEN RAPE BOYS?

A thoughtful newspaper account of the trial of a thirty-seven-year-old woman charged with the statutory rape of a thirteen-year-old boy captures societal attitudes about sexual behavior between women and boys. Writing in *The Boston Globe*, Karen Aronoso (July 9, 1996, pp. 15–17) describes "an age-old double standard: Men who have sex with children are criminals; boys who have sex with women are lucky. . . . Sex with any female—particularly a mature, experienced one—is perceived as good fortune for a boy. Intercourse is rarely considered unwanted."

Aronoso quotes neighbors and others familiar with the case:

"I'm sure the boy wanted this. He knew what was going on. He could tell people, 'Hey, I had sex with an actual woman.' "

"She's just a little immature, not violent or anything like that."

"It's definitely rape, but we all kind of accept it because of the way society says boys should be sexually active at a young age."

"[For an adolescent boy] it's like a dream to have sex with an older woman."

These comments reveal the pervasiveness of cultural attitudes that tacitly or openly condone sex between boys and women. Ganzarain and Buchele (1990) note how difficult it is to convince a jury that a woman has molested a boy. This was summed up in the remarks of the chief of the child abuse prosecution unit in the case Aronoso describes. Noting that only once in five years had she previously prosecuted a rape involving a woman and a boy, she is quoted as saying, "The reaction in these cases is usually winking and nodding and saying boys will be boys and that this is all part of the learning experience. . . . It's very hard for boys to come forward because they feel ashamed at admitting they've been victimized."

About this last point, Aronoso notes: "When a boy does say he has been raped, both his peers and his elders may express disbelief. . . . Traditionally viewed as strong and self-sufficient, males are expected to escape any situation they find unpleasant." And, further, "When a stereotypically maternal figure seduces a child, society may cast her aggression as no more than poor judgment and not harmful."

Maloney (1995) describes the myths about men and women that make it difficult to imagine women as sexually abusive. Among the cultural illusions he enumerates about men and women are that men are responsible for all sexual activity, including sexual abuse; that sex with a woman is always an enjoyable rite of passage for a boy; that all sexual abuse is overt; that boys and men can protect themselves from the "weaker sex" and therefore if they are assaulted they are fools; that if a male victim doesn't enjoy sex with a female abuser he is homosexual; that men enjoy kinky and aggressive sex; that all men's orgasms and erections are voluntary; and that a woman can do no harm sexually because she has no penis.

More notorious than the Massachusetts case is the story of Mary Kay LeTourneau, a thirty-five-year-old Seattle schoolteacher who was impregnated by her thirteen-year-old sixth grade student, a boy she had also taught in second grade. A married mother of four, LeTourneau gave birth to a baby girl, who is being raised by the boy's mother. She was convicted of two counts of child rape and sentenced to seven and a half years in prison. According to *People* (March 30, 1998), at her sentencing "she expressed remorse and pleaded for leniency. 'I did something I had no right to do. Morally and legally it was wrong. Help me. I give you my word it will not happen again'" (p. 47). Accordingly, she was given parole for all but six months of her sentence, and was released on condition that she attend a program for sex offenders and not see the boy again. Days after her release from prison, however, she had stopped taking the medication prescribed for her bipolar disorder and was rebelling against her psychological treatment. She was soon rearrested for being in a parked car with the boy (*New York Times*, February 4, 1998, p. A17). Her parole was revoked, and shortly thereafter it was discovered that she was six weeks' pregnant by him. At the time she was rearrested, it appears she was getting ready to flee the country with the boy (*People*, March 30, 1998). There was no further prosecution of LeTourneau. She gave birth to a second daughter while in jail, and this child is also being raised by the boy's parents, who are said to be accepting LeTourneau as a member of their family (*New York Times*, October 18, 1998, p. A30, and October 24, 1998, p. B18).

While this woman's behavior was recognized as sexually abusive and she was brought to trial, she was penalized far more leniently than a man in her position might have been. Imagine what would have followed had a thirty-five-year-old married male teacher impregnated his thirteen-year-old student. Is it likely he would have been given a six-month sentence and let out on parole based solely on his word not to recontact the girl? The answer, I think, is self-evident. Without going into the appropriateness of one sentence over another for any abuser, I believe that the sentencing in this case embodies the different societal attitudes about men and women as sexual abusers.

Meanwhile, the boy in the case maintained that "he had initiated the sexual relationship, and that LeTourneau had tried to resist before finally giving in" (*People,* March 30, 1998, p. 47). Insisting that there was nothing wrong with what had happened, the boy told a reporter, "All that matters was that we loved each other" (*New York Times,* November 9, 1997, p. IV3).[1]

But *is* that all that matters? Can any thirteen-year-old, no matter how mature, be ready to make the life decisions this sixth grader was encouraged to make by his teacher? Thinking that love is all that matters might in itself be considered a sign that he is not ready to make such a complex choice about his future. In Chapter 1, I noted that there may be some occasions when early sexuality is nontraumatic for a given child. This is more likely to be the case for an adolescent nonviolently involved with an adult whose gender is appropriate for his own object choice. However, I also commented that a boy may have little capacity to judge the effects of premature sexuality on himself, or even to name it as troubling or agitating.

Because of the cultural myths that women cannot be sexually exploitative, the traumatic impact of abuse of boys by women is particularly minimized in our culture (see Mendel, 1995).[2] Indeed, one sexual abuse researcher has gone so far as to say that "sexual abuse by women is virtually nonexistent" (Crewdson, 1988, p. 70). Consequently, a boy

---

[1] In a related case where there was no pregnancy, a female high school teacher in Minnesota was sentenced to nearly seven years in jail for having sexual relations with a fifteen-year-old male student. She was also ordered to register as a sex offender and submit her blood sample for DNA testing. She said she loved the boy, but he testified that she was a "monster" whom he never wanted to see again. His father described him as a formerly carefree young boy who became angry and depressed because of his relationship with the teacher (*New York Times,* August 2, 1998, p. A23).

[2] For discussions of female sexual abusers of boys, see Sarrel and Masters (1982); Marvesti (1986); Condy, Templer, Brown, and Veaco (1987); Johnson and Shrier (1987); Banning (1989); Krug (1989); Shengold (1989); Kasl (1990); Mathews, Matthews, and Speltz (1990); Baron, Burgess, and Kao (1991); Harper (1993); Bachmann, Moggi, and Stirnemann-Lewis (1994); Elliott (1994); Siegel (1996); and Miletski (1997).

is likely to feel he is "supposed" to enjoy sexual encounters whether they are welcome or not, especially if the initiator is female but not his mother. As Johanek (1988) says, "[T]he boy who is molested or abused by a woman is often unaware he is being victimized. . . . If a boy discusses such events with his peers, he is often congratulated for his luck, with no one paying any attention to his uneasiness or feelings of being used or exploited" (p. 108).

For example, Ramon, a man who as a child and teenager was molested primarily but not exclusively by men, used his experiences with women to "prove" that his experiences with men did not mean he was homosexual. He was therefore initially unable to encode his experiences with women as abusive in any way. As Ramon initially portrayed it, he had been sexual with women because he wanted to, but he was more ambivalent and ashamed about his activities with men. He said that he felt reassured by the pleasure he felt with the women, that being with them even at age ten "made up for" being sexual with men as well. When I suggested that whatever his desires at the time, he had been molested as much by the women as by the men, he was surprised. But when I asked what he would think if he heard about a ten-year-old boy engaging in sex with an adult woman, he nodded vehemently and said, "Of course! It shouldn't happen!"

CINEMATIC DEPICTIONS OF SEXUAL INITIATION OF BOYS BY WOMEN

As Johanek (1988) notes, "Popular literature is replete with stories of boys who are introduced to adult sexuality by older women" (p. 108). Boys who look to such popular media as film for information about premature sexuality with women (for example, *Tea and Sympathy, The Graduate, Harold and Maude, The Last Picture Show,* and *Summer of '42*) find virtually no support for any feelings of anxiety or discomfort. Such experiences are almost universally portrayed in a positive light, as the sexual initiation of an adolescent into manhood by an experienced, caring, and/or attractive older woman (even, in the case of *Murmur of the Heart,* his mother[3]). There is virtually no sense in any of these films that a boy may not always be happy to be sexually involved with an older woman. Although in some cases the boys initially react to their seductions with embarrassed fumbling, often they become magically skilled lovers, reinforcing the idea that a relationship like this transforms

---

[3] A darker view of maternal incest is depicted in *Spanking the Monkey.*

them into "real men." Any long-term negative consequences for them are ignored or minimized.

Conversely, the women are generally portrayed as nonexploitative and nonmenacing. Indeed, they may be depicted as noble and self-sacrificing, even as victims for whom we feel compassion when the boys eventually abandon them. They are never seen as adults sexually molesting children. However, if we look closely, many of the women are needy and have personal agendas that influence their decision to become sexually involved with the boy. For example, they may have shaky marriages, feel neglected or old, or be in mourning for a former lover.

Even if we accept the premise of each individual film that in the particular situation being portrayed there was no abuse or trauma involved, we must also consider the overall cultural effect of film after film in which sex between a boy and an older woman is seen as positive for him. There is no model for a boy in such a situation to feel it is acceptable not to welcome, enjoy, and take pleasure from the relationship. This is the crucial point I wish to make: portrayals in this popular medium *only* support the idea that boys are happy to be offered sex with older women, and virtually *never* endorse the view that such situations are or can be sexual betrayals.

Such depictions reinforce and perpetuate attitudes toward sexual victimization that make it difficult for boys to process and heal from traumatic sexual experiences with women. A boy cannot help but deduce that feeling anxiety, dread, or apprehension about these situations makes him different from other boys and perhaps even unmanly. He learns to ignore these sensations, deny them, or never allow them into awareness.

ENCODING FEMALE SEXUAL BEHAVIOR WITH HETEROSEXUAL BOYS

I got a call one day with an unusual and urgent request from a young woman named Doreen. She said she had been in treatment with another therapist for several years, in part because of a history of childhood sexual abuse by her brother, Ed. Having decided to confront Ed about the abuse, she had asked him to fly in from the distant state where he lived. She had told him only that she needed to talk to him about something very important to her. Ed was arriving that afternoon, and she was planning to talk to him that night about the abuse. She wanted to know if I could be available to meet with him if he felt he needed to talk to a therapist afterward. Almost in passing, she mentioned that she wondered if Ed had also been sexually abused as a child.

I said I would be willing to meet with Ed. After hanging up the phone, I considered the interesting nature of their relationship. Doreen knew Ed would drop whatever he was doing to come a long distance to talk to her if she said she needed him. And, although Doreen was convinced that Ed had abused her, she obviously loved him enough to try to find him psychological support in the midst of preparing herself for what clearly was going to be a difficult confrontation. Or had her abusive history prepared her to take care of her abuser no matter what? I could not tell.

Ed telephoned me the next morning and we arranged to meet. He was an open-faced, likeable man in his late twenties, dressed casually, with the long hair and beard of an outdoors man who would never have to punch a time clock. He seemed bright and articulate, though not particularly psychologically minded.

Ed was still in shock from his confrontation with Doreen. He had no recollection of the events she described, although he did not deny they had occurred. As Doreen recounted the story, on several occasions when he was eight and she was five Ed tickled her while she was in bed. The tickling had gone beyond the bounds she was comfortable with, involving rubbing of her chest where breasts would be, and also stroking of her thighs and vagina. She protested, but he just laughed and continued.

Ed did remember childhood sexual activity with Doreen, but from a later age, when he was about fourteen and she was eleven. They had gone into the woods with friends who were also brother and sister and of the same ages as Doreen and Ed. There, the four of them had undressed, looked at each other, then played together without any overt sexual touching involved. He remembered this occasion as one that involved excitement and guilty pleasure because they thought they would be punished if they were caught. His overall sense, though, was that it had been a "lark." Ed said he told Doreen about this episode, but she did not recall it. Her explanation, which he accepted, was that she probably had not remembered the incident because it had apparently been consensual and therefore not traumatic.

At first, Ed was mainly interested in talking about how he should discuss the memories with Doreen so as to be as healing and helpful to her as possible. In this context, we talked about his need to be open, to allow expressions of anger, and to accept responsibility for the kind of brother he had been and continued to be. It was clear that there was much in the relationship that was mutually positive and supportive.

We talked about their family and upbringing. Nothing sounded particularly remarkable: the family was middle class, there were two other siblings, there had been family separations, and there seemed to have been basically positive relationships among the siblings and between the children and their parents. I asked what it had been like between him and Doreen as children. Ed said they had been close but then he laughed and said he had "loved to tease her and drive her crazy, like any brother liked to do with a younger sister or brother." He supposed "there might have been a competitive streak" between them.

Then I mentioned that Doreen had said she wondered if Ed had also been abused as a child. Ed chuckled amusedly, saying he had not been. Later, however, Ed mentioned having had an eighteen-year-old female baby-sitter when he was about seven who encouraged him several times to touch her bare breasts under her sweater. Laughing again, he said he wished he'd been older when it happened because he would have enjoyed it. As it was, he was "dumb enough" to tell his parents not to hire her any more.

I stopped him and inquired further. Why did he think it was "dumb" to have her fired? Startled, he said, "Because I'm sure it felt very nice to touch her breasts, and I'd love to do it now." We had to go over the events several times before he acknowledged the difference between an adult man imagining with pleasure fondling a young woman's breasts and a boy of seven feeling uncomfortable with the guilt-inducing and frightening stimulation of fondling the naked breasts of his caretaker. I said, "You certainly behaved like someone protecting himself from abuse when you asked your parents not to use her any more." His laughter vanished, and he nodded uneasily, obviously troubled, saying he had never thought about it that way.

As we retraced the events of that period, it became clear that the incidents with the baby-sitter had stimulated Ed considerably. Additionally, I think it plausible that they had encouraged him to add behaviors into his already rough but probably normative treatment of his little sister so that it became abusive. He had been taught that intimate touching is acceptable in a hierarchical relationship even if the less powerful participant is uncomfortable with it. Not surprisingly, he took this new knowledge to the relationship in which *he* wielded the power, began to touch Doreen intimately, and did not stop when she protested. In addition, of course, Ed shifted the balance of power with the baby-sitter and had her fired.

This vignette highlights important aspects of the experience of childhood sexual abuse, including some of the potential differences between how boys and girls ultimately understand what happened to them. Both Doreen and Ed were sexually abused as children. From an external standpoint, neither had encountered profound or even malevolent violation, yet each had a sense of having been invaded and feeling helpless in the face of a more powerful person's sexual wishes. But

Doreen understood that she had been abused. Ed, on the other hand, while uncomfortable at the time, later thought of himself as "dumb" for not having enjoyed what "should" have been an exciting sexual awakening. Like many men, he had over time apparently revised a sexually abusive boyhood experience with a woman so that it became retrospectively defined as normative (Holmes and Slap, 1998).

What about Doreen and Ed's different memories of their childhood sexual experiences? I believe Doreen was correct when she said that she remembered the earlier episodes because they were traumatic and forgot the later one because it was consensual. An alternate explanation, that the later experience was dissociated or repressed because it was traumatic, seems much less persuasive to me. On the other hand, even though Ed was the guilty party in the earlier occurrences, he did not recall them. Perhaps his nonrecall resulted from a repression of guilt feelings about what he had done to Doreen. Or perhaps these events were not as important to him as the incidents with the baby-sitter, to which the abuse of Doreen was a reaction. They certainly seem not to have been as exciting to him as the episode with the other brother and sister. In any case, it appears that both Ed and Doreen selectively remembered experiences that were pivotal as they grew up, pivotal particularly in relation to feelings about burgeoning sexuality and boundary violations.

The differing attitudes of Ed and Doreen illustrate one way men and boys may encode their sexual abuse by women differently than women and girls encode their abuse by men. In addition, we can see in them the different societal norms about sexual activity with girls and boys. Sexual abuse of girls is more common than abuse of boys, but it is also more universally condemned when discovered (Groth, 1979). And, while I do not doubt that girls are traumatized by abuse as much as boys, girls may be readier than boys to recognize their abuse *as* abuse. This recognition helps girls come to terms with the abuse as adults.

WHEN THE ABUSER IS MOTHER

In general, then, it is difficult for boys to encode sexual behavior with women as molestation. Encoding sexual mistreatment by a mother is far more complicated. Mothers are often thought to be their sons' primary object of erotic desire. The Freudian concept of the Oedipus complex conveys the powerful longing sons have for their mothers. Its resolution is insurance that sons do not act upon these strong wishes. But the deep sense of erotic connection boys want with their mothers is rarely thought to be a wish for actual genital union.

Mother–son incest is perhaps the most taboo incestuous relationship in American society. I have often been greeted with blank stares of horror and disbelief, even in professional settings, when I bring up overt mother–son incest even as a theoretical possibility (see Welldon, 1988, for a discussion of attitudes toward mothers as desiring, erotic individuals). The traditional focus of psychoanalysts on the mother–son incest taboo highlights its ubiquity in our culture as well as the power of the wishes it is thought to restrain.

Maloney (1995) enumerates some of the cultural myths that underlie and/or result from this taboo: every woman loves her children unselfishly; mothers have their children's best interests at heart at all times; mothers are altruistic and loving; mothers are there to meet the needs of their husbands and children; a mother may be sexual as a spouse but is asexual as a mother; and a mother is never sexually attracted to her children. These myths are powerfully entrenched in our culture and buttress the strong cultural prohibition of incest by a mother.

On the rare occasions that overt incest between a mother and son comes to light, it is more likely than covert incest to be considered wrong. Siegel (1996) reminds us that incestuous mothers have been regarded by mental health professionals as more deeply disturbed than incestuous fathers, though neither she nor I agree with this assessment. I myself have heard it stated flatly that only a psychotic mother could abuse her son.

Maternal sexual betrayal of a son often occurs covertly, in the guise of some aspect of caretaking and nurturing, as when a mother gives her son unneeded enemas or spends too much time washing his genitals. Kyle, for example, was lined up, along with his sisters, for weekly anal examinations by his fanatically meticulous mother. She claimed to be checking for worms, and scrutinized each of them with metal probing instruments while the other children watched. Such situations are rarely recognized as either sexual or abusive. If the behavior is noticed at all, it is at worst likely to be considered the result of the mother's overcompulsivity or overzealousness in her maternal role.

Gabbard and Twemlow (1994) explain the denial of maternal sexual abuse, as well as the denial of abuse of boys by any woman, by arguing that "deeply ensconced gender-based stereotypes play a role in minimizing the traumatic impact of maternal seductions on male children. Within our culture we have clear gender biases regarding who is the seducer and who is seduced, who is the victimizer and who is the victim, and who is likely to be damaged by the sexual act" (p. 172).

There have been some reports of mother–son incest in the psychoanalytic literature. Margolis (1977, 1984) and Shengold (1980, 1989), for example, both remark on the heightened sense of specialness and entitlement felt by adolescent boys they treated who had been abused by their mothers (see also Siegel, 1996). Gabbard and Twemlow (1994) also note this sense of specialness, but add: "The sense that their exalted status is tenuous, contingent, and provisional leads these men to develop a pervasive anxiety related to the perception that a disaster may occur at any moment" (p. 183). One possible explanation for this pervasive anxiety is the boy's guilty and ambivalent pleasure in the incest. However, anxiety is often explicitly engendered by the interpersonal dynamics of the abusive situation. For example, the mother of the patient Gabbard and Twemlow describe would abruptly interrupt their sexual activity, leaving him overstimulated and bereft. In addition, she threatened to hurt him if he "let go" and ejaculated when they were together. Not surprisingly, as an adult he developed the symptom of ejaculatory inhibition. Finally, the mother made it seem as though her son was the aggressor in their sexual activity and that she was relieved when his father appeared and pulled him off her. Thus, she organized the incest in such a way that her son could never be sure that his special relationship with her would continue.

Given the extreme taboos about mother–son incest, recognizing such behavior as both incestuous and abusive can be cataclysmic for the son. The inner consciousness that he was excited by erotic contact with his mother can be especially devastating and confusing. He may be proud on some levels of his sexual "prowess" (Siegel, 1996), and this may lead to a sense of grandiosity about his abilities to seduce women (see Chapters 8 and 10). At the same time, however, the incestuous activity was likely to have been suffused with distortions by the abusing mother, as when Gabbard and Twemlow's patient was told by his mother that he had been the sexual aggressor. In turn, the son may need to create distortions of the situation, either then or later, in order to bear thinking about it at all.

Silber (1979) relates how his patient's distortions of reality stemmed from his early maternal abuse. This man was abused by his mother at nap time over an extended period during his preschool years and later. At first, she invited him to explore the scar from the caesarean section she had had at his birth, telling him he was entitled to do so because he had been the cause of it. Then she extended downward the area he could explore until he was rubbing her vulva. Over time, she shifted his body to be on top of hers and rubbed him against her genitals by holding on to his hips. At other times, in the guise of play, she forced his face to her genitals and rubbed his abdomen. Silber hypothesizes a series of defenses that his patient developed in response to the trauma of this abuse, including an ability to enter hypnoid states and a pervasive denial of reality, especially in his interpersonal relationships, that extended into his adult years. (See Chapters 7 and 8 for a more extended discussion of these dissociative defenses and their effect on an individual's ability to relate to others.)

Brooke Hopkins (1993) has written a moving account of his sexual victimization by his mother at a very young age. At the time, he understood the abusive events to be wrong and, in some unarticulated way, simultaneously abusive, yet powerfully inviting. He describes how at about age six he waited after bedtime for his mother to get into bed with him and spend the night. He thought at the time that perhaps it would have been better if he had been a girl, because then he wouldn't have to worry about "that thing of mine" (p. 34) and all the erotic urges he felt toward his mother:

> Somehow, I felt, it would have been easier with another kind of body, one more like hers, because what was happening was, I knew, not supposed to be happening, and very dangerous, even though I yearned for it every night, had become completely addicted to it, and could hardly have imagined myself living without it. But by the time she slipped into bed with me, her six-year-old son, all these thoughts vanished in the sheer pleasure of having her body next to mine. (p. 35)

He describes the intense sexual excitement he felt for his mother, the nearly unbearable desire that he simultaneously loved and feared:

> [I was] almost unbearably excited by being so intimately in bed with her, by exploring her body with my hands . . . , feeling her warmth and her smell. Sometimes my penis would be so stiff from rubbing against her that I was afraid it would break off, literally like a stick. . . . [T]here were moments when I could hardly contain myself with the desire to be touched as well. It was about this time that I began to anticipate my mother's coming down the hall with a combination of the most intense longing and an almost equally intense dread. (p. 43)

He touched her body everywhere, and, seemingly passive, she allowed such contact without ever openly acknowledging what was happening. The only exception was when he once tried to touch her vagina and she "said sleepily, 'No, I'm sorry. You can't touch me there. That place is saved for your father'" (p. 44). Hopkins then relates how his father put an end to the overt sexuality between him and his mother by suddenly coming into his room one night and violently pulling his mother out of Hopkins's bed.

Richard Berendzen (Berendzen and Palmer, 1993) has written another compelling personal description of the extreme confusion of a boy in an overtly incestuous relationship with his mother. Berendzen is the former president of American University in Washington, DC, who resigned in disgrace after it was discovered that he had compulsively made telephone calls suggesting he was committing child sexual abuse. After undergoing extensive psychotherapeutic treatment, he wrote a book linking his bizarre behavior to his own severe history of childhood sexual abuse by his mother (and on one occasion being included in sexual intercourse with both parents). In the book he writes about his disorganizing responses to the overt sexuality with his mother:

> What happened . . . came in a dizzying blur, feelings of confusion, disgust, and terror slamming into each other, toppled by momentary convulsions of nausea, excitement, and shame. *A hurricane overtook my small boat.* I tied myself to the mast, closed my eyes, and tried to survive the storm. I felt a deep revulsion, a revulsion buried under my skin. My body knew a secret, hidden from the world. Yet within this awful revulsion, I experienced momentary pleasure ripples of tingling sensation. To experience pleasure and disgust for the same reason and almost simultaneously created overwhelming confusion and torment. If I knew I hated what happened between my mother and me, how could my body respond as it did? Arousal led to pleasure, which capsized instantly in shame and disgust. It sickened and bewildered me to hate my body for making me feel good. (p. 21; emphasis added)

Hopkins and Berendzen thus encapsulate the all-encompassing ambivalence of the survivor of sexual abuse by a mother, and perhaps, in a heightened form, the reactions of any child victim of sexual abuse by a caretaker. The child experiences desire and excitement along with disgust and revulsion. His inner world is deeply immersed in a civil war that would have terrible long-term effects on the psyche of any child.

The boy thus must somehow reconcile the paradox of his own warring emotions. But, as Berendzen dryly, and bleakly, concludes, "Paradox does not fascinate a child" (p. 21).

ENCODING MALE ABUSE OF HOMOSEXUAL BOYS

Like a heterosexual boy abused by a woman, if a boy growing up to be gay is abused by a man, he may think of it as something he deliberately sought or at least liked. This situation is especially complicated because being involved in erotic same-sex behavior may itself be experienced as shameful, and may give cause for others to consider the boy himself depraved or wanton. Wright (1995) describes how a thirteen-year-old boy, not a hustler, was arrested along with the adult man who was having sex with him. Instead of being treated as a victim of a crime, however, the boy was *himself* charged with sexual immorality. This makes sense only if we believe that boys, whether gay or straight, are in charge of themselves, sexually and otherwise, and therefore are totally responsible for all their actions. This is a concept whose other implications I will examine in Chapter 3.

I will further discuss the subject of abused men's sexual identity and sexual orientation struggles in Chapter 4. For the moment, however, consider the reactions of one gay man to his early sexual experiences with an older man.

Coming to treatment with me in his retirement years, Owen was a man with complex reactions to his homosexuality, to being exploited by his family, and to his sexual misuse by an older man throughout his adolescence. The complexities of these experiences led him to believe for the rest of his life that he had not been sexually abused, even though he freely acknowledged that if he were to hear of a child going through experiences identical to his own he would try to protect the child from them.

Owen grew up in a family whose roots in its midwestern community went back many decades before his birth. His family was respectable and hardworking, though never wealthy. Indeed, during Owen's formative years in the Great Depression they were quite poor, although never in an absolutely disastrous financial situation. The oldest of six, Owen was raised with a strong sense of duty to his family, and in particular was given considerable responsibility for his younger siblings. This became more pronounced when a younger sister was invalided for several years by a life-threatening debilitating disease requiring frequent hospitalizations and constant special care.

Owen's interest in other boys was well established by age eight, when he was involved over a period of time in consensual sex play with a ten-year-old friend. At age twelve, Owen began a long-term "affair," as he called it, with Calvin, a twenty-nine-year-old man.

Calvin was a man of some wealth, a member of the town's most prominent family. He openly courted Owen, though the sexual nature of this courtship seems not to have been apparent to others, and showered him and his family with various gifts and favors. He was a constant visitor in Owen's home. He owned a car, something of a rarity in the town at that time, and willingly gave rides to various members of the family. Owen recalled his father requesting him to ask Calvin if the father could use the car, so it appears that the specialness of the relationship between Owen and Calvin was clear and openly acknowledged. Owen was ashamed of having to ask Calvin to do such favors for his family, but only in therapy nearly sixty years later did he begin to think about how the family used him to get what they needed from Calvin. Owen's father once asked him if Calvin ever did anything with Owen that "he shouldn't." Owen quickly answered "No," and the question was never brought up again, even when Calvin took the family on vacations at his own expense and shared a room (and bed) with Owen while the rest of the family shared another room.

When Owen went away to college, the sexuality in the relationship with Calvin ended at Owen's request, though a friendship continued until Calvin's death. After Owen married, Calvin also married, and even asked Owen to be his best man. Owen declined because he was afraid that somehow people would know that he and Calvin had been sexually involved if he filled this role. Calvin later had children of his own, and only in his treatment with me did Owen begin to wonder whether Calvin had abused his own children.

It was in the context of our exploring Owen's attitude toward his homosexuality that he told me about his "affair" with Calvin. Owen never considered the relationship to have been abusive, even though, as I have said, he acknowledged that if he heard about such a relationship between a twelve-year-old boy and a twenty-nine-year-old man he would feel it was inappropriate and exploitative. But he maintained that there was no abuse from Calvin because Owen knew how interested he was in sex with men and with Calvin. Owen insisted that since he had always loved sex and was delighted to be sought out as a sexual partner by nearly any man, he could not have been abused by Calvin. Equally important, and not unrelated, Calvin was very loving in manner to Owen and emotionally supportive in a variety of ways. This support was largely lacking elsewhere in Owen's life, where he was expected to nurture his younger siblings while much of the parental attention was focused on his dangerously ill sister. In addition, for many years Calvin was the only person Owen knew who seemed content about being homosexual. I will further discuss Owen's feelings about his homosexuality in Chapter 4.

It was almost an afterthought for Owen that he never felt he loved Calvin, and was far more interested in boys his own age. That Calvin loved him was sufficient for them to have a six-year "affair." This seems to be primarily related to Owen's inner sense, which lasted all his life, of being homely and perhaps unloveable. He experienced himself simultaneously as highly sexual but unattractive, and learned that sexualized responses from men, starting with Calvin, ultimately made him feel both loved and sexually fulfilled. He therefore could not imagine that such attentions could be abusive.

PRIMARY OBJECT CHOICE
AND GENDER OF THE ABUSER

We have seen many demonstrations of how men are likely to encode their abuse as "sexual initiation." This is particularly true if the abuser is not a parent and is of the same gender as the boy's eventual primary object choice. Thus, a straight man who was abused by a sister or a female baby-sitter, or a gay man who was abused by an uncle or a male camp counselor, often thinks of the episode as one he should have liked or actually did like, rather than as anxiety-laden or abusive.

In the example of Ed earlier in this chapter, this dynamic was demonstrated in a heterosexual man abused as a boy by a female baby-sitter. We will also see that Ira, another heterosexual man abused by women, felt that he was lucky to have an affair with his college professor, and never recognized that the downward spiral of his life afterward might have been related to this relationship.

Owen, the gay man just described, similarly maintained that at age twelve he could not have been abused by an older man because he was already interested in sex with men. And as a boy and adolescent Jared thought he was not especially affected by what he considered excited, willing, and pleasurable participation in sex at age five with a teenage boy. In his case, however, he realized later that the experience had severe effects on his adult relationships.

Thus, none of these men initially encoded premature sex as betrayal, and all considered the sexual events they experienced to have been pleasurable, even though each demonstrated sequelae that suggest the experiences had abusive and traumatizing aspects. The picture is very different when the abuser's gender does not match the boy's eventual predominant primary object choice. Elsewhere in this book, especially in Chapters 3, 4, and 8, I will discuss the troubling implications for boys in such situations. I will also note problems for some gay boys abused by men, especially boys whose abuse occurred before they had any understanding of their homosexuality.

For the moment, however, I will briefly illustrate the likely reactions of boys abused by adults of the opposite sex from their eventual predominant primary object choice. Yale, for example, was a gay man who was abused by a nun as a second grader. His scornful attitudes toward others, especially the women in his adult life and the presumably straight boys he seduced in high school, were closely connected to his continuing clear inner sense of having been abused and exploited by her. He openly loved "getting back" at heterosexuals, whom he considered to have mistreated him in many ways all his life. Conversely, Quinn, a straight man who was abused by his grandfather for years from the time he was a preschooler, and Harris, a straight man abused by his father during his latency years, both felt victimized and continued to harbor both rage and dread about men, particularly those in authority. Each felt a mixture of fear, yearning, and contempt about the possibility of intimate relatedness with other men.

CHAPTER 3

Struggles about Masculinity

A fundamental obstacle for many sexually abused men involves a struggle to reconcile abuse with their inner vision of what it means to be a man. Cultural concepts and expectations about men and masculinity generate uncertainty about his manhood if a man cannot live up to them. These problematic views are perpetuated and culturally reinforced in the popular culture. They are the underpinning for the likelihood that men will encode premature sexuality as sexual initiation (see Chapter 2). In other ways as well, they present major difficulties to the man trying to come to terms with a history of child sexual abuse (see Lisak, 1993; Khairallah, 1995).

In particular, a man sexually abused as a boy is likely to feel challenged about his "masculinity." While he may not doubt the actual biological fact of his maleness, his experience of his masculinity may be compromised in two interrelated areas: the *self-perception* of whether he is a man and the *socially constructed ideal* of a masculine self. These ideas are often used interchangeably. This blurring of definitions can be confusing, however, since the concepts are vastly different and have diverse ramifications for men.

At issue here are the prevailing myths that victimhood is the province of women and that men cannot be victims. A man who has been victimized, therefore, must often combat an inner conviction that his victimization is a sign that he is not male. The ways in which he struggles to reconcile his attitudes about manhood with his sexual victimization create inner turmoil and may result in a wide range of symptoms.

Before analyzing the specific struggles sexually abused men may have about masculinity, I will put these struggles into context by defining and clarifying several relevant concepts. I will first consider the concepts of gender and gender identity, including the development of masculine gender identity. In particular, I will explore the idea that masculine gender identity is a social construction. Having laid this groundwork, I will go on to discuss specific questions about the convergence of masculine gender identity and male sexual victimization. I will then clarify the consequences internalized ideas about masculinity have for sexually abused men. In that discussion, I will focus on the meaning to men of being victimized and penetrated; on hypermasculine reactions to being victimized; on the seductive appeal of remaining a psychological boy; on multiply gendered self-representations; on sexually abused men's fears of being around other men; and, finally, on their need to redefine masculinity in order to heal from sexual abuse.

WHAT IS GENDER?

In the next two sections, I will summarize some of the contradictory theory about gender identity in general and masculine gender identity in particular. First, however, we must understand what we mean by gender itself. Dimen (1991) defines it this way: "Conventionally, 'gender' denotes *the psychological and social dimension of the biological category of sex*" (p. 336; emphasis added). Since the difference between the sexes seems obvious, the concept of gender appears equally simple at first glance. As Dimen adds, however, "This characterization sounds like a clear enough division of epistemological labor. But it is not. What gender seems to denote is one thing; what it actually connotes is another" (p. 336). The male/female binary is given added arbitrary, culturally determined meanings that may have nothing to do with bodily differences or with gender in its literal sense. Thus, we slide in discourse from talking about sex, to talking about gender, to talking about culture. These three concepts become intertwined, and we may refer to gender or sex when we are really talking about cultural definitions of what is "masculine" and what is "feminine."

For example, to talk of farming, or composing music, or piloting an airplane, or teaching physics as masculine pursuits is to imply that men, by the fact of their maleness, are uniquely suited or qualified to do these things. Of course, these activities have nothing to do with a man's biological sex, so perhaps we might think of them as gender-appropriate behaviors for men, since they involve psychosocial facets of maleness.

But the psychosocial gender-based aspects of these pursuits ultimately derive from dated male-dominated cultural ideas that men can do them and women are incapable of doing them. Thus, ideas that emanate from the culture become inextricably attached to gender stereotypes. By extension, they seem to become characteristics of one sex and not the other, even though the attributes in question have nothing to do with actual maleness or actual femaleness.

This example leads us to an important debate about gender: To what extent are gender-based characteristics immutably tied to the essence of one sex or the other (the *essentialist* view), and to what extent do they derive from social constructions about maleness and femaleness that are internalized as children grow up (the *social constructivist* view)? These are important questions, and arguments based on both positions can be made in relation to specific aspects of gender. For example, Corbett (1996) criticizes the essentialist theories about homosexuality underlying the work of Stoller (1968, 1985), Green (1987), and R. C. Friedman (1988). Anne Fausto-Sterling, in her book *Myths of Gender* (1985), analyzes the socially and politically constructed beliefs framing gender myths that at first glance seem rooted in biology and genetics.

As D. Schwartz (1996) points out, essentialism and social constructivism are not simply opposing perspectives. Rather, they relate to different kinds of assumptions about the world: "Essentialism consists always of a set of specific and content-laden claims about human nature and experience, while constructivism is a method of critical analysis, of showing how supposedly scientific claims about human nature are almost without exception unverifiable" (p. 250). Arguments about these positions are additionally complicated by the uncertainty, ambiguity, and shifting, contradictory qualities of gender (Dimen, 1991; Harris, 1991; Benjamin, 1996). As Harris puts it, "[G]ender is neither reified nor simply liminal and evanescent. Rather, in any one person's experience, gender may occupy both positions. Gender may in some contexts be as thick and reified, as plausibly real as anything in our character. At other moments, gender may seem porous and insubstantial" (p. 212). Thus, she says, to see sex or gender as grounded in biology or "what is real" misses the importance of psychology and social context in our understanding of personality.

In sum, the seemingly simple idea that gender refers to the psychological and social qualities that correspond to the biological differences between the sexes is actually a knotty one. It is entangled in concepts of culture and biology, as well as in psychology and social structure. Its meaning is not stable or neat, yet it has deep resonance and profound implications for any maturing individual.

GENDER IDENTITY

Gender identity is, broadly speaking, a person's self-identification as belonging to one gender or the other. It is a complex construct and has increasingly been a focus for theorists and clinicians in recent years. Understanding the theories underlying the concept of gender identity helps us clarify the process by which boys and girls learn to differentiate characteristics identified as male and female. In most cases, they eventually define a crucial aspect of their core individuality from either their male or female gender identity.

Gender identity has different meanings to different writers and often refers to different phenomena. Brooks and Silverstein (1995) point out that a problem with the concept of gender identity is that it has been used at times to refer to gender constancy, that is, the ability to comprehend the immutable differences between the sexes, and at others times to refer to what it means to be male or female in a particular cultural context. Much of modern psychological and psychoanalytic theory has added to the confusion by not differentiating sufficiently between anatomical sex and gender identity (Dimen, 1997).[1]

Money and Ehrhardt (1972) attempt to clarify the meaning of gender identity by differentiating it from *gender role*. They define the two terms this way:

> Gender Identity: The sameness, unity, and persistence of one's individuality as male, female, or ambivalent, in greater or lesser degree, especially as it is experienced in self-awareness and behavior; gender identity is the private experience of gender role, and gender role is the public expression of gender identity.

> Gender Role: everything that a person says and does, to indicate to others or to the self the degree that one is either male, or female, or ambivalent; it includes but is not restricted to sexual arousal and response; gender role is the public expression of gender identity, and gender identity is the private experience of gender role. (p. 4)

Despite making this differentiation, they note that in common usage a semantic problem arises from not having a single term that encompasses the overarching concept of "gender identity/role." They therefore sug-

---

[1] For the sake of precision, wherever possible in this chapter and throughout this book I use the word "gender" to refer to culturally and socially determined characteristics usually thought of as "masculine" or "feminine." When referring to an individual's biological maleness or femaleness, I use the word "sex."

gest using gender identity to connote gender identity/role unless the context indicates otherwise, but acknowledge the conceptual confusion that may result from this use of language.

It is likewise problematic that gender identity is often equated with sexual orientation. These concepts may overlap in their meaning, but their focus is very different. Gender identity, as noted, refers to the individual's self-identification as either male or female through self-concept and behavior. Sexual orientation, which I discuss at length in Chapter 4, refers to predominating erotic desire for either men or women. A homosexual man, then, may be male-identified (for example, Owen, Jared, Greg, and Abe, among other gay men described in this book, were clearly male-identified), while a heterosexual man may be female-identified (see my discussion of Cory later in this chapter).

Contemporary concepts of gender identity involve looking at masculinity and femininity in a manner first formulated by feminist and gender theorists who have developed their ideas since the 1970s (for example, Money and Ehrhardt, 1972; Chodorow, 1978, 1989; Gilligan, 1982; Benjamin, 1988, 1996; Butler, 1990, 1992; Dimen, 1991, 1995a, 1995b, 1997; Goldner, 1991; Harris, 1991). They have focused on the development of female identity in our society, criticized it in a variety of ways, and/or advocated for change. This has led to a more recent focus on complementary theorizing about the development of masculinity. I will discuss this theory in the next section, but for the moment I want to emphasize again that his internal concept of masculinity complicates how a boy or man deals with his sexual abuse and indeed may deeply influence his innermost sense of whether he is actually a man in any but the biological sense.

THE DEVELOPMENT OF MASCULINITY

Several writers have proposed theories explaining how gender identity evolves in a developmental process throughout childhood. Object relations theory, for example, posits that every infant has an initial primary attachment to its mother. After an extended period of being merged with the mother, the infant begins to separate and individuate from her. Greenson (1966, 1968) and Stoller (1968, 1973, 1985) propose that a boy, as he gradually realizes that his biological sex is different from his mother's, feels compelled to give up his attachment to her and to disidentify with her as he establishes a male gender identity that matches his biological sex. This differentiation process is an interpersonal one in which the mother, in complementary fashion, is also pushing her son out of the early stage of attachment to her in order to start the differentiation process. At this point, the son becomes threatened by his former strong attachment to his mother, and looks to his father for his masculine identity.

An aspect of this process hypothesized by Chodorow (1978; see also Abelin, 1980) is that, because fathers are often physically and/or emotionally absent in contemporary families, the male role a father personifies may be incomprehensible to the son. Indeed, she says, boys may not have a personal identification with their fathers, but rather may develop an identification with the *absent position* of men in relation to families to establish primary masculinity. This has implications for their own relatedness later in life, since it makes them more likely to take absent or distant positions with their own families. For Chodorow, men's needs to be dominant arise from the fragility of the core gender identity thus established. Or, as Kaftal (1991) puts it, "[T]he first core gender identity is female, and maleness is a difficult and perhaps never quite successful renunciation of that 'protofemininity' " (p. 317).

Irene Fast (1984), in *Gender Identity: A Differentiation Model*, has written more comprehensively about the development of gender identity in boys and girls. She argues that the classical Freudian model is insufficient to explain the phenomenon. This model (Freud, 1905) posits that all children consider themselves boys in early childhood. As girls and boys begin to comprehend their differences, according to this theory, girls feel incomplete while boys find validation of their maleness. In Fast's differentiation model, by contrast, boys and girls prior to age three believe that everyone is the same and that therefore all possibilities are open to them. As they learn, between the ages of three and four, that there are differences between boys and girls, they also realize that their own possibilities are limited. Both boys and girls experience a sense of loss about this discovery, but then go on to develop a differentiated sense of self in which their possibilities are demarcated, but therefore restricted. This process, the development of gender identity, "involves renunciation of early gender-indiscriminate self representations and identifications now found to be physically impossible or gender-inappropriate" (p. 12). Fast furthermore believes that the development of a consistent and enduring core gender identity is a prerequisite for any individual's psychological health.

Masculinity and femininity, of course, can be defined in many ways. Fast observes:

> Subjective definitions of masculinity and femininity must be distinguished from objective ones. Objectively defined, individuals' characteristics are masculine or feminine to the extent that they are typical of one or the other sex in a particular social group. Subjective definitions

refer to personal constructs of masculinity and femininity, individuals' own notions, applied to themselves and others, of what it is to be masculine and feminine. (p. 77)

Specifically, how does masculine identity develop? According to Fast's gender differentiation theory, boys and girls differentiate themselves from one another as "masculine" or "feminine" in ways that correspond to societal models that may have little to do with actual biological differences: "It is the social meaning of the anatomical differences that is determinative, not the differences themselves" (p. 72). As a boy develops, he learns to delineate various behaviors as "masculine" or "feminine." A process of masculine identification begins before he has any awareness of sex differences between his parents. He may begin to try out a range of masculine and feminine behaviors, discarding those he perceives as not conforming to a masculine gender identity. During this process, as time goes on, he incorporates masculine behaviors and makes feminine behaviors ego alien. Weeks (1985) notes that masculine identity is "achieved by the constant process of warding off threats to it" (p. 190). In this process, it becomes especially important to exclude that which is perceived as not masculine, especially those qualities experienced as feminine or homosexual (see Nasjleti, 1980, and Chapter 4 in this book).

But most men never completely banish all their feminine characteristics. Decades ago, Jung (1933) proposed an inevitable balance of masculine ("animus") and feminine ("anima") archetypes in any adult. Thus, a psychologically balanced man will eventually be comfortable with characteristics in himself that he has defined as feminine. Indeed, according to Fast (1984), a "'dis-identification' or 'repudiation' [of identification with the mother] signals failure in optimum development of masculinity, an organization too exclusively phallic, denying the actual procreative capacity and nurturing possibilities in men" (p. 73). Fast notes that "the man who perceives his own retained femininity as infantile, indicative of passivity, or incomplete masculinity may see these as actual characteristics of women" (p. 73). To this, I would add that such a worldview in itself implies a man's lack of openness to his own psychic experience.

Michael Diamond (1997b) addresses this need for men in mature adulthood to reembrace the "feminine" characteristics they have previously rejected. Diamond describes the process by which this occurs: "The mature man consolidates his gender identity by developing his capacity to contain the tension that is inherent between his *core sense of who he is* and the fundamentally *fluid, shifting nature of his multifaceted self*" (p. 3). Such a mature man no longer needs to rely on the black-and-

white, bifurcated constructs of masculinity and femininity that were necessary in his childhood, adolescence, and young adulthood. "In the end,
the fully becoming man who has access to both the genderized and
nongenderized *multitude* within, has largely transcended the need for a
clearly defined, well-bounded masculine gender identity" (p. 19).

Building on these theories, William Pollack (1990, 1995, 1998) proposes a scenario like Greenson's and Stoller's in which the realization
that he is biologically different from his mother forces a boy to develop
an identity separate from hers. Agreeing with Fast that this happens at
about age three, Pollack suggests that at this age boys can only give up
their attachment to their mothers with traumatic consequences. As a
consequence of this early interpersonal trauma, boys have a "gender-
specific vulnerability" (Pollack, 1995, p. 41) to feelings of loss and abandonment in relationships, and are likely to have "a continuing need to
defend against urges toward affiliation and intimacy because of the
repressed trauma of shameful and premature separation" (p. 41). Such
tendencies lead to the interpersonally isolated and nonempathic modes
of relating that have been stereotyped as masculine, with men learning to
communicate through "action, symbol, and symptom" (Kaftal, 1991, p.
308).

SOCIALLY CONSTRUCTED MASCULINE
IDENTITY AND ITS CRITIQUES

Fast's differentiation theory for the development of gender identity is a
valuable conceptual framework, but the work of more recent writers
brings in to question some of her assumptions. Brooks and Silverstein
(1995), for example, argue that Fast's theory does not "distinguish
between *socialized characteristics*, such as activity level and tenderness,
and *biological attributes*, such as the ability to have a baby or a penis"
(p. 300). More significantly, Brooks and Silverstein challenge Fast's
assumption that the development of a consistent and coherent gender
identity is a necessary prerequisite to adult psychological health. Indeed,
they argue that a view of masculinity and femininity as a collection of
separate and mutually exclusive characteristics creates severe psychological problems:

> This theoretical position accepts the cultural mythology that gender,
> like sex, is a binary concept. Since gender is culturally, rather than bio-
> logically, constructed, it is not limited to only two possibilities. We
> would argue that the cultural prescription to achieve a coherent and
> consistent gender identity is, by definition, psychologically dysfunc-

tional. We believe that the attempt to achieve a consistent gender role identity pressures an individual to conform to a gender role that is restricted to one of only two possibilities. (p. 301)

The feminist psychoanalyst Virginia Goldner (1991) speaks to this issue when she questions whether for either men or women an internally consistent gender identity is desirable and even whether it is possible. She believes that gender coherence, gender consistency, gender conformity, and gender identity are all culturally mandated normative ideals, norms that are themselves pathogenic. In addition, she argues that these normative ideals have been accepted uncritically by therapists as well as by the general population. She suggests that gender in this sense is a necessary fiction, a defense that allows a person to navigate some aspects of life but also creates confusion and conflict because of its fundamental artificiality. A crucial goal of psychological treatment, therefore, is to allow an individual to tolerate ambiguity and instability in relation to gender concepts, in order to develop a more rounded and less pathological sense of self.

Goldner's argument, then, like Chodorow's (1978), seems to be that there is no such thing as core masculinity, that it is entirely a cultural idea inculcated through socialization. Lisak's (1995) view is less sweeping, but he agrees that "whatever biological roots may underlie some of the behavior and characteristics that we call 'masculine,' these roots are enormously elaborated by culture" (p. 259).

Whatever the proportion of biological, social, and cultural components of masculinity, at present our society promotes internalized normative gender ideals, and most men are affected by them. Boys whose development into men does not reflect these normative masculine ideals are often marginalized or pathologized. We see this in the story of Beau, an effeminate boy who was teased, mocked, and later raped by his peers. Coates (1990, 1992; Coates, Friedman, and Wolfe, 1991) writes about such boys as having gender identity disorders in which they try to resolve severe separation anxiety by using cross-gender behavior to reclaim their mothers' presence. Green (1987) also pathologizes this "sissy boy" behavior, calling it central to the development of homosexuality in some boys. Corbett (1996), on the other hand, argues cogently for another point of view. He describes these children as "girlyboys" having alternative but not necessarily pathological masculine gender characteristics, wanting neither to grow up as women nor to deny their male bodies.

Among the expectations that boys (and girls) in our society are commonly socialized to have about men is the belief, conscious or unconscious, that "real" men are in charge of themselves and therefore cannot be victimized. Related beliefs are that masculine men don't express emotions, are "independent" rather than "needy," are competitive and resilient, and welcome sexuality whenever it is offered, particularly from women. These internalized beliefs present specific problems for sexually abused men (Finkelhor, 1984; Gerber, 1990; Lew, 1990; Isely, 1992, Etherington, 1995; Mendel, 1995). Even men who rationally believe that these values are artificial and damaging are nevertheless influenced by them, often enduring unconscious negative reactions if they feel they have not upheld them. Running through these perceptions of masculine gender identity are the (usually) "unconscious views of masculinity as a good substance and femininity as lack of that substance" (Blechner, 1998, p. 601). Thus, if a man perceives that he is unmasculine or feminine, he sees himself as lacking an important and necessary positive element in his nature.

In the postfeminist era, theories about masculinity have described and begun to critique socially constructed masculine ideals (for example, Brod and Kaufman, 1994; Levant and Pollack, 1995). Levant (1995) writes about the nearly universal socialization of men to be alexithymic, that is, to be unable to put emotions into words. In this process, he says, "men become strangers to their own emotional lives" (p. 237) and frequently channel their vulnerable emotions into anger and their caring emotions into sexuality. Crowder (1995) observes that "[s]ome homophobic men believe that only homosexual men express emotion and they develop a stoic persona to confirm their 'masculinity'" (p. 23). This is what Perchuk and Posner (1995) have aptly termed the "masculine masquerade."

Pollack (1995), citing his own research, notes that boys and girls are both endowed with an inborn physiological capacity to experience vicariously the affective states of other human beings. Like Levant, he concludes that gender-tracked socialization enhances this resource in girls but suppresses it in boys. Pollack further argues that men and women are both done a disservice if they confuse the binary bedrock of what he calls core gender identity (biologically based maleness versus femaleness) with a more elastic diversity of gender role possibilities, which he calls "engendered identity." But men have a tendency to see themselves in dichotomous, black-and-white terms, especially in hierarchical relationships where gender is a factor (Kupers, 1993).

Socially rooted models of masculinity create what Pleck (1981, 1995) has termed "gender role strain" (1995, p. 11) for men. Pleck delineates three areas in which cultural standards for masculinity, implemented in gender socialization, have potential negative effects on men: First, there may be *gender role discrepancy,* that is, low self-esteem because a man sees the difference between who he actually is (his real self) and who a man should be (his gender ideal). Second, Pleck describes *gender role trauma,* declaring that the socialization process itself is traumatic. Third, he discusses *gender role dysfunction.* This occurs because a man who has successfully integrated masculine role expectations is now by definition behaving in ways that have inherent negative side effects, either for himself or others, such as maintaining a low level of family participation.

Thus, while masculine identity often entitles men to positions of power and privilege in the larger culture, it also has severe drawbacks. Devastating to all men (Pollack, 1995), socially constructed masculine ideals culminate in what Levant (1995), citing infant research, calls the "ordeal of emotional socialization [through which boys, who] start out life more emotional than girls, . . . learn to tune out, stifle, and channel their emotions" (p. 236). As Stephen Mitchell (1996) observes, "Many men, perhaps all men . . . , long to be free of socially constructed male gendered identity" (p. 61). Pollack (1995) goes further, asserting that "only as men come to see that the present gender role-based expectations for masculinity in our society are impossible to achieve and lead only to pain, loss, and a false, too vulnerable sense of self-esteem[, will they] be able to recognize that change is necessary, that there must be a reframing of our concept of what it means to 'be a man' " (p. 58).

Despite these deeply traumatic and abusive aspects of masculine socialization, however, it does not necessarily follow that everything that results from it is negative (D. Lisak, personal communication). As Lisak (1998) points out, there may also be tremendous use on a societal level in having men socialized into masculinity. A culture in which many individuals conform to the masculine ideal has an adaptive advantage because it is better equipped to compete for limited resources in less harsh environmental circumstances. On a more personal level, the less rigid and harsh forms of masculinization can instill a deep sense of responsibility and loyalty. Such personal qualities as strength in adversity, persistence, determination, and the ability to suppress pain in the pursuit of an important goal, are all potentially valuable to an individual. However, as Lisak (personal communication) further argues, these attributes can be instilled without linking them to gender role and without forcing people to renounce so much of their basic human potential in order to attain them.

Several writers propose far-reaching changes in the male socialization of men and boys (Brooks, 1995; Levant and Kopecky, 1995; Levant and Pollack, 1995; Levant and Brooks, 1997). One prominent family therapist, Olga Silverstein, has written a book directed at mothers (Silverstein and Rashbaum, 1994), to guide them in raising sons who have nontraditional masculine identities. Radical feminist John Stoltenberg (1993), on the other hand, declares that there is no positive way to redefine masculinity, that it must simply end. Lisak (1994), Real (1994), and Pleck (1995) do not go this far, but they do conclude that the gender socialization of men is itself a form of abuse and traumatization. And Morris (1997) concludes that "[t]he new real man will scoff at myths of masculinity" (p. 216).

SEXUAL ABUSE AND MASCULINE IDENTITY

We have seen that achieving the masculine gender ideal can involve a betrayal of self that creates severe psychological and social stress for a man. In combination with a history of sexual abuse, this betrayal is excruciating. Influenced by unrealistic internalized ideals of manhood, a boy may be even more reluctant than a girl to report sexual abuse, feeling he has more at stake—his masculine identity—in being identified as a victim (Finkelhor, 1986; Gartner, 1994, 1996b, 1997a). And if masculinity is at the core of a man's psychic identity, then to lose his masculine identity is to lose himself, to suffer a kind of psychological death (Lisak, 1998).

Lisak (1994; Lisak et al., 1996) reports a study in which he interviewed men who were sexually abused as boys. He found the following common psychological themes in their responses: anger, betrayal, homosexual concerns, helplessness, isolation, alienation, shame, humiliation, loss, worries about masculinity, negative peer relationships as boys, negative schematas about people in general, and problems related to sexuality, self-blame, and guilt. Lisak notes that most of these internal states violate the rules of masculinity that the sexually abused man had already internalized, so he feels permanently branded as "not a man." Paradoxically, the path of recovery from abuse must go through exactly the territory of emotionality that culturally he is not supposed to feel. Apparently, men who do allow themselves to counter this masculine ideal and experience the emotions related to their abuse have more positive outcomes than those who do not; Lisak reports that men who acknowledged the most distressing childhood experiences tended to be the most empathic men in his sample.

Lisak proposes that in this contradictory situation a sexually abused man has three possible basic adaptations: First, he can strive forever to be the masculine ideal that internally he knows he cannot be. An example of this is the action-oriented man who does not permit any self-reflection about his externalized way of dealing with the world. Second, he can relinquish the struggle, become passive, and so give up such aspects of himself as the capacity for anger. This stance is typified by the isolated, meek nonachiever who does not allow himself to engage in interpersonal relationships except on a superficial level.

The third adaptation posited by Lisak involves an endless struggle with the dilemma of attempting to "be a man" while simultaneously trying to deal with abuse. Lisak believes most men are caught up in this last conflictual adaptation. In this effort, however, many of them resolve their inner discord by becoming either more empathic or more hypermasculine, a stance I will discuss later in this chapter. Those who become more empathic are usually more open to psychological intervention. They may be readiest to engage in psychotherapy because they are already wrestling openly with the issues involved. This seems to occur when they are in their thirties or forties, a time when in my experience sexually abused men are most likely to begin therapy and attempt to confront their histories directly (see Horsley, 1997). In essence, these empathic men create a fourth adaptation to their abuse: they redefine their masculinity.

One factor that influences the underreporting of male sexual abuse is the sense that the sexual victimization of boys may not be sufficiently acknowledged by adults even if it is reported. Such denial by others may arise from the same gender expectations that cause boys themselves not to acknowledge their victimhood. Unfortunately, the women's movement, despite its many positive effects, has also reinforced the view that men are perpetrators and never victims and that women are victims and never perpetrators (Wright, 1997b). Men are generally seen as offenders rather than victims, not only in the rape literature but also in rape intervention centers, which "have often alienated, tokenized, or rejected" male victims (Sepler, 1990, p. 76). Indeed, one man described to me his call to a rape hotline, an attempt to talk for the first time about his boyhood abuse. Tellingly, but chillingly, an obviously insufficiently trained counselor snapped, "We don't work with perpetrators," before she hung up on him.

Even if he is believed, a boy may be insufficiently shielded from further abuse by the service system designed to protect him (Dimock, 1989a). Upon disclosure of abuse, a male juvenile is more likely to be referred to the police than to child protection agencies (Finkelhor, 1984). If he is reported to such an agency, he is less likely than a girl to be placed in protective custody outside the home and less likely to be referred for counseling. If referred, he is likely to have shorter treatment than a girl (Vander Mey, 1988; Finkelhor, 1984; Pierce and Pierce, 1985; Crowder, 1995).

Johanek (1988) gives an example of how internalized masculine ideals interfere with sexually abused men's ability to process their own experience. He notes that men are more likely than women to offer a wealth of details about their victimization if they talk about it at all. He emphasizes, however, that men's descriptions are not accompanied by the intense affect often displayed by women. Men, he says, speak of their abuse in a "robotlike monotone, . . . [having] learned to avoid experiencing and displaying emotions at all costs" (p. 112). The therapists Crowder (1995) surveyed likewise reported that abused men are more likely to dissociate emotions while abused women are more dissociated from the cognitive aspects of their abuse: "Male survivors often tell the story of their abuse quite matter-of-factly, describing in detail the behaviors involved in the abuse. However, they talk about these events as if they had happened to someone else, expressing little affect or compassion" (p. 38).

In my own experience, this male/female dichotomy between dissociation from emotion and dissociation from cognition is not as clear-cut as these writers imply. However, although there are many reverse examples, I have indeed found a *tendency* for men to dissociate feeling and women to dissociate cognition. Thus, Gene spoke of his eleven years of regular molestation by his father as though he were describing a mildly problematic academic difficulty. He smiled and described his abuse and severe social isolation in removed, slightly amused terms. Likewise, Willem spoke politely about his abuse as though he were describing a scene he saw momentarily from the window of a moving train.

In reacting to trauma, the male victim is threatened with emotional overarousal, an intensity of nonmasculine emotions he tries to but cannot regulate. In reacting to this threat, he tries to stop the possibility of having such emotional experiences or stops the experiences themselves. Either he deadens himself emotionally or else he does indeed become emotionally hyperaroused. In this dynamic (which of course can also occur for women), his internal defenses disconnect him from his emotional life, or else he resorts to external forceful actions against the perceived source of his discomfort. Thus, as Sepler (1990) notes, male victims often appear "aggressive, violent, masterful, commanding, and threatening. These postures are the socially determined means for males to accommodate victimization" (p. 79), and are seen less frequently in female victims. Andreas, for example, described his years as the victim of a child-molesting ring in flat, deadened tones. He maintained a nearly complete amnesia concerning his childhood and adolescence, and kept a tight rein on what he allowed into consciousness, for he knew how easily he could become flooded with emotion. Yet in work situations he seemed assertive, competent, and powerful.

Because of differences in the socialization and cultural expectations, men and women may also have different reactions when coming to terms with any acquiescence to the abuse they suffered. While both men and women may feel rage and guilt for having acquiesced, compliance is more acceptable for women in terms of their societal roles. In that *ste-*

reotyped sense, complying means to a woman that she *has been* female, while to a man acquiescence means he *has not been* male (Neilsen, 1983). Thus, Andreas could not forgive himself for obeying the men who commanded that he return weekly for sessions of abuse. For him, this represented an unmanly participation in his own abuse. I will discuss later in this chapter how some men react counterphobically to experiencing such demasculinization by becoming abusive themselves.

The feminist psychoanalytic theory I cited earlier that has made us reconceive our ideas of gender also helps us understand men's experience of victimization on another level (Benjamin, 1988; Dimen, 1991; see also Hepburn, 1994). According to this view, in sexual situations, men expect to be *desiring subjects* who initiate and take charge of sexual activity. Sexual abuse attacks a boy's internalized social structure so that he becomes instead a *desired object*, as women usually are. If he allows himself to experience this turnabout, he is likely to feel shame and therefore to protest this feminization of his socially constructed masculine identity, on the one hand, or to have profound doubts about his gender identity, on the other.

In the rest of this chapter, I will look at specific motifs that affect sexually abused men as they try to integrate sexual abuse with masculine identity.

VICTIMIZATION AND MASCULINITY

Most men cannot even visualize themselves as victims (Morris, Hunter, Struve, and Fitzgerald, 1997). Lew (1988) explains that "our culture provides no room for a man as victim. Men are simply not supposed to be victimized.... If men aren't to be victims ..., then victims aren't men" (p. 41). Or, as Crowder (1995) puts it, "Our culture has no mythology to identify the process of male victimization and boy victims are emasculated by this bias. They are either seen as being like a woman and therefore feminized, as being powerless and therefore flawed, or as being interested in sex with men and therefore homosexual" (p. 12).

The inability to live up to the unrealistic expectation that men cannot be victims leads to male gender shame for many men. As Kyle put it, "I have a sense of being ruined, a *foundation* of shame I take with me everywhere." If a man equates victimization with femininity, any acknowledgment that he has been victimized may shame him about his inability to be masculine. A sexually abused man quoted by Mendel (1995) stated flatly, "The abuse tells me that I'm not a man" (p. 205), while Lisak (1994) cites a man who bitterly described himself by saying, "I'm not a man, I'm a victim."

Olson (1990) writes about this self-devaluation: "Boys still experience shame about their abuse and deny the emotional impact on them. It is difficult to expect children or adults to estimate the impact of so socially denigrated and shameful an experience on the full development of one's life as a man" (p. 149). In a study conducted by Dean and Woods (1985, cited in Dimock, 1989a), 75 percent of the men in their sample felt shame because they failed to stop their abuse from occurring. Paradoxically, blaming themselves for the abuse allows them the continuing sense that they had control over what happened, and also serves the important function of preserving "an idealized image of their caregivers or people around them in a position of power" (Horsley, 1997, p. 74).

Because of such internalized ideals of masculine identity, a boy who has been sexually victimized has to do considerable internal work to keep his view of himself as a masculine being intact. Often, this inner work involves defining the sexual victimization as something he sought out and over which he therefore had mastery, as I discussed in Chapter 2. Finkelhor (1984) found that boys are more likely than girls to initially encode their abuse as positive, more likely to say that they were interested and felt pleasure in the sexual activity. This comes at a cost, however. Finkelhor's research also demonstrates that abuse has a more negative impact on boys' sexual self-esteem than on girls'.

The feeling that he had mastery over his abuse situation may be easier to accomplish if the victimization was enacted by a woman, since, as we saw in Chapter 2, boys tend to be admired for premature sexual activity with women. If sexual victimization was committed by a man, whether the boy was previously heading for a predominantly heterosexual or a predominantly homosexual orientation, the boy's reactions to it are likely to be more complicated, as we will see in Chapter 4.

Even boys abused by their mothers may feel they were in charge of the situation. Silber (1979) writes about a man who was abused by his mother as a young boy. In fantasy, the patient makes himself the more active participant in the molestations. Silber believes his patient mentally manipulated what actually transpired in order to console himself for the horror of his actual experience. In my view, this was probably not a "manipulation" in an active sense, since the molestation may have been instantly dissociated and thus may never have entered his internal experience at all. (See Chapter 7 for a discussion of dissociative processes.) Silber notes that as a result his patient developed a characteristic defense through which he consistently distorted his experience. This defensive posture caused him to replace his participation and interest in the outside world with a heightened and potentially disabling concentration on his fantasy life.

This removal of focus from his external to his internal world also affected Isaac, a boy with multiple male abusers who as an adult was underemployed and had a sparse social life. Yet his mind was quick and he was interested in ideas. He read many psychologically oriented self-help books. When he first came to therapy, he frequently fantasized about career possibilities and relationships with women, neither of which he was able to pursue.

When the victim is male, the interpersonal atmosphere between victim and abuser often bears the trappings of consensuality (Sepler, 1990). Victims quickly make and reinforce the psychological, physical, and social adjustments necessary to make themselves believe that they willingly participated in the abuse. This adjustment camouflages the underlying coercion and manipulation, but "the existential reality of sexual victimization for a male victim may well be a sense of ownership and participation" in the sexual activity (Sepler, 1990, p. 77).

Thus, Ed as an adult saw fondling his baby-sitter's breasts as a delicious act, even though he had her fired at the time. Jared claimed that he had felt happy and loved when he engaged in sexual activity with a teenager ten years his senior. Yet his abuser put him out a window to wander home alone at night when he was only seven—hardly a sign that he cared for Jared.

Such distortions of reality about who initiated his molestation create further difficulty later when the man is considering whether he was abused. Having earlier reached a conclusion that he was the instigator rather than the victim of his premature sexual experiences, he now must question what had been a bedrock of his beliefs about himself and his masculinity.

Brooke Hopkins (1993) describes his struggle about these issues in his narrative account of abuse by his mother. Noting that most accounts of sexual abuse describe perpetrators who are men and victims who are girls, he writes that in his case, "[T]he standard roles were reversed. *I* was the active party, while my mother's role was almost completely passive" (p. 49). This was because his mother had come into his bed and sleepily "allowed" him to touch her sexually. Hopkins goes on, painfully, to question this interpretation: "[W]ere the roles we played . . . really as straightforward and unambiguous as all that?" (p. 49). He reminds himself that he did not choose to sleep with her; that his mother actively came into his bed, surely knowing better than to do so; and that his father allowed his wife to sleep with their son for weeks. But his need to force himself to rethink the circumstances of his abuse in this manner illustrates how deeply ingrained is the pressure for a boy or man to consider himself the active partner in all sexual activity.

How do those men who accept that they were sexually abused deal with the abuse from the point of view of their gender identity? Since, stereotypically, in our society, victims are seen as feminine, men are likely to experience their sexual abuse as meaning they are not really men. Feminist critiques have shown us that we tend to consider the binary concept of masculinity/femininity as roughly equivalent to the binary of predator/victim; that is, we see predators as masculine and victims as feminine. Therefore, the man who has been sexually abused may consider himself feminized because he has been victimized.

Another way to look at this is that by being victimized the man has lost his sense of *agency*, his ability to feel that he is in charge of himself as he moves through his world. Slavin (1997; see also Slavin and Pollock, 1997) defines "agency" as "the capacity to experience oneself as an agent of one's actions, feelings, and interpersonal relationships that enables the individual to feel not simply at the mercy of other internal urgencies or the will of others" (p. 227). He argues that it is the capacity to feel agentic that allows an individual to describe life events as though they pertain to that person's own self. I would further contend that, while both men and women need a sense of agency in their lives, for men *not* to feel such agency exacerbates any doubts they may have about their masculinity. This is because they must struggle not only with the need every individual has to feel agency, but also with culturally determined integrations that to be a man is to be agentic. Therefore, to lose such a sense of control of oneself is by definition feminine. In any case, an individual who has been abused, especially when the abuse has been chronic, is less likely to feel capable of agency in his life, less able to be in charge of the forces that impinge on him in his world. Andreas's chronic suicidality was a paradoxical way of maintaining his sense of agency. He said that having the option to kill himself was a comfort that allowed him to endure his life; he felt curiously empowered by the knowledge that he could end his misery if he so chose.

BEING PENETRATED AND MASCULINITY

Yet another way to understand men's unique reactions to abuse is to consider how they feel about being penetrated. Being penetrated, whether physically or psychically, carries meaning for men well beyond the acts or relationships involved. Most classical psychoanalytic papers about men's fear of penetration have focused on anxiety about possible homosexual wishes. This is an inadequate explanation of the ubiquity of these fears. At heart, the fear of being penetrated, like many fears related to masculine gender identity struggles, is a fear of forfeiting a self-definition as a man. This self-concept was achieved through *disidentify-*

ing with qualities that signify being either female or homosexual. The disidentification with femaleness seems to originate in a very young boy's need to define himself as different from the mother with whom he identified in his earliest years (see the theoretical discussions of this process earlier in this chapter). In this schema, homosexuals are seen as men who have not successfully differentiated themselves from their female identity. Since women and homosexuals are seen as passive and penetrable, men must experience themselves as active and impenetrable to maintain a sense of themselves as men.

A masculine sense of self, then, "is based on, *dependent upon*, an impermeable psychic boundary which is *not* to be penetrated. . . . [I]t may be basic enough to be seen as a threat to core *identity* (from which masculinity is seen as inextricable). . . . [I]t is not primarily the penetrability of the body, but *of the mind*, that influences sense of self, gender, sexuality and relational dynamics" (Elise, 1997, pp. 2–3). Men are likely to reject any sense of being penetrated as a means of maintaining adulthood and masculinity.

Being a penetrator, rather than being the one penetrated, thus becomes a defining characteristic of manhood. Sexually abused men, whether or not physical penetration has taken place, are challenged in this area. They must go to great lengths to protect themselves from the fragmentation of identity that would follow a recognition of their having been penetrated. This need has many negative effects on them, as we will see in examples presented throughout this book. Of course, women also feel penetrated by abuse, whether psychically or physically, and are traumatized by the nature of this penetration. Again, however, recognition of the penetration does not make them question whether they are women, although their violation may make them hate being female.

Men's fear of penetration seems rooted in classical Athenian culture (Halperin, 1989). For the Greeks, sexual relations between men and boys were common. What was important, however, was neither the homosexuality nor the intergenerational nature of these relationships. According to Halperin, sex was not relationally based at all, in the sense of two partners engaging in sexual relations for mutual pleasure. Rather, sex served to further differentiate participants according to class and social stature. The man of higher social stature was the penetrator in sexual acts, while the person of lower social stature was the one penetrated. Social stature could derive from age, gender, class, or citizenship. An Athenian citizen took his pleasure by penetrating a boy, a woman, a slave, or a foreigner. These were people who did not have access to his political and legal privileges and rights, and their sexual pleasure was therefore unimportant:

> Phallic penetration . . . is construed as sexual "activity"; even if a sexual act does not involve physical penetration, it still remains polarized by the distribution of phallic pleasure: The partner whose pleasure is promoted is considered "active," while the partner who puts his or her body *at the service* of another's pleasure is deemed "passive." . . . Sexual penetration, and sexual "activity" in general, are, in other words, thematized as domination: The relation between the "active" and the "passive" sexual partner is thought of as the same kind of relation as that obtaining between social superior and social inferior, between master and servant. (Halperin, 1989, p. 49)

Most Western societies live in some measure with a legacy from this aspect of ancient Greek culture. This further helps us understand men's phobias about being penetrated. In the context of a belief system like this, to allow penetration is to say, "We are not equals. You are my master." It is therefore an act of self-abasement and self-abrogation.

Likewise, in many cultures, including contemporary Latin societies, masculinity is defined by penetration (Blechner, 1998). In such a tradition, a man will not consider himself unmasculine or homosexual if he has sex with other men, as long as he is performing the act of penile penetration. Heterosexually identified men may "regularly perform penetrative anal and oral intercourse with other men, but consider themselves masculine and not gay" (Blechner, 1998, p. 602). This is similar to how men in New York treated same-sex sexual activity until the 1940s (Chauncey, 1994). If a man was sexually serviced by other men, always taking the penetrating role, then he was considered "trade," a masculine-identified term. By contrast, "queers" or "fairies" allowed themselves to be penetrated and were considered feminine.

HYPERMASCULINE REACTIONS TO ABUSE

One alternative to experiencing victimization is to deny abuse. We have seen how some men deal with molestations by believing they desired and invited the premature sexuality and were therefore "in charge" of it. Such a man may go further in his search for a sense of power and control. Identifying with his abuser, he becomes "hypermasculine" in a reactive overcompensation to his perceived feminization (see above). In such a counterphobic, hypermasculine reaction to fear that as a victim he has been unmasculine, he may therefore become aggressive following abuse (Sepler, 1990). This helps him "avoid an enormously painful state of victimization and helplessness" (Mendel, 1995, p. 17). Such men often are diagnosed as having antisocial personality disorders.

As Struve observes (Morris et al., 1997), men are socialized to act out feelings rather than to experience or verbally express them. Briere (1995) likewise postulates that women are trained to be good at feeling and men to be good at behaving. Men are therefore generally more likely to try to reduce tension through behavior like sexual compulsivity, predatory exploitation, gambling, drug addiction, alcoholism, workaholism, or overexercise. Taking this tendency much further may unfortunately lead to the action-oriented mode of dealing with feelings that is most likely to result in the man becoming sexually abusive himself (Conte, 1985; Gilgun, 1990; Urquiza and Capra, 1990). Such a man is resorting in the extreme to the defensive externalization that is frequently observed in boys anyway.

According to Lisak et al. (1996), "Male gender socialization, like childhood abuse, is implicated in the genesis of interpersonal violence" (p. 723). Lisak et al. address the intense conflict for a boy who is simultaneously dealing with sexual abuse and the gender norm not to express emotion. They note that, to achieve this norm, abused boys often neutralize affect. This dynamic conflicts with any attempt to deal with the intense feelings of helplessness and fear that accompany trauma.

Thus, at exactly the moment the boy is learning to control emotions in order to feel masculine, he is being flooded by the very emotional states that are considered nonmasculine by the culture. He must find a path toward resolution of this conflict, and may accomplish this through rigid adherence to cultural norms of masculinity. Such an adherence requires a forceful suppression of feelings and in particular causes a general constriction of vulnerable emotions like sadness, shame, embarrassment, fear, and loneliness. This narrowing of his ability to experience affect results in a diminution of his capacity to empathize with others. Alternatively, he may convert his feelings of helplessness and fear into anger, one of the few emotions sanctioned by masculine gender norms (Bruckner and Johnson, 1987; Lew, 1988; Struve, 1990; Isely, 1992). He particularly feels the need for power and control (Bruckner and Johnson, 1987; Lew, 1988; K. Singer, 1989; Isely, 1992).

Note, however, that these are the choices made by men who cannot encode and process their abuse. The preponderance of sexually abused men are actually more empathic and less constrained about gender role and emotion than nonabused men, and so are not likely to become abusers themselves (Lisak et al., 1996; see also Briggs and Hawkins, 1996). Apparently, boys who have been able in some measure to symbolize their victimhood have a comparatively enhanced potential for compassion and flexibility. Thus, contrary to popular opinion, most do *not* become victimizers.

A significant minority of sexually abused men do indeed become perpetrators of abuse, however (see Groth and Oliveri, 1989; Vasington, 1989; Sepler, 1990; Briggs and Hawkins, 1996). In Lisak et al.'s sample of nearly 600 randomly selected college men, 23 percent of the men acknowledged being perpetrators of physical or sexual abuse. The average age of the first incident of being an abuser was 17.0 (*SD* = 4.0). This is probably an underestimate of the number of abusers in the general population because the sample was relatively young, with an average age of late twenties (the study was done in an urban campus with many older students). Presumably, the percentage of victimizers rises with an older population, as many men may victimize for the first time at a later age.

Approximately one-third of those who abused sexually also abused physically, and approximately one-third of those who abused physically also abused sexually. Of the abusive men, 79 percent had themselves been abused as children. However, when the researchers looked at the men who were themselves abused as children, only 19 percent later went on to abuse children. Thus, for this group of men still in young adulthood, *although four out of five abusers had themselves been abused, only one out of five abused children had later become abusive.* More studies need to be done with wider populations to see if these figures hold up.

Lisak and his colleagues add that the subpopulation of sexually abused perpetrators is more likely than the subpopulation of sexually abused nonperpetrators to be emotionally constricted and stressed by gender issues. While traumatized women (and some men) often need help in getting in touch with their rage, many sexually traumatized men present anger as their sole affect (Sepler, 1990; also see Chapter 8 in this volume for a discussion of rage in sexually abused men). In addition, a sexually abused perpetrator's propensity to anger combines with his lowered empathic response. Together, as Lisak and his colleagues (1996) note, they increase his likelihood for aggressive action and decrease his ability to deal with trauma:

> [G]ender rigidity, with its resultant constriction in emotional experience, is also likely to interfere with the individual's capacity to constructively integrate his traumatic experiences. The gender-rigid, emotionally constricted individual is less likely to be able to tolerate approaching the negative emotional states evoked by trauma, and more likely to avoid them, either by using psychological defenses, or by converting them to aggressive action. (p. 725)

Some male victims may become hustlers as a way of unconsciously channeling this aggression and attempting to resolve their betrayal

(Wright, 1995). Robbed by his abuse of feeling powerful, in control, and sexually aggressive, as he has been socialized to believe men always feel, such a boy tries to right his sense of unbalance by finding a sense of pseudopower though prostitution. As a prostitute, he believes he can set his price, say what he will or will not do, and find men who ask him for sex. Consider the teenage hustler protagonist of the novel *Mysterious Skin* (Heim, 1995): "He smiled, the pained, divided smile a person would make while being tattooed. . . . 'I stay in control,' he said" (p. 196). A hustler's delusion of being in charge, with an ability to turn men down, often turns out, of course, not to be the case, as the boy in *Mysterious Skin* eventually discovers. If men are coercive with him or bargain down his price, his low self-concept is reinforced.

The overuse of externalizing defenses means that as the boy develops he has a diminished capacity to monitor and experience his inner, more emotional life. This is further reinforced by the many traditional concepts of what it means to be a man that limit most men's ability to experience the full spectrum of their emotional life. It is essential to redefine and critique masculinity during psychotherapy in order to overcome a sexually abused man's sense of demasculinization and help him heal (Lisak, 1995). Such a process may involve allowing what has been previously defined as feminine to be redefined as masculine. This includes an ability to acknowledge fear, vulnerability, and emotionality. Thus, Willem's increasing capacity to tolerate his emotional life enabled him to weather crises without resorting to such behaviors as the impulsive but nearly lethal suicide attempt that had first propelled him into therapy.

In addition to openly aggressive external solutions to conflicts, there are nonviolent predatory outcomes. A man may become a tyrannical boss at work or a demeaning dictator at home. Externalizing on a more limited scale may also lead to the nonpredatory acting out we see in some of the men I describe in this book. Attempting to prove their masculinity, they resort to hypersexuality, invulnerability, and continuous efforts at control and mastery. Alternatively, they define themselves as everything they believe their abusers were not, avoid behaviors and interests traditionally thought of as masculine, and develop qualities typically encoded as unmasculine (Dimock, n. d.). On the positive side, these qualitites may include tenderness, cooperativeness, and caretaking. On the negative side, they may include nonassertiveness, overcompliance, and fearfulness.

Thus, on the one hand, Abe compulsively allowed himself to be picked up by men as a young teenager and was sexually compulsive as an adult. Yale developed a subtly exploitative attitude in human relationships. Keith became a workaholic, a stance that protected him from intimate relationships. On the other hand, Cory, Seth, and Xavier took the opposite tack: all retreated far into an internalized way of dealing with the world that led to emotional constriction and being an overly "good little boy."

Unfortunately, and ironically, it is the man with the most fragile and insecure self-concept—and this often includes sexually abused men— who has the most trouble acknowledging the need for help. Instead, he may embrace action-oriented modes of dealing with his chaotic emotions. Many of the men I have seen originally took refuge from their psychic pain in numbing behaviors that tend to be encoded as masculine (see Chapter 7). These include numerous compulsive and addictive activities, especially behaviors related to alcohol and drugs. A large proportion of the men whose histories I describe throughout this book (for example, Abe, Devin, Greg, Harris, Isaac, Keith, and Patrick) had prolonged periods in their lives when such behaviors were used extensively as a means of trying to cope with overwhelming inner worlds. While these addictions almost inevitably served to make their lives deteriorate in the long term, in the short term they tended to soothe and numb the man's problems without challenging his self-concept as a man.

THE SEDUCTIVE APPEAL OF REMAINING A BOY

One solution to the problems of accepting a societally informed identity as a man is to retain an internal sense of oneself as a boy who does not need to conform to the demands made on men. In doing so, a man is able to remain less aggressive than he perceives men must be, while still not experiencing himself as feminized. This position is associated in our culture with the character of Peter Pan, the boy who wouldn't grow up. It has particular resonance for some sexually abused men.

Isaac exemplifies this unconscious strategy. He had a history of twelve separate molestations as a boy. Radiating a boyish sweetness and diffidence that belied his well-hidden aggression and fury, Isaac attended college on and off for over twenty years before finally graduating in his early forties. Throughout this period, and even afterward, he remained underemployed in a low-level service industry job that did not require a high school diploma. Dependent on his stepfather for financial assistance as well as emotional support, his relationships with male and female friends lacked complexity and depth. His discussions of his interpersonal interactions often involved puzzled questioning of what people intended by their behaviors or quotations from self-help books he had consulted to help him discover how people relate to one another. At times, these discussions were of a nature and at a level that I might expect from a young adolescent.

One day Isaac was late to a session and apologized. I noted to him that he seemed like a young boy who was expecting to be punished as he bashfully made his excuses. He agreed that he felt very young at that moment. As we explored his feelings about this we both realized that he often felt and seemed far younger than his age. He said he did not really know how to be older than a teenager. In his own mind, most adult men were like the many older boys or men who had abused him, all of whom he assumed were straight, and he felt he would have to behave abusively if he were a "regular" heterosexual adult man. On the other hand, he conceived of gay men as societal victims. He wanted to be neither gay nor a victim, but was terribly afraid he was both. So he retreated to a seemingly asexual and innocent adolescent posture and self-concept, even though he was now in his forties. With time, he warily began to give this up, and explored in therapy his continued passive, eroticized, "feminine" longing for men, which coexisted with his measured, "masculine," cautiously pursued interest in women.

MULTIPLE GENDERED SELF-REPRESENTATIONS

Evolving perceptions of masculinity and femininity translate into a parade of self-representations on the masculine–feminine continuum, some primitive and some much more sophisticated, each incorporated at some point during the development of a man's masculine identity. We have seen several such self representations in the preceding sections of this chapter: the inexpressive self, the active self, the needy self, the victimized self, the agentic self, the feminized self, the Don Juan self, the hypermasculine self, the boy self.

Any of these gendered identifications may be available to an individual at a given moment, so, according to this way of understanding gender identity, *all* adults have the capacity for multiple gendered self-representations. Thus, a person may instantly switch from neediness to violence, or from sexual predator to dependent child, in the course of a given interaction. Depending on the degree to which that individual is psychologically integrated, this can either result in a heightened capacity for gender flexibility or in severe gender confusion (see Chapter 7 for further discussion of the concept of multiple self-states).

Greg was sexually betrayed by his father and grandfather in boyhood as well as by his pastor in young adulthood. He discerned at one point that his bewilderment about his gender identity as a boy might have been related to a similar confusion on his father's part. He revealed that his father used to say to him when he was small, "When I was your age, I was a girl." At first, Greg interpreted this as an example of his father's inauthenticity. But as we investigated the meaning behind the father's words we both began to wonder what the father's fantasy had meant. Given his father's general inexpressiveness and rigidity, it seemed impossible that he was playfully conveying a flexibility about his own gendered self-states. Our exploration of his mysterious statement was an example of how multiple possible layers of meaning may be uncovered in the analysis of an interpersonal communication.

We wondered whose "girl" the father had been. His mother's? His father's? Was the father ever allowed by them to be a girl, whatever that meant to him? Or did he have to hide his fantasy from the adults in his life? Had the father himself been abused? Did he feel like a girl because of such childhood sexual abuse? Greg noted that when he was a child his father had often acted in hypermasculine ways. For example, he used to do handstands on the beach and show off his physique. Greg now wondered whether this was a counterphobic reaction to a "girlness" he felt inside. He also remembered that, unusually in their culture, his father had not minded when Greg dressed up in girl's clothes as a little boy, though the father later seemed ashamed of this behavior. Was Greg living out unresolved gendered fantasies for his father?

We then wondered about his father's reactions to Greg's homosexuality. Did the father himself have secret homosexual wishes as represented by the fantasy that he had been a girl when he was young? Had he communicated these wishes to Greg by saying he used to be a girl? Had whatever sexuality that went on between Greg and his father, whether overt or covert, been an acting out of such homosexual desires on the father's part? Or was it a representation of the power relationship between the two, as sexual abuse and rape often turn out to be? This parade of questions represent how thinking about multiple gendered self-representations and self-states can help move treatment along for a sexually abused man who is capable of addressing such issues.

CORY: A FEMALE-IDENTIFIED HETEROSEXUAL MAN

Cory's story illustrates some aspects of these multiple gendered self-states. A female-identified man, his sexual betrayal by his mother seemed to have no effect on his heterosexuality. He identified strongly with this seductively abusive mother, who believed that men and male sexuality are terrifying. Interestingly, despite this highly feminized identification, his sexual orientation seems never to have been in doubt. (See Chapter 4 for a discussion of whether sexual orientation is affected by sexual betrayal.)

Cory was a gifted academician in his early thirties whose betrayal was subtle and can only arguably be defined as sexual abuse. He came to therapy after suddenly experiencing dissociated terror during sex with his wife when she caressed his back in a certain way. He saw his mother's face on his wife and bolted upright in bed, weeping and shouting, "Don't touch me!" Depressed, unable to work, and feeling suffocated in his marriage, Cory did not have specific memories of sexual abuse, and did not regain such memories while in therapy. Nevertheless, he identified himself before beginning treatment as a survivor of sexual abuse by his mother and continued to feel that his memories of abuse remained maddeningly just beyond his conscious level of awareness. He felt nauseated when he was near his mother or even when he spoke of being touched by her. He remembered spending most of his childhood puttering in the basement workshop because it was the one place in the house his mother never came.

Cory's father was a manic–depressive civil servant, undiagnosed until Cory was an adult. Cory recalled him as a passive nonpresence in the household except occasionally when his manic episodes would precipitate a family crisis. The family included three sisters in addition to Cory, and he reported that his mother controlled them all through strict rules and fearful warnings about the outside world, particularly about the untrustworthiness of men, including Cory's father. This recurring attack on all men ultimately became a psychological betrayal of Cory by his mother. She also made consistent sexualized violations of his psychological and physical boundaries. A prime example is the one overt behavior of his mother's that Cory classifies as sexually abusive, which involved telling him in extravagant detail the horror she felt during sex on her wedding night and thereafter. In addition, paradoxically, she complained of the lack of sex with his father and his inability to satisfy her sexually.

Cory and his sisters all toed the line and grew up exceptionally well-behaved and high-achieving in school. About this Cory bitterly said, "My mother brought us all up to be ladies. She taught me over and over that men were scary and awful. Then one day I was fourteen and I had hairy knees and broad shoulders and I was fucked—I was one of Them." Cory felt his mother was repelled by him now: by his smells, by his sweatiness, by his bulk, by the sexual thoughts he might be having. He likewise disgusted himself, and considered entering the priesthood as a solution to his agony about his burgeoning male sexuality.

By late adolescence, Cory found himself unable to relate to most men or women, though he seemed more capable of establishing uneasy alliances with women. He never had a date in high school and in college managed to room in an otherwise nearly all-female dormitory after his freshman year. Thus, he continued an existence in which he had few meaningful contacts with men, but instead "remained one of the ladies." Somehow, he was able consecutively to develop his friendship with two women in his dormitory into more intimate relationships. He married the second woman after graduation.

One man who did befriend him in college had been Cory's senior dorm advisor. This man once made a sexual advance toward Cory, who felt frozen and numb. When Cory's body was physically unresponsive to his overtures, the man stopped. Nevertheless, Cory talked about this incident with shame. He felt that had he not gone into a state of physical semiparalysis (which he did not experience as self-induced), he would have acceded to his friend because of his own passivity and expectation that he must give in when demands are made of him.

As he began psychotherapy, Cory was wary of possible sexual interest from men or women, consciously dressing in odd old clothes to make himself less attractive. Deeply frightened of all sexuality, his closest friends aside from his wife were all lesbian women, the only people with whom he felt truly safe sexually.

In his treatment, Cory voiced the anger he repressed as a boy, the anger he felt would have made his mother label him "a rough, hairy killer." Eloquent expressions of feeling about intrusion alternated with anxious explorations of how even to conceive of interpersonal boundaries and then later of how to build such boundaries in his relationships.

Haltingly, with anguish and anger, Cory started to break through his paralysis and proceed with his life. As we confronted his feminine identifications and his fury about them, he began to go to a gym, develop his physique, and wear clothes that revealed his attractiveness and maleness. This work on his gender confusion helped him feel stronger, more "manly," and far less reactive to the needs of his mother and the many people he perceived as being like her. This enabled him to participate more actively in his marriage and to discover how different his wife and mother were.

His wife, who very much wanted the marriage to work, was exceptionally willing to listen to his concerns about boundary violation once he found the words with which to articulate them. All their intimate interactions became a grid on which they consciously tried to slow down the action so they could pinpoint the moments when Cory got anxious and started to dissociate. This led to painful confrontations about his fears of spontaneity and closeness. As he ironically put it once, "I don't want any spontaneity unless I know what's going to happen." She, in turn, voiced her needs for reassurance when he froze or turned away from her. That she was capable of having such conversations with him was a revelation to him and helped him see that she was not, in fact, like his mother. This made him feel safer during succeeding intimate moments so he could sustain their closeness without instantaneously closing off. The couple's relationship improved dramatically over Cory's five years of treatment.

ABUSED MEN'S REVULSION AND FEAR OF OTHER MEN

It is common for sexually abused men to be reluctant to associate with other men. They may be fearful and isolated, and may consequently be uncomfortable undressing in locker rooms, urinating in public lavatories, participating in traditional masculine activities, or even being alone in a room with other men (Dimock, n. d.).

Elsewhere in this book I talk about sexually abused men's fears of men in authority and of men who may be sexual predators. For many men, this has generalized to an unconscious belief that they are in constant danger of one kind of victimization or another from other men. This leads them to lead isolated and lonely lives, with few if any same-sex friendships. The wariness and revulsion about being with other men is closely related to the unarticulated fear that victimization has made them into semi-eunuchs whose nonmale status will subject them to further humiliation, ridicule, and shame from other men. (I discuss these issues further throughout this book, particularly in Chapters 8, 10, and 11.)

Seth recounted with pain the continual sense of contempt he felt from men in groups. He was therefore phobic about being around men. Yet he desperately needed and longed for a positive experience with other men, never having had the chumship relationships in preadolescence that Sullivan (1953) describes as necessary for same-sex intimacy. He did eventually get such experiences in an all-male group therapy situation. Until then, he was caught up in an escalating and unrelenting cycle with men: he felt vulnerable to them, behaved in ways that probably communicated this vulnerability, then was easily mistreated by them, thus making him feel all the more threatened and insecure.

For example, his job required him to go by car from one venue to another to do his work. One day he discovered that his car was missing from a company parking lot, and the group of men working there seemed to be smiling knowingly at one another when he asked where his car was. Nevertheless, these men, colleagues with whom he worked on a regular basis, all claimed they did not know what happened to his car. He realized they were lying, and tried to treat the situation as a joke, but they started to get nasty, especially when he began to flush and, eventually, to weep in exasperation and helplessness. The men derisively mimicked his crying as he got angrier and angrier, before finally telling him that one of them had lent Seth's car to another worker who needed to take his wife to the hospital. It was not clear to Seth how much of an emergency the situation was, or whether another car might have been available whose owner was there to give permission. Seth was left feeling that once again he had been made a victimized fool by men who considered him odd and unmale. This was a feeling he had had since childhood, particularly because of his interest in solitary and artistic activities and his aversion to team sports; but it was far more pronounced after his sexual victimization in his early teens. Not surprisingly, it took an enormous effort for Seth to come to a group therapy for sexually abused men. It was a long time before he could even begin to let down his guard in the group, particularly about his rage toward other men, his accompanying fear of them, his longing to overcome his isolation from them, and his sense of not belonging to any group, particularly groups of men.

REMASCULINIZATION
OF SEXUALLY ABUSED MEN

When I initially wrote about this topic, the title of my first paper was "The De-Masculinization of Sexually Abused Men" (Gartner, 1996b). I was referring at that time to the likelihood that men feel demasculinized by their abuse while women seem less likely to feel defeminized by theirs. But the complexities of the treatment of sexually abused men make me think of another meaning for that title. Here I refer to the need to deconstruct masculinity, to talk proactively with the sexually abused man about how his ideas about what it means to be a man inhibit his ability to address the consequences of his abuse (see Lisak, 1995).

A man I worked with once called this process the *re*masculinization of sexually abused men. He was alluding to what he felt was the absolute need of sexually abused men to redefine their ideas about what it means to be a man in order to heal from their sense of victimization. While most men would gain greater health and flexibility through redefining their masculinity, sexually abused men often have been specifically blocked by their masculine gender ideals from coming to terms with their trauma.

The process of redefining what it means to be a man involves questioning whether it is unmasculine to be a victim, or to turn down sexual offers, or to express emotional pain. If a man succeeds in doing this, then he will be better able to experience and own his childhood experiences. He will encounter his sexuality, his sexual orientation, and his gender identity without going into dissociated states. In short, he will develop more functional concepts of what it means to be a man.

But engaging in this process is a complicated and challenging task. Coming to psychotherapy itself is difficult for many men because they feel that doing so is a sign of their incompetence in navigating life. (Remember that part of the internalized masculine ideal is to be competent.) Most psychotherapists have worked with many men, sexually abused or not, who were initially very reluctant to enter treatment for this reason. Indeed, according to one study (Baraff, 1991), only 15 percent of patients in psychotherapy are men (see also Levant, 1990). To acknowledge weakness by going for help, and to develop a relationship with a therapist whom the man worries will observe and judge his ineptitude, is humiliating for many men. On the other hand, overcoming this reluctance may be a man's important first step toward redefining himself and his manhood.

CHAPTER 4

Same-Sex Abuse

Same-sex abuse is often interpreted as a sign of the victim's or the abuser's homosexuality. Yet victims are frequently headed for predominantly straight sexual orientations at the time they are abused, and virtually all male abusers consider themselves heterosexual. Confusion of same-sex abuse with homosexuality gets further complicated when considered in the context of masculine gender ideals, as discussed in the previous chapter. In turn, they both interact with a man's understanding of his own sexual orientation and any ambivalence he feels about himself as an erotic, sexual being.

These are all are complex, interrelated subjects for a male victim of childhood sexual abuse. As these themes emerge in treatment, both therapist and patient may be unclear about which is the crucial thread at any given moment. For example, a man may easily confuse shame about victimization with shame about same-sex behavior, or shame about homosexual wishes, or even shame about feeling sexual desire. It is important to track the patient's subtle shifts in focus as he moves from one of these feelings to another.

Sexual victimization brings up concerns about sexual orientation when a boy equates victimization with passivity, and passivity in turn with homosexuality (Nasjleti, 1980). Ignorance, prejudice, and misinformation about homosexuality permeates our culture, influenced by socialized masculine gender ideals. Therefore, when a boy's abuser is a man, the betrayal is apt to be regarded by the boy or by anyone who hears about the molestation as something to hide, specifically, a worrisome indication that the boy is gay (see Johanek, 1988; Sepler, 1990; Struve, 1990).

Thus, fears of homosexuality may especially interfere with the ability to process same-sex abuse. In this chapter, I will consider the history of homosexuality as a concept. I will then focus on homophobia and heterosexism, analyzing their effect on how sexually betrayed men come to terms with their abuse histories. In particular, I will address the common fear that childhood sexual abuse makes a boy gay. I will also focus further on boys' and men's shame about same-sex victimization, and how our culture reinforces their sense that silence and revenge are the only acceptable responses to such victimization.

UNDERSTANDING SEXUAL ORIENTATION

What is homosexuality and why is it worrisome?[1] These appear to be obvious questions with obvious answers, but to properly understand the relationship between male sexual victimization and fears about homosexuality, we need to examine each of the relevant concepts in turn. In this and the following section, I will address sexual orientation, homophobia, and heterosexism, as well as the history of psychological theory in relation to them.

Sexual orientation may be defined as the predominating erotic desire for a particular kind of sexual partner. Usually, this includes romantic and affectional attachment as well. In contemporary usage, the term is usually used to denote same-sex or opposite-sex attraction. Like gender identity, sexual orientation is a complex construct with multiple meanings. Further, it is shaped, created, and perceived through a cultural lens.[2] Individuals may be attracted to both sexes in different degrees at the same time, or they may be primarily attracted to one sex or another at different points in their lives. For this reason, common but erroneous binary concepts of heterosexuality and homosexuality (see Blechner, 1995a), by which men are thought to be entirely heterosexual or entirely homosexual, further confuse the integration of a sexual abuse history.

Sexual *orientation* is often confused with sexual *behavior*. Kinsey and his associates, in their classic study *Sexual Behavior in the Human Male* (Kinsey, Pomeroy, and Martin, 1948), used largely behavioral mea-

---

[1] I am specifically referring to male homosexuality in my discussion, although many of the themes are also relevant to female homosexuality.

[2] For discussions of the meaning of same-sex sexual behavior in different cultures over time, see Duberman, Vicinus, and Chauncey (1989).

sures to infer *degrees* of sexual orientation. In doing so, they attempted to move away from binary assessments of sexual orientation to take into account the diversity of men's actual sexual experiences. They assigned men numbers on a seven-step scale based on the frequency of homosexuality and heterosexuality in their behavioral histories, as well as in their dreams and waking fantasies. They then categorized gradations of sexual orientation from exclusive heterosexuality through varying proportions of heterosexuality and homosexuality to exclusive homosexuality. As they wrote:

> The world is not to be divided into sheep and goats. Not all things are black nor are all things white. It is a fundamental taxonomy that nature rarely deals with discrete categories and tries to force facts into separate pigeon holes. The sooner we learn this concerning human sexual behavior, the sooner we shall reach a sound understanding of the realities of sex. (p. 65)

Kinsey et al. thus argue for a view of sexuality in which bisexuality and complex multiplicities of sexual attraction are normative. But their great insight about the inadequacy of binary, dichotomous formulations for sexual orientation has yet to be fully integrated into theoretical and clinical discussions—though in recent years it has become a more commonly espoused idea. In common discourse, it is nearly impossible to discuss sexual orientation without falling into an either/or binary of homosexuality versus heterosexuality that does not capture the range of possible sexual attractions.

A man's self-concept as a gay, straight, or bisexual individual is the best reflection of his predominating sexual orientation.[3] It is instructive to consider behaviorally based models of sexual orientation like Kinsey's. But same-sex or opposite-sex *behavior* is not necessarily an accurate predictor of an individual's eventual enduring erotic *desire* for individuals of either the same or the opposite sex, or for both sexes. Nor is sexual behavior necessarily a sign of whether the individual identifies himself as gay, straight, bisexual, transgendered, or otherwise. Predominant erotic imagery and fantasy is another reflection of sexual orientation. A man may engage exclusively in heterosexual behavior while having sexual fantasies exclusively about men, or vice versa. Indeed, for some men, fantasy may be a more powerful indicator of sexual orientation than behavior.

---

[3] For ease of expression, I usually refer to sexual orientation in this chapter as predominantly gay or predominantly straight. However, I note that this ignores the full possible spectrum of sexual orientations and also may misleadingly convey that sexual orientation has a static nature.

Self-concept, behavior, and fantasy thus all contribute to a man's consistent sense of his sexual orientation. However, the categorizations of homosexuality, heterosexuality, bisexuality, and transgendered sexuality have in recent years been widely criticized as constituting a narrowing of experience that catalogues individuals into inaccurate and static sexual orientations (see, for example, Corbett, 1993; D. Schwartz, 1995). It is not unusual for individuals at various points in their lives to have shifting thoughts, fantasies, behaviors, self-concepts, or preferences about their own sexual orientation (see Gonsiorek and Weinrich, 1991; Domenici and Lesser, 1995). In that sense, sexual orientation may be a shifting concept for any given individual. Nevertheless, as adults, most people do seem to identify on a conscious level with a single predominating sexual orientation, whatever the complexity or variety of their fantasy lives, behaviors, or self-concepts.

HOMOPHOBIA, HETEROSEXISM, AND SCIENTIFIC EXPLORATIONS OF THE ORIGINS OF SEXUAL ORIENTATION

In Chapter 3, I noted the need of boys endeavoring to establish traditional masculine identities to disidentify with women as they develop. Femininity and homosexuality are often equated in this process. The struggle to define oneself as "not female" frequently leads to a disparagement of qualities seen as feminine, and often to a (usually disguised) antagonism toward women. Hatred of homosexuals, who are often viewed as men who did not succeed in disidentifying with women, is usually more open. The widespread fear and prejudice against homosexuality in the United States has been well documented and discussed elsewhere (Isay, 1989; Sedgwick, 1990; Herek, 1991, 1998; Martin, 1991; Moss, 1992; D. Schwartz, 1993; Domenici and Lesser, 1995; Katz, 1995; Drescher, 1998). It is usually called *homophobia*, literally meaning "fear of homosexuality" but usually used to connote hatred of it. In most cases I prefer the term *heterosexism*, which implies an unconscious predisposition to view life from a heterosexual viewpoint, and therefore to be intolerant or prejudiced against alternate sexualities. D. Schwartz (1993) has proposed using the term *heterophilia* for these phenomena.

Homophobia and heterosexism are ubiquitous throughout North American society. They were unfortunately prevalent in writings about psychiatric and psychological diagnosis and treatment for many years, although to some extent this has changed in recent years (but not entirely; see Blechner, 1993, 1995b; Drescher, 1996). In this section, I will briefly review the history of how homosexuality has been portrayed in the clinical literature. This will serve as a backdrop to understanding sexually abused men's fears that they may be gay.

Homosexuality itself is a relatively modern idea, having first appeared in writing as a scientific term in 1869 (Wiedemann, 1962). Heterosexuality is likewise a relatively contemporary idea that was itself "invented" (Katz, 1995). Homosexuality was almost invariably thought to be pathological by psychological, psychiatric, and psychoanalytic writers from the late nineteenth century until at least the 1970s and, to a lesser extent, continuing to the present (see Bergler, 1956, 1959; Socarides, 1968, 1978, 1995; Nicolosi, 1991). The hypothesized pathological nature of homosexuality has at various times been viewed as stemming from moral, biological, and psychological sources. For decades, it adversely affected the psychotherapeutic treatments of many gay individuals. Martin Duberman, in his book *Cures* (1991), and Paul Monette, in *Becoming a Man* (1992), each chronicle harrowing histories in which he was thus affected in his own psychotherapy (see also the case of Owen later in this chapter).

A rare exception to this trend to pathologize homosexuality is represented by the work of Evelyn Hooker (1957), a psychologist who devised a double-blind study of Rorschach responses of apparently well-adjusted homosexual and heterosexual men in the general population. She found that there was no reliable way to discern any difference in their Rorschach responses, and therefore concluded that though homosexuality may be atypical it is psychologically within the normal range of sexuality.

Initially far more influential than Hooker's work, *Homosexuality: A Psychoanalytic Study of Male Homosexuals,* the 1962 study by Irving Bieber and his associates, is perhaps the prime example of scientific work that pathologizes homosexuality. A ten-year study of homosexuals and heterosexuals undergoing psychoanalytic treatment, it was, in the years following its publication, nearly universally cited by writers who considered it to have confirmed traditional psychoanalytic ideas about the pathology of homosexuality (see Lewes, 1988, for an extended discussion of this issue). Bieber concluded that homosexuals were likely to have been involved in overly close, often seductive relationships with their mothers, and distant or hostile relationships with their fathers. The Bieber study claimed a 27 percent rate of conversion from homosexuality to heterosexuality through psychoanalysis, although details were not given about the treatments or the quality and duration of these conversions. This is close to the 35 percent conversion rate cited by Socarides (1968, 1995), a contemporary advocate of so-called reparative therapy to convert homosexuals to heterosexuality.

Questions have been raised about whether these conversions reflect true changes in orientation. Even if we accept the figures Bieber and Socarides offer, however, their studies yield a failure rate of 65–73 percent, hardly convincing evidence for the validity of the treatment they advocate (Drescher, 1998).

Subsequent empirical studies have consistently not differentiated homosexual and heterosexual adults on measures thought to indicate mental health (Lichtenberger and Buttenheim, 1998). In 1973, only eleven years after the publication of the Bieber study, the American Psychiatric Association voted to delete homosexuality from its list of psychiatric disorders. This was the result of a sea change in the psychiatric community, with mostly nonanalytic psychiatrists successfully challenging the dominance of the mostly psychoanalytic psychiatrists who had previously held sway. While the change itself did not stop the controversy (see Lewes, 1988), and still has not been accepted by some parts of the professional community, the depathologizing of homosexuality has gradually generalized to some degree in scientific writing. In recent years, a number of observers have documented and discussed the (often unconscious) homophobia and heterosexism prevalent in the clinical literature (Mitchell, 1978, 1981; Kwawer, 1980; R. C. Friedman, 1988; Lewes, 1988; Isay, 1989, 1991; Blechner, 1993, 1995a, 199b, 1996; Corbett, 1993; Lesser, 1993; MacIntosh, 1994; Dimen, 1995b; May, 1995; Schafer, 1995; Drescher, 1998).

In the 1990s, there has been increasing evidence offered by scientists for a biological model of homosexuality (Money, 1988; Hamer, Hu, Magnuson, Hu, and Pattatucci, 1993; LeVay, 1993; Byne, Hamer, Isay, and Stein, 1995; Zhang and Odenwald, 1995). This model has relieved many homosexuals from anguished feelings that they have somehow unknowingly "chosen" to be homosexual, and are therefore responsible for hurting their families or for what they may think of as their own "degeneracy." But the biological explanation of homosexuality can itself be used in the service of unconscious heterosexism. This is because the very question of why someone becomes homosexual, a question rarely asked about heterosexuality, can be an expression of nonaccepting and pathologizing hatred (Blechner, 1995b).

In sum, homophobia, or heterosexism, has constituted a dominant societal attitude about sexual orientation. It is a bias that in itself has been called sexual abuse (Fitzgerald, in Morris et al., 1997). It has affected all homosexual individuals in our culture, as well as heterosexuals, and its effect on psychological theory and treatment has at times been devastating. Now let us look at its effects on boys who have been sexually abused.

THE INTERNALIZED MEANING
OF HAVING A MALE ABUSER

Self-concepts in relation to both sexual orientation and gender identity
have not yet coalesced for boys and adolescents, and therefore they tend
to understand concerns about their own or others' orientation in a literal
and concrete way (see Shapiro, 1994, and Chapter 10 of this book).
Fears, prejudices, and misinformation about both sexual orientation and
gender identity are particularly prominent in adolescence, when both are
being consolidated. Such preconceptions about orientation create great
confusion and internal turmoil for boys sexually abused by men. Sexual
abuse may cause boys to remain caught up in the black-and-white views
of homosexuality and heterosexuality that are characteristic of childhood and adolescence, when they were first abused. Thus, Bruno and
Isaac both had simplistic, behaviorally oriented ideas about whether
their same-sex sexual activity with abusers, and later with other men,
meant that they were "actually" gay.

Molestation by a man is likely to undermine a boy's sense of his
gender identity and orientation, whether he is predominantly heterosexual or homosexual (Bruckner and Johnson, 1987; Dimock, 1988; Lew,
1988; Bolton et al., 1989; Gonsiorek, 1993, cited in Mendel, 1995;
Mendel, 1995). This is particularly likely if he encodes his experience as
a "feminizing" victimization (see Chapter 3), especially one that goes
counter to his own object choice (see Chapter 2). The problem is made
even more complicated when we take into account how far the boy's
conscious understanding of his sexual orientation and identity has developed at the time of the abuse.

We saw in Chapters 2 and 3 that a boy who has been headed for a
predominantly heterosexual orientation is likely not to consider molestation by a woman to be abusive. If, however, he is abused by a woman
and is not sexually aroused, he may take this as a sign that he is gay
(Mendel, 1995). If he is abused by a man, he may perceive the very fact
of his molestation as a shameful sign of "queerness" or femininity
(Sepler, 1990; Struve, 1990). He may fear that he somehow invited the
abuse and therefore is "really" interested in men. Or he may wonder
why he was chosen by a man as a sexual target, and whether having
been chosen means he is "truly" homosexual. Whether he is aroused or
not, then, he may fearfully assume he is "really" gay.

Meanwhile, a boy with even a partial awareness of being headed
toward a predominantly homosexual orientation may be repulsed and
frightened by sexual activity with a woman. When the abuser is a man,
however, he may feel excited by what he considers a "sexual initiation."
On the other hand, sexually abused boys who are predominantly homo-

sexual may feel the experience prematurely hurried them into defining themselves as gay.

As I outlined in Chapter 2, men are especially likely to think of their abuse as "sexual initiation" if the abuser is not a parent and is of the same sex as the boy's eventual primary object choice. But for nearly *any* boy molestation by a man brings up questions about his gender identity and sexual orientation, as well as worries about why he was chosen as a victim (Nasjleti, 1980; Finkelhor, 1984; Dimock, 1988; Lew, 1990; Struve, 1990; Mendel, 1995). Usually, sexually abusive behavior is fundamentally about power and aggression rather than about sexuality (see below). Even when homosexual desire is not the motivating force in a molestation, however, as Pescosolido (1989) notes, "[T]he victim's *perception* is that of being involved in homosexual behavior. As a result, [he] is left with emotional confusion regarding his developing psychosexual identity. Essentially the victim may believe that something within himself almost magically communicated a homosexual invitation prompting the molestation" (p. 89; emphasis added).

Pescosolido adds that there is even more uncertainty for the victim if he becomes erect or ejaculates during the abuse (see also Ehrenberg, 1992). While these are the normal physiological responses to stimulation, he may feel they provide proof of his participation in the act. Thus the boy, and later the man, may ask himself, "Was I chosen because I seemed interested? *Was* I interested? Did he know I was not man enough to resist? Did my 'femininity' or 'sissiness' show enough to attract his attention?"

RAMON: SEXUAL ORIENTATION CONFUSION WHEN A MALE ABUSER IS ALSO NURTURING

When a male abuser is also a source of nurturance and pleasure, the boy's confusion about the implications of the abuse for his sexual orientation is especially painful and bewildering, as Ramon's case illustrates.

Ramon returned again and again in therapy sessions to his feelings about the neighborhood puppeteer who first abused him. He was initially afraid to voice his internal experience, afraid I would censure his positive feelings about their relationship, afraid that he or I might decide he was gay or bisexual if he put his obsessive thoughts into spoken words. Finally, though, he sputtered that this man had been tender, that he had known how to make Ramon feel good, that the sex had been sensuous and arousing, and that he never felt pain, even when he had bled. He said, miserably, "It's never been so sweet, so nice with anyone again. What does that mean? Who am I?" I remarked that with this man he had felt safe and cared for, that he had felt this was the one person who focused on him and was attentive to him at a time when his world was coming apart.

Later in treatment, Ramon revealed ashamedly that when he thought about his experiences with the puppeteer he felt an erotic "tingling" throughout his genital and rectal areas. He then talked about how during the period he had been abused by this man he woke up every morning waiting for the moment he could go visit the puppeteer and feel his tender lovemaking. He said, "I've been looking for that again ever since. I wish every day I could feel so good. But I don't think I'm gay—I never look that way at men on the street, and I like being with women. And if I tell anyone, my girlfriend, my friends, how I feel turned on when I think of being with him, they'll think I'm indecent—they won't take care of me any more."

Ramon thus revealed that, for him, a prime motivation for being sexual at all was to feel cared about and to enjoy someone allowing him to be dependent. Ramon said he didn't really want to have sex with the puppeteer or someone like him again, although it was not clear to me whether he was saying this because he meant it or because he was trying to allay his own fears about being homosexual. Either way, he was obsessed with the sensations of safety, nurturance, and eroticism that had accompanied his abuse.

We talked about this many times, and finally arrived at a model for thinking about it that seemed to pacify his intense anxiety. I likened the abuse experience to Ramon's thumb sucking as a very young child. In both instances, he felt comforted and calmed by the activity. He could remember those feelings with some longing in both cases, and yearn to have them again, but this did not automatically mean he as an adult actually wanted either to suck his thumb or to be penetrated again by a man like the puppeteer. That could be a separate decision for him. Ramon held on to this idea. At one point he actually resolved that to distract himself from his fears of homosexuality he would substitute sucking his thumb for the tingling in his rectal areas when he felt it again. Making this plan seemed to free him considerably, and he reported with relief some receding of his constantly recurring erotic sensations. While he remained confused about his sexual orientation, this confusion no longer interfered in the same way with his day-to-day life.

ARE MALE ABUSERS GAY?

Complicating the belief that abuse turns a boy gay is the related common folkloric myth that men who abuse boys are homosexual predators. This myth particularly extends to pedophiles who abuse large numbers of boys over time. While some pedophiles may consider themselves gay, it is far more often true that boys are abused by men who consider themselves heterosexual. Some of these men do not really differentiate between boys and girls, choosing whoever is most vulnerable and/or available (Dimock, 1989a).

Groth and Oliveri (1989) studied sexual victimizers of children, focusing on pedophiles rather than incest offenders. They divide abusers into three categories: First, there are *those with an exclusive fixation* on children. Some of these are only interested in boys, some are only interested in girls, and some are interested in both or do not discriminate between boys and girls. Second are *those with a nonexclusive fixation*. While primarily drawn to children, they have a secondary interest in adults. A third category of abusers includes *those whose pedophilia constitutes a regression*. They are primarily oriented to adults, but during some periods of their lives they regress and are drawn to children.

Groth and Oliveri report that if homosexuality is defined as being primarily oriented to *adult* men, then there are virtually *no* homosexual pedophiles. Among over 3,000 offenders they studied, they did not encounter a *single* man who had regressed from an orientation to adult men to an orientation to children. On the contrary, the men they studied who were nonexclusively fixated on children or who regressed from an adult orientation *universally* described themselves as heterosexual in their orientation toward adults, and indeed were usually homophobic (similar findings are reported by Jenny, Roesler, and Poyer, 1994).[4]

Pedophiles preying on boy victims often report that they are uninterested in or repulsed by adult homosexual relationships and are attracted to young boys' feminine characteristics and absence of such secondary sexual characteristics as body hair (Groth and Birnbaum, 1979). This supports the accepted clinical picture of sexual offenders and pedophiles as people who are psychosexually immature and who therefore in some way identify as psychological and psychosexual peers of the children they molest (Groth, 1982; Pescosolido, 1989).

A related view of pedophilia, sexual abuse, and rape is that they are not primarily expressions of sexual desire but rather are abuses of power and expressions of aggression (Burgess and Holstrom, 1979; Groth, 1979; Pescosolido, 1989). This is congruent with the classical Greek concept of sexuality described in Chapter 3, in which sexual penetration

---

[4] Note, however, that in some cultures and subcultures, as described in Chapter 3, men who take a penetrating role in sexual activity may consider themselves heterosexual even if the person being penetrated is male.

was a means of further establishing the dominance of the penetrator over the person being penetrated (Halperin, 1989).

These are further arguments that in most cases when a man abuses a boy homosexuality is not fundamentally the issue. This is why I use the term "same-sex victimization" rather than "homosexual victimization" to refer to situations in which perpetrator and victim are of the same sex (see also Pescosolido, 1989). To talk about "homosexual molestation" or "homosexual incest" implies that homosexuality is what caused the offense, rather than the many complex possible dynamics that are actually associated with child sexual abuse.

THE FEAR THAT SEXUAL ABUSE TURNS A BOY GAY

A boy with a consciousness of being gay may welcome aspects of his sexual experience with male predators, especially if he has felt isolated and freakish in relation to his sexual desire. I discuss this attitude more fully below. On the other hand, as I said, such a boy may feel hurried into considering himself gay. For him, there are complicated questions beyond those of heterosexual boys might ask themselves, such as: "Did I ask for it? Was my interest in men so obvious? Did I really want it? If I found it exciting does that mean it was not a molestation?" and, finally, "Is this why I'm gay?"

Any boy growing up gay in our society is likely to endure painful psychological and social struggles as he comes to understand his orientation and deal with people's reactions to it. In reacting to these struggles, he will probably go through a period of wondering about how he came to be homosexual. At such a time, he will look everywhere for an answer to the question "Why am I gay?" And, if he has been sexually abused by a man, it is easy for him to "blame" his sexual orientation on the abuse.

Many boys or young men who have been sexually abused share the commonplace view that sexual abuse by a man makes a boy gay. Beau, for example, took it as a matter of course that any man sexually abused in childhood was molested by men, as he had been, and grew up to be gay, as he had. He was astonished to hear that some men in the group for sexually abused men he was joining considered themselves straight and that some (not always the same ones) had been abused by women.

Paradoxically, however, a young gay man abused by a woman in childhood may use the reverse logic to account for his homosexuality. In that case, he may assume that fearful reactions to his female abuser generalized to all women, and made him later turn to men for sexual pleasure. Thus, whether the abuser is male or female, the betrayal complicates how the homosexual victim deals with being gay, and he may view abuse as the origin of his orientation.

But if we were to assume sexual orientation is changed or directed by sexual abuse, similar logic could be applied to heterosexual men. Thus, straight men abused by women would think their early sexual experience with women turned them heterosexual. If abused by men, they might assume that fears of men made them turn to women. But heterosexual men do not seem to consider these possibilities, nor is there any reason for them to do so. By the same token, there is no reason for gay men to believe sexual abuse caused their orientation.

Note that I am talking here about how the individual encodes experiences that coincide in his life. A boy or man knows he has been sexually abused and also knows he is attracted to men. As he puts together this knowledge, he is likely to add a causality between the two that is in fact logically specious. Interestingly, this conflict seems to get resolved for many sexually abused gay men by their mid- to late twenties. Most gay men I have seen at this age no longer link their orientation to sexual abuse, a finding also reported by Lew (1988, 1993) and Gonsiorek (1993, cited in Mendel, 1995).

Is there indeed a link between sexual molestation and subsequent predominant sexual orientation? As Mendel (1995) says, "The relationship between factors associated with childhood sexual abuse and sexual orientation is complex and controversial" (p. 169). In discussing the higher incidence of childhood sexual abuse among homosexual men, Finkelhor (1981, 1984) considers the possibility that boys growing up to be gay are more likely to be vulnerable to sexual victimization, but he favors the explanation that abuse fostered the homosexuality. This is contradicted, however, by the fact that most researchers believe predominant sexual orientation is established before latency, while most sexual abuse of boys occurs later (Gonsiorek, 1993, cited in Mendel, 1995; Mendel, 1995). Nor does it explain Simari and Baskin's (1982) finding that most of the abused gay men they studied had a clear sense of a homosexual orientation before their abuse or incest. I will return to the issue of gay boys being especially vulnerable to sexual abuse later in this chapter.

The sexual confusion and homophobia seen in boys who were sexually abused by men is also discussed by Bolton et al. (1989). They conclude that there is no reason to believe that sexual abuse alone fundamentally changes or shapes sexual orientation, despite the conventional wisdom that premature sexual activity with a man can "turn" a boy homosexual. Whether a man's orientation is homosexual, heterosexual, or bisexual, however, sexual abuse often affects the *quality* of his sexual relatedness (Rosenberg, 1995; see also Chapter 8). I am referring here to such aspects of sexuality as sadomasochistic fantasies or activities, various erotic obsessions and compulsions, and the capacity for intimacy.

Like Lew (1988, 1993), Bolton et al. (1989), Gonsiorek (1993, cited in Mendel, 1995), and Rosenberg (1995), my clinical impression is that sexual orientation is nearly always determined for reasons other than premature sexual activity. On the other hand, it is not at all uncommon for a straight man who suffered same-sex abuse to go through a period of sexual acting out with men, sometimes of a compulsive nature, while he struggles to answer for himself whether the abuse either means he was always gay or turned him gay. Andreas, for example, at one point in his thirties experimented sexually with men because of the numbness he felt during sex with his wife. Eventually, he decided he had even less interest in sex with men than in sex with women.

I will now consider several other men described at greater length elsewhere in this book whose boyhood sexual abuse by men seemed not to affect their predominantly heterosexual orientation, although their capacity to relate intimately was often compromised: Ezra was a socially shy heterosexual man; as a child, he was lured to a wooded area by a neighborhood teenager who masturbated on his bare chest. Harris was repeatedly abused by his father; as an adult, he was sexually interested in women, often picking them up for one-night stands but unable for years to be available for a relationship. In his early teens, Julian had an ongoing relationship with a priest; as a man, he was troubled by his compulsive, time-wasting interest in heterosexual pornography. Quinn was abused by his grandfather starting as a preschooler; he grew up to be a heterosexual man who had severe problems with self-esteem and depression. Teo, a heterosexual man who as a boy was abused by his godfather for an extended period of time, had two troubled marriages before meeting the supportive woman who became his third wife. Willem was apparently abused by more than one of his mother's lovers and husbands; he grew up to be a heterosexual man with severe problems of emotional detachment. Zak also grew up heterosexual following horrendous and prolonged emotional, physical, and sexual abuse at the hands of his adoptive father.

By way of contrast, I will now describe Bruno, a single man in his mid-sixties who suffered physical, verbal, and sexual abuse from several sources as a boy. Bruno is one of the very few men I have treated whose sexual orientation seemed fundamentally disordered by his reactions to same-sex abuse (a somewhat similar case is discussed by Gilgun and Reiser, 1990).

Bruno came to treatment hoping to discover his sexual orientation so that he could pursue either men or women with a vigor that had eluded him all his life. In the eight months we worked together, it gradually became clear to me that his multiple abuse experiences with his father, brother, teachers, and doctor had left him afraid to expose himself to any possibility of further abuse or ridicule. This was true in all interpersonal situations, but especially true in the sexual arena. Bruno enjoyed socializing with women, flirting mildly with them, and escorting them to social events. In more intimate situations, however, he was terrified they would make sexual demands on him. He had some mild sexual interest in them but was sure he could not perform adequately and would be subject to ridicule from even the kindest women he knew.

The youngest in a large immigrant working-class family, Bruno had been severely beaten as a boy by his father and one of his older brothers. His mother was overworked and passive, though apparently she herself was not abused. In describing his family, Bruno seemed to accept physical brutality as expected and acceptable, not unlike what happened in other families from his culture. The greater part of his conscious rage was reserved for the nuns in the parochial schools he attended. In memory, Bruno experienced these nuns uniformly as critical, derisive, terrifying, and cruel, particularly about what apparently was his undiagnosed dyslexia. He had numerous memories of humiliations he suffered from these women.

When he was twelve, Bruno was taken to the family doctor for treatment of a mild illness. During the examination, the doctor engaged in mutual oral sex with Bruno, and told his parents to bring him back every week, which they did for *three years*. Bruno protested, but did not tell his parents about the abuse. They angrily told him he was ungrateful for the doctor's interest in him. Not coincidentally, the doctor did not charge any of the family for medical attention given in the years he was molesting Bruno. Finally, when Bruno was fifteen, the doctor lost interest in him, and, as Bruno later understood it, he became similarly attached to a younger boy.

I have described Bruno's near-phobic reactions to the possibility of intimacy with women. He did have homosexual encounters, but we came to understand that his main interest seemed to be in attracting the other man rather than in having sex with him. While he often followed through and completed sexual acts with men, this appeared to be more out of a wish to placate them than from his own sexual desire. Indeed, as he got older, Bruno found that, more often than not, he would walk away from the other man once he knew the man desired him.

Bruno went through his entire adult life in this manner, only coming into therapy in late middle age, never having had an intimate relationship, uncertain about his sexual orientation. He sometimes thought of himself as a homosexual who did not enjoy sex with men, and at other times considered himself a closet heterosexual who was afraid to have sex with women.

My initial impression of Bruno was of a closeted gay man with low self-esteem whose cultural background made it impossible for him to accept his homosexuality. As we explored the nature of his sexual fantasies, I therefore felt it was crucial to distinguish his feelings about homosexuality from his own homosexual wishes. Bruno certainly shared some of the homophobic and heterosexist attitudes of the working-class Catholic family he grew up in during the 1920s and 1930s. On the other hand, he said he had reached a point in his life where he was more afraid of staying confused about his sexuality than of discovering that he was indeed gay.

Having declared this, Bruno noted that, while he was enraged about the doctor's molestations, they had provided him with the heady experience of feeling attractive and desired. This was what he tried to repeat with men as an adult. These interludes with men were never really gratifying, he said, but they did sometimes result in completed sexual acts, which had not been the case with women except for a few prostitutes when he was a very young man. Bruno believed that his molestations by the doctor had turned him into an "unwilling homosexual."

I was now confused about how to understand his sexuality and sexual orientation, and unfortunately had only meager fantasy material from him with which to support my various hypotheses. I felt his experiences with men supplied him with a way of functioning sexually, while his psychological paralysis with women prevented him from acting on the heterosexual impulses he also had. Yet his sexual desire never seemed to center clearly around men, and so, despite my initial impressions, I had trouble seeing him as fundamentally, or even predominantly, homosexual.

We began to clarify Bruno's sense of inadequacy and his feelings about men and women, and to connect both with his abuse experiences in childhood. It became more and more evident that his ability to relate to anyone sexually was very limited. Indeed, the undeveloped quality of his interpersonal functioning indicated that in many ways he had never reached a level at which mature sexual relating was even possible. Instead, he was stuck at a preadolescent stage of psychosexual development. To the extent that he even wanted sexual relationships, the main desire seemed to be to find companionship and have his considerable dependency deprivations assuaged.

As we delineated his need to be pleasing to women as well as to men, Bruno seemed to lose interest in both, at least for the time being. At this point, he told me a prevailing sexual fantasy had emerged of a partner who was a virginal hermaphrodite: young, feminine, and naïve. He pictured this person as having breasts and female genitalia, but with small male genitals as well. The male genitals would calm his anxiety about being with a woman, while the virginal naïveté would make it unlikely that Bruno's sexual performance would be criticized.

Bruno actually contacted a hermaphrodite who seemed to fulfill this fantasy. However, he broke off treatment before they met. The premature termination was not fully discussed. It could have been because of anxiety about the material he had uncovered; or because experiencing his sexuality felt dangerous; or because of a feeling I was leading him too quickly down a path of discovery about sexuality, whether gay, straight, or otherwise; or because of material he never hinted at, such as an erotic transference to me. I do not know whether any of my impressions about his orientation would have held up over time. Possibly his cultural background, combined with his abuse, did indeed make it impossible for him to acknowledge his homosexuality. Possibly he was right that his combination of abuse experiences had changed a fundamentally heterosexual orientation into a defensively homosexual one. Possibly he was neither gay nor straight nor even bisexual or transgendered, but rather of some unusual sexual orientation or gender identity as represented by his wish for a hermaphrodite partner (see D. Schwartz, 1995). Certainly his repeated traumas in early relationships left him functionally nearly asexual, disabled in all relationships because of his primeval terror of feeling closely connected to another person.

Bruno suffered multiple abuses in the context of a brutal family system that demanded unquestioning compliance from him. Perhaps because of these complexities, Bruno, almost alone among the sexually abused men I have treated, was affected by his history so that on all these levels the directions of his sexual orientation became thoroughly confused.

GAY BOYS AS TARGETS OF MALE ABUSERS

Among men with histories of sexual abuse, homosexual men are more likely than heterosexual men to have had male abusers (Simari and Baskin,1982; Finkelhor, 1984; Johnson and Shrier, 1985, 1987; Mendel, 1995). On the surface, this finding supports the common belief that boys with male abusers grow up to be homosexuals. But the reasons gay boys are abused by male predators are tangled and complicated. Sensing themselves as different or "other" than their peers, they may project an air of vulnerability (Lew, 1993). Or they may have developed some awareness of their interest in boys and men, whether conscious or unconscious. And potential sexual predators, whether from inside or outside the family, are skilled at recognizing and taking advantage of such vulnerability or incipient sexual interest. Interestingly, the results of research investigating whether straight men are more likely than gay men to have had female abusers are not as clear-cut (see Johnson and Shrier, 1985; Mendel, 1995).

Some boys whose gay orientation is at least partly conscious at the time of their abuse may welcome aspects of the molestation. Many boys in this situation feel very isolated in their developing gay identities. Indeed, they may have no idea that any other boys or men have similar sexual interests. In such a case, the boy may pay far more attention to the escape from this feeling of total isolation than to the abusive aspects of his experience (Myers, 1989). As Uri said about his concurrent abuse and personal devaluation at age thirteen by the twenty-two-year-old brother of his best friend: "I felt such joy discovering that I wasn't the only one who was aroused by men that I didn't care who showed me or how. As far as I was concerned, I had been liberated. I was no longer alone in the world. The sex itself felt good, and up till then having sexual thoughts had always been terrible for me. At the time, I hardly realized how horribly he was treating me—I didn't care about anything but my relief at not feeling like a total freak any more."

Greg, on the other hand, used aspects of his early knowledge of his homosexuality to confirm for himself that he had indeed been abused. He was a boy growing up gay who had already in some ways integrated or accepted his sexual interest in men before he was abused by his father and grandfather.

Greg remembered being interested in boys and men from early childhood. As an adult, he recalled his earliest pubescent fantasies and came to feel that they were confirming evidence of sexual abuse by his father. Although he had clear memories of his grandfather exposing himself to Greg when Greg was of latency age, his memories of abuse by his father were more shadowy. But he told me, with great embarrassment, that as a young adolescent he had had overwhelming, frank, consuming sexual fantasies about his father. Later, he began to think this was abnormal, and said, "I used to think it was because I was gay—yet another shameful thing about being gay—that I had sexual fantasies about my father. Then, as I grew up, I suddenly wondered—Do straight men have sexual fantasies about their mothers? I don't think so—not like I did, not all the time. Something was definitely going on between us if I was having fantasies like that. But I always thought it was just me and my dirty, evil mind."

GAY BASHING AS SEXUAL ABUSE

Sometimes when boys developing gay identities are sexually abused, the attack is a direct reaction to the abuser's recognition that the boy is homosexual. This abuse has a different character from incestuous abuse or molestations by pedophiles in that the victimization arises from hatred and prejudice about homosexuality itself. Violent antipathy to homosexuality is common among some heterosexuals. It appears to represent an attempt at mastery over fears about what is perceived as a threat to both masculinity and heterosexuality. This is especially likely among those who have never evolved beyond the concrete and simplistic views of homosexuality often held by adolescent boys whose sense of their masculine identity is not yet consolidated.

Hatred for homosexuals in such cases may result in what has come to be known as "gay bashing." Its virulence can lead to particularly ugly outcomes. Witness the case of Beau, a gay man who suffered multiple abuses and a multiple rape as a teenager. Beau's effeminate mannerisms appear to have preceded in time any conscious consolidation of his homosexuality. His traumatic introduction to homosexual behavior through a severe gay bashing incident in early adolescence further eroded his already shaky sense of himself.

An introverted boy, small for his age, Beau grew up in a conservative small town whose population included many rednecks and members of the religious far right. Both parents were well educated. He described his mother as vicious and verbally abusive and his father as fussy and fastidious, a man who spent time on intricate, isolating hobbies and was passive with his wife and nonresponsive to his son. Beau was often teased for his effeminacy. In addition, on a number of occasions in his preadolescence and teenage years he was groped or otherwise approached sexually by adult married men. On one occasion, he was fondled at his grandmother's wake by a professional man well known in the community. These incidents led him as an adult to be sneeringly infuriated at what he felt was the common hypocrisy of married men who were regarded as pillars of the community.

As a ninth grader in high school, Beau was anally raped by three student athletes. They took him under the athletic field bleachers for the assault. An assistant coach passed by and saw what was happening. According to Beau, he said, "I want some of that too," and also raped him. At the time of this violation, Beau had already known he was emotionally drawn to men, but he had only the vaguest sense of what physical acts of sex involved. His rape trauma was therefore particularly profound, since it also served as his introduction to even imagining overt sexuality with men.

School officials knew of the rapes, but never punished the assailants. Indeed, the assistant coach was eventually made head coach at the school. Beau said that when school officials called his father to tell him about the assault—it is not clear that they conveyed the news that his son had actually been raped—he told them to send Beau back to class. According to Beau, when he got home that day his mother called him a "little bitch" for having caused so much disruption.

After the rape, Beau became an object of rampant abuse and derision on a daily basis at school. Boys would force him to choose either to fellate them or give them payoff money to leave him alone. Girls knew about this and openly called him a faggot and a sissy. He was miserable, frightened, and endangered till he graduated from high school and went away to college, never to return to his hometown again except for brief visits to his parents. I will come back to the sequelae of Beau's abuse in Chapter 8.

THE INTERSECTION OF ABUSE
AND SELF-DISCORDANT HOMOSEXUALITY

I have discussed boys who were already moving in some way along a path toward confirming their homosexuality. What happens to a boy like this whose homosexuality is unacceptable to him?

Many boys developing a homosexual orientation are bewildered by the meaning of their orientation. This confusion can last a lifetime if the boy never comes to terms with his sexuality. Homophobic and heterosexist biases are nearly omnipresent in our culture, although this is less true now than it was even a decade ago. These introjected societal convictions about homosexuality intersect with a man's developing attitudes about sexual abuse. Together, they may complicate a man's views of both his gayness and his abuse history. Sometimes a preoccupation with changing or hiding a gay sexual orientation distracts him from even thinking about the abuse.

Let us return to Owen, the sixty-eight-year-old man whom I discussed in Chapter 2 with regard to his not encoding as abuse his "affair" starting at age twelve with a twenty-nine-year-old man, Calvin. Owen was a boy developing a homosexual orientation who before his "seduction" by Calvin had found at least one other boy with similar sexual interests. While apparently certain of his interest in men, he had extremely negative feelings about homosexuality, and was sure he would be ostracized by family and friends if he revealed his homosexual interests. Like many men, especially of his generation, he hid his homosexuality throughout most of his life. He sought treatment to "cure" his homosexuality, and apparently in his earlier therapies the focus on changing his orientation superseded any analysis of the meaning of his childhood "affair" with Calvin. Such a focus, as I have said, was common in the psychological treatment of homosexuals at that time. Yet we discovered that the subtle effects of his having been exploited by both Calvin and his family, and his willingness to be so exploited, were also central to his psychology. He never felt that his early sexuality with Calvin constituted molestation, but with time he agreed on the importance of analyzing his susceptibility to being manipulated.

Owen called me for a consultation two months after walking out of his previous analyst's office in a rage. He had been in treatment with this analyst for most of the previous thirty years, at frequencies of one to three times a week. A major focus in that treatment, and in Owen's life up till then, was his conflicted feelings about his homosexuality.

Even when involved with Calvin as a preadolescent and adolescent, and throughout college and a period in the armed services, Owen maintained and acted on the interest in boys and men he had evinced before meeting Calvin. He fell in love with other men several times. Some of these relationships were with heterosexual friends and were never completely enacted. Others were with more openly willing partners and included sexuality and, at times, living together, though never publicly as lovers. Most of these men eventually entered marriages with women, though Owen believed that many of these were basically marriages of convenience, as his own turned out to be. As was common in Owen's generation, these men, like Owen himself, seem to have been profoundly uncomfortable about homosexuality and appear not to have faced directly whether they were indeed gay. Indeed, for many years Calvin was the only person Owen knew who seemed content about being homosexual.

Much of Owen's adult life struggle was about his sexual orientation. He lived a conservative life, sure that his interest in men was pathological and that revealing it, particularly the "wanton" relationship with Calvin, would mean rejection by his family. In his mid-twenties, he married, at her insistence, a woman who accepted his lack of enthusiasm for sex with her. He was recurrently depressed and started to see a psychiatrist a few years after the marriage. His depression continued and deepened. When he was about thirty, his wife called his psychiatrist, who met with her alone and, with Owen's relieved permission, told her that Owen was homosexual. She immediately told Owen that everything was "all right" and she wanted to stay married. Feeling that he could not bear to disappoint her further, Owen agreed. The couple, who remained childless, divorced after twenty-five years when his wife fell in love with another man.[5]

Shortly after his wife learned of his homosexuality, Owen began to work with the classical psychoanalyst he saw for most of the next thirty years. According to Owen, this analyst confirmed his belief that homosexuality is a disease, and they set out to cure Owen of it. In general, Owen said, the analyst interpreted his homosexuality as an expression of anger toward women and maintained that he could get beyond this

---

[5] For further discussion of gay men in heterosexual marriages, see Isay (1998).

anger if he worked hard enough in treatment. Owen felt positively in many ways about his work with this analyst, and particularly felt helped during periods of major depression, when medication was effectively used in addition to an intensification of the psychotherapy. But it appears that the relationship with Calvin was never addressed except as a prime example of his early homosexual experience. Its exploitative aspects seem never to have been recognized.

Nor did the efforts to "work through" Owen's "anger toward women" result in any shift in Owen's sexual orientation. He never understood or accepted the idea that he was basically hostile to women. After his divorce, Owen began to live a relatively open homosexual life, though he never came out to any of his family members. He remained convinced that they did not know about the sexual nature of his relationship with Calvin, and he felt certain they would be horrified by this knowledge. He had a few relatively brief but serious relationships with men who seem to have been needy and dependent. In each of these affairs, Owen ultimately felt used by the other man, and the relationships all ended badly. In his treatment, the thrust of the work until the 1990s continued to be an analysis of the lower level of psychic adjustment supposedly represented by his homosexuality.

When Owen was in his early sixties, his analysis apparently shifted gears. He and his analyst began to focus on Owen's accepting his homosexuality and trying to develop a relationship with a man after all. But Owen and the analyst continued to have major ongoing arguments. The analyst said they disagreed "profoundly" about the origins of homosexuality, while Owen began to say more confrontationally that he never felt he had "chosen" one way or another to be gay. In addition, Owen felt he was being treated shabbily by his analyst, who sometimes called Owen several times over the course of a week, or even in a single day, to change appointment times for the convenience of the analyst's schedule. He also became aware of some ethically shady practices the analyst engaged in with regard to insurance billing. During one such argument, Owen left in the middle of a session and never returned.[6]

Two months later, Owen came to see me at the suggestion of a friend. He felt emotionally shaky, depressed, and bereft. Much of the beginning work with me focused on coming to terms with the way he

---

[6] It is, of course, difficult to make judgments about a lengthy psychoanalysis on the basis of the reports of a disappointed patient. Nevertheless, Owen's treatment, as he described it, appears to be an example of an analyst using his authority to ally himself with a patient's compliance and convince the patient of the analyst's views about homosexuality. This may change a patient's behavior, but does not address the internal conflicts or confusions a patient may have about his sexual orientation (see Drescher, 1998).

terminated with his previous analyst. Despite my encouragement to do so, he did not feel he could go back and end the relationship more completely. Instead, he used those early sessions with me to articulate the ways he felt his analyst had failed him, his sense of loss over leaving that treatment, his positive connections to his analyst, and the ways he had allowed himself to feel used without confronting his analyst. Also, Owen's deep fears of interpersonal abandonment were delineated as we explored his relationship with his previous analyst. It was only much later that the earlier precursors of these patterns became clear to us both. He had been exploited by Calvin and his parents, and this pattern became the template in his adult life for his relationships with lovers and his analyst. I will further discuss this aspect of Owen's treatment in Chapter 8.

We also began to approach Owen's internal conflicts about being gay. As he talked about his conviction that he had not chosen to be homosexual, he realized that I was not arguing with him, as he expected me to. He began to read, with my support, contemporary psychological and psychoanalytic texts in which homosexuality is depathologized. While he felt great relief at finding such validation for his own conscious beliefs, he continued to experience shame about being gay, and was unable to shake completely the internalized heterosexist and homophobic attitudes of a lifetime. In particular, he remained very fearful about revealing his homosexuality to his family or to his many old heterosexual friends. He was unwilling to risk being abandoned by them, even though his conscious belief was that most of them already knew he was gay. Thus, despite a partial amelioration of his shame about his homosexuality, he continued to suffer from internalized homophobic views. These were compounded by internalized shame about having been used sexually by a man as a boy, and having felt erotic pleasure in those early experiences.

CINEMATIC PORTRAYAL
OF ABUSE OF BOYS BY MEN

Sexual situations between boys and men are cinematically portrayed in a very different light from sexual activity with women (see Chapter 2). In contrast to the sense that women are offering boys sexual education and pleasure, men are usually seen as humiliating and hurting boys through sexual activity (for example, *The Prince of Tides, Sleepers, Porky's, Powder, The Boys of St. Vincents*), sometimes for humorous effect (for example, *My Life as a Dog, Porky's, Powder*). Sexual scenes between boys and men are usually coercive and brutal, often involving outright rape if a sexual act is completed.

In addition, these incidents are inevitably portrayed as shameful, and the boys in the movies are depicted as believing they must never discuss what happened to them. This silence usually has disastrous effects on them (*The Prince of Tides, Sleepers, The Boys of St. Vincents, The Celebration*).

Boys abused by men are often portrayed as antisocial in later life. This is indeed often the case, but rarely do the movies show that, as is also frequently true, an abused boy may grow up sensitive and compassionate, although depressed, anxious, or agitated in one way or another.[7] There is virtually no model for this relatively more positive outcome should he be able to talk about what happened to him, even though it has been demonstrated, as we will see in Chapter 5, that having a confidant ameliorates some of the worst effects of childhood sexual victimization.

A boy abused by a man, therefore, can easily conclude from the movies he sees that he should be silent about a shameful experience, even though the effect of his silence spreads far beyond the specific betrayal situation and is likely to lead to devastating results. He views his experience as something that may cause ridicule or social ostracism if it is known. He learns he should keep quiet about same-sex sexual abuse in order to avoid derision and humiliation. Silence has terrible effects on the boys portrayed in movies, but the only action allowed them by filmmakers is hypermasculine revenge.

I am, obviously, not advocating either censorship or limiting artistic freedom of expression in any way. I believe, however, that consciousness raising about male sexual victimization is as appropriate for creative artists as for all other members of society. In *Mysterious Skin*, a novel by Scott Heim (1995), when two boys sexually abused by their Little League coach reencounter one another in early adulthood, they are finally able to articulate the experience that led one to become delusional about being taken away by aliens and the other to become a sexually compulsive hustler. As one of them says afterward, "If we were stars in the latest Hollywood blockbuster, then I would have embraced him, my hands patting his shoulder blades, violins and cellos billowing on the soundtrack as tears streamed down our faces. But Hollywood would never make a movie about us" (p. 283).

---

[7] *The Boys of St. Vincents*, which portrays the sexual, physical, and emotional abuse of boys in a Catholic orphanage and its aftermath fifteen years later, is one notable exception. In it, the boys grow up with a variety of severe problems, but none has been abusive as an adult, although their chief victimizer is revealed to have had a boyhood history of severe abuse.

CHAPTER 5

The Familial and Cultural Context of Abuse

Sexual abuse occurs within a family, a culture, and a life. The trauma of childhood sexual abuse devolves not only from physical, verbal, and/or psychological violations that have taken place. The traumatic impact of these events is equally influenced by the interpersonal and familial setting of the betrayal and by the way the abuse has been treated in that context.

Family dynamics are most obviously relevant in abuse situations where the sexual betrayal is incestuous in nature. In these cases, the abuse has developed in some way *from* the family dynamics. When the abuser is outside the immediate family, however, a boy's reactions to it are also affected by his family experiences. For some of these boys, the family situation is much more relevant to the abuse and its aftereffects than for others. It is certainly possible, for example, that a boy abused by an outside predator has come from a family that is neither neglectful nor abusive. Even here, however, the nature of the family dynamics may affect—either positively or negatively—his reactions to abuse. Some families support a child who has been traumatized, while others do not. Thus, there are families that are capable of protecting a child from further abuse and supporting him as he deals with his experiences. Other families are more likely to ignore the child, blame him for the abuse, or further shame him in some way.

Analyzing and treating childhood sexual trauma therefore requires understanding this interpersonal environment. Some families set the stage for abuse to occur, even abuse from outside the family, while others create a sense of safety that enables the child to weather abusive or potentially abusive situations. Thus, abuse can be either a single event occurring in an otherwise supportive environment or one of many recurring traumata in a chronically assaultive life. A case of the former circumstance might involve a molested boy who tells his sensitive parents, who then deal promptly with the situation; a case of the latter might involve a boy who is molested repeatedly by a parent in a dangerously dysfunctional family where there is no recourse and where the boy himself is blamed for the abuse.

Many clinical researchers have looked at families in which incest occurred to try to determine how they differ from other families. For example, Maddock, Larson, and Lolly (1991) developed a protocol for assessing incest family functioning, using a clinical population of families in treatment for incest problems and comparison families in treatment for other problems. (They do not say whether the incest families included any in which boys were abused.) They looked at families both before and after treatment. In their comparisons, they found pretreatment incest couples tended to present their marriage in a more idealized fashion than did comparison families or posttreatment incest families. The comparison families had parents who were more willing as a group to differ openly with one another and to reveal their conflicts. Not surprisingly, incest families, in addition to their characteristic denial of problems, tended to exhibit boundary difficulties (see Chapter 7).

Maddock et al. go on to warn, however, about a tendency to overgeneralize about family dynamics in incest families. They point out that many people, including professionals, tend to make simplistic blanket statements regarding them, for example, that they are enmeshed or that the mothers have colluded in the incest. They note, however, the variability and complexity among incest families. Even characteristics that are predictable in these families may not actually contribute to the incest dynamics. Also, features commonly found in families with incest, like boundary problems, are not necessarily indicators of incest, since they may also appear in families where incest does not occur.

In this chapter, I will describe the literature on families with abused girls before going on to speculate about families with abused boys. In the literature on girls, typical paradigms for incest families have been proposed, and I will summarize the dynamics hypothesized for families in which father–daughter incest has occurred. However, I believe that there is a real danger that the uniqueness of each individual and each family can get lost in attempts to develop such prototype families. I also believe that there may be more variability in the families of the abused men I have treated than in the families of abused women described by researchers. Instead of attempting to develop such models for families where boys are abused, therefore, I will describe in the latter part of this chapter the specific issues and themes that I believe are important to consider when thinking about families in which abused boys have grown up.

FAMILY DYNAMICS WHEN GIRLS ARE ABUSED

The literature on sexually abused women contains a number of rich descriptions of their families. Price (1994), for example, notes the chaos, secrecy, boundary violations, and role confusion common in these families. Overinvolvement and neglect alternate, and "[a]ll of this may be masked by a sense of normalcy, family superiority, and idealization" (p. 214).

The women's literature suggests typical patterns for families in which the incestuous abuse of girls takes place. Most often the families described are families in which incest has occurred between a father or stepfather and a daughter or stepdaughter. Herman (1981), for example, in her groundbreaking book *Father–Daughter Incest,* studied forty women who had had sexual contact with an adult in paternal authority. Their families tended to be conventional to a fault, frequently maintaining a perfect facade of respectability. Fathers were typically traditional patriarchs in the sense that they ruled their families with absolute authority. Their intimidation was often backed up by a hovering possibility of violence, often exacerbated by alcohol abuse. These fathers tended to isolate the women in the family from social contact. Feared tyrants within the family, they were frequently admired by outsiders as sympathetic, reputable men who took their familial responsibilities seriously. At the same time, however, the fathers tended to be perceived as meek or inadequate in outside social situations. Mothers were most often homemakers who completely depended on their husbands for financial support. Sex roles were rigidly defined and adhered to, and mothers and daughters were considered inferior to fathers and sons. Mothers were seen as incompetent or disabled, sometimes from too many enforced pregnancies. They were likely to be depressed, alcoholic, and/or psychotic. Daughters were given the role of keeping their fathers occupied and happy; many also took responsibility for parenting their siblings. Herman also describes the milder form of this essential family dynamic that she believes is characteristic of families in which fathers are seductive and erotic with their daughters without overt incest occurring.

Kirschner, Kirschner, and Rappaport (1993) offer a historical perspective on how father–daughter incestuous families have been treated in the literature. They note that in family therapists' writings in the 1960s mothers tended to be given responsibility for incest because of their psychological distance or coldness. This misogynistic view gave way as a feminist perspective on abuse emerged in the 1970s and the responsibility of male perpetrators for their behavior was emphasized. Daughters were then seen as victims of the men in their families and of a male-dominated culture, and so were given little or no responsibility for their victimization. The authors try to use the strengths of both approaches as they develop a way of looking at incestuous families through both family systems and individual dynamics points of view. They note the dysfunctional marital relationship they have invariably seen in families with father–daughter incest, with recurring poor communications and inferior conflict resolution skills. These poor skills prevent parents from forming an effective parental team. Daughters frequently act as go-betweens in the marriage, and in general children are made into parental caretakers as well as caretakers of other children. Unlike Herman, who essentially describes one family pattern, Kirschner et al. go on to describe three patterns in father–daughter incestuous families: father-dominated, mother-dominated, and chaotic. This matches my own perception that incest families, like men involved in incest as boys, have varied qualities, capacities, dynamics, and dysfunctions.

FAMILY DYNAMICS WHEN BOYS ARE ABUSED

The literature on boys who have been abused has not yielded composite family patterns analogous to those described for girls by Herman and others. This may be due to the fact that the population has not been as widely studied as families in which girls are abused. Another factor, however, may be the reality that most sexual abuse of girls originates within the family, while a greater proportion of sexually abused boys seem to be subject to extrafamilial abuse (Lisak et al., 1996). Because boys are subject to abuse both from inside and outside their families, we must search in their families not only for characteristics that lead to incest, but also for patterns that make it likely that a boy will accede or be vulnerable to molestation from abusers outside the family.[1]

In my own work, I have not encountered either a single dynamic pattern or a group of patterns that recur again and again in the families of the men I have treated. Nevertheless, some generalities do seem to be

---

[1] No literature I know of relates to families of girls whose abuse was extrafamilial.

true of many of these families: the parental relationship is usually defi-
cient, particularly in the area of communication; boundary difficulties or
violations are common; and sexuality tends to be either avoided altogether in conversation or to be ever present, with an overstimulating
effect. These characteristics are consonant with the prototypic families
posited for abused girls. However, they do not necessarily distinguish
families with incest from other families.

Bolton et al.'s (1989) work has an implicit finding that typical family dynamics cannot be developed and ascribed to families in which boys
are abused. Rather than generating such a universal picture of the
dynamics of the abusive family, they describe various environments that
do or do not lead to abuse. In their descriptions, they focus primarily on
a continuum of family attitudes toward sexuality in what they call the
Abuse of Sexuality Model for families. This is a useful model, which they
elaborate as a way to look at how families may abuse sexuality, whether
or not overt sexual abuse occurs.

Bolton et al. first write about *ideal* and *predominantly nurturing
environments,* in neither of which is much potential for abuse. These
environments, in varying degrees, include models for appropriate expression of nonaggressive sexuality, prevent children's exposure to inappropriate sexuality, and, in general, make accurate information about sexuality available.

They then describe environments in which the abuse of sexuality
and possibly (but not necessarily) sexual abuse become more likely: The
evasive environment provides little or no accurate sexual information.
Instead, the adults' anxiety about sexuality leads them to communicate
in euphemisms and, at times, to act out sexual myths and misinformation. In the *environmental vacuum,* by contrast, there is a void about
sexual matters. In the guise of protecting children, adults deliberately
convey no information about sexuality. In a *permissive environment,*
adults allow children free exposure to sexual matters. Though this may
arise from well-meaning motives, the effect may be to overwhelm and
therefore overstimulate a child with material he does not have the capacity to process. In a *negative environment,* sexuality is seen as bad, and
the child is told in countless ways that sex is harmful, evil, and a sign of
weakness. Little sexual information is provided the child, and his
attempts to find out about sex may be blocked or punished. In a *seductive environment,* on the other hand, one or more adults directly communicate to a child, either verbally or behaviorally, their sexual interest
in him. While overt abuse may not result, the child is constantly aware
of his attractiveness to the adult, who may "inadvertently" expose him-
or herself to the child. This is part of the general titillating atmosphere
that also surrounds any sexual education of a child in this kind of family.

Finally, the authors describe the *overtly sexual environment,* which includes sexual abuse as well as sexual misuse of the child. In this environment, there is overt sexual contact between the child and one or more adults. Sexual information is communicated for exploitative purposes, as, for example, when a child is shown pornographic material in the guise of sex education. In addition, adults may covertly encourage sexual contact between children.

This model for understanding how families deal with sexuality gives the clinician a framework within which to consider the environment from which an abused patient has emerged. It includes many points along a continuum of family functioning in relation to sexuality. As the authors note, traditionally clinicians have focused solely on the overtly sexual environment when describing incest families. They emphasize, however, that in *any* of these environments there exists a possibility that the sexual misuse or abuse of children will occur. Understanding these different environments can provide clinicians with a range of frameworks within which to understand abuse and help place an abused child in his familial context. It is important, for example, for a therapist not to assume that incest only occurs in an overtly sexual or a rigidly puritanical family.

DO ANY CONTEXTUAL FACTORS
MEDIATE THE EFFECTS OF ABUSE IN BOYS?

A widespread belief about sexually abused boys is that they grow up to become sexually abusive men. I noted in Chapter 3 that, while it is true that four out of five abusers were themselves abused, it is also true that only one in five abused boys goes on to become an abuser (Lisak et al., 1996). In this section, I will consider contextual influences that may mediate the worst effects of abuse.

I want first, however, to emphasize how the widespread but fallacious logic that abused boys inevitably grow up to become adult abusers leads to added pain for sexually abused men. Some of them are disturbed by the thought that they themselves could become abusive, despite having no history of abusing or inclinations to do so. Others feel further stigmatized and intimidated if others discover their abuse history.

Willem volunteered time in an abuse-oriented project run by a non-profit children's agency. When he told a supervisor that he had been abused as a boy, he noticed that he was never again permitted to spend time alone with a child, and was slowly moved to administrative work.

Likewise, when Andreas, a respected lay figure in his church, once alluded obliquely to having a history of abuse, a church elder pursued the topic until Andreas confirmed that he had been sexually abused. The elder said, "Then it's a good thing you don't work with children." Andreas replied, "Nothing would ever happen if I were with a child, but I stopped working with children because I wanted to make sure I never embarrassed the church." Afterward, Andreas was alternately depressed and furious. The fury was not only directed at the man who made the comment, whom he felt was well meaning though ignorant, but at himself for answering in a docile manner that seemed to validate the elder's mistaken opinion that abused boys always become abusive men.

Why do some sexually abused boys grow up to be sexually abusive men, while most do not? The circumstances of the abuse themselves do not seem to be the best predictor of outcome. Instead, the boy's social group is a critical factor in "determining who becomes a psychiatric casualty, who pursues a life of criminal behavior, and who is spared" (Bloom, 1997, p. 9).

In Chapter 3, I discussed how masculine gender role rigidity, with its concurrent emotional constriction and deficits in empathy, leads to a greater likelihood that an abused boy will become abusive later in life. In addition, as Crowder (1995) points out, "having a strong sense of self prior to the abuse experience, having a relationship with positive male role models, having supportive interpersonal relationships, and developing an awareness of healthy sexual expression are some of the factors that reduce the likelihood of a victim becoming an offender" (p. 30).

What specific familial factors mitigate the effects of incest and other child sexual abuse on boys? In a study of 369 sexually abused children (24 percent were boys), Conte (1985) found that 21 percent demonstrated no symptoms following their abusive experience. The single most important factor in reducing the negative effects of abuse was the presence of at least one supportive adult relationship. Similarly, Gilgun (1990, 1991) studied the effects of childhood sexual and other maltreatment on boys, searching for what might prevent the child from acting out violently as an adult. Confirming Conte's work, she found the most crucial positive factor to be "the presence of confidants and other supportive persons in the abused child's life" (1990, p. 182). Such individuals could come from within or outside the family; were usually, but not always, male; and could be peers, but were more likely to be older people in positions of authority. The presence of such supportive relationships, often with caretakers, meant that the boys did not grow up to be men who raped, molested children, or committed violent nonsexual acts. This was true even for boys who had other major negative factors in their history, such as physical abuse. Psychological resiliency was almost invariably associated with the ability to confide in others, especially about the abuse.

While it is intuitively obvious that the presence of interpersonal support in the child's environment will lead to relatively benign outcomes, Conte's and Gilgun's research suggest ways to prevent molested boys from becoming victimizers later in life. It supports the need for early psychological intervention in such situations. Abused boys and boys at risk for abuse might be offered relationships in which they have the potential to confide in a trusted other. Such a relationship could be established with a teacher, guidance counselor, Big Brother, therapist, or other responsible and caring older person.

The Conte and Gilgun findings that the boy can cope better if he has a caretaker who is emotionally attuned to him must be understood, however, in familial contexts where the caretaker *is* the abuser. Childhood incestuous or abusive relationships are very complex, and the same person or the same familial circumstance may have both positive and negative effects. An abusive parent or caretaker may also be the sole source of nurturance, while a nonabusing parent may be neglectful and psychologically (or physically) absent. Relationships with abusive parents who are also caretakers lead to complex internalizations of the parent and subsequent expectations from other authorities. Nurturers will be viewed with suspicion, while exploiters will be expected to be giving. (See the discussions of Ramon in Chapter 4 and of Quinn and Isaac in Chapter 8 for illustrations of the ambivalence a boy may feel about an abuser who was also a nurturer.)

Conte's and Gilgun's work argues for a number of possibilities as a boy's personality develops while he is suffering abuse. Consider again the boys in the two situations hypothesized in the opening section of this chapter. The first is in a seemingly more benign situation, where there are sensitive parents and the molestation is a single act. But, if, because of shame or other factors, the boy is unable to talk about his abuse to anyone, there may be worse sequelae than otherwise expected (see my descriptions of Seth, pp. 129–132, and Ezra, p. 32). The second boy is in a more malignant situation, where he is chronically abused by a parent and is blamed for it. But, if he is able to confide in a trusted individual, perhaps a teacher or guidance counselor, even this boy may grow up troubled, but not violent.

RELATING ITSELF BECOMES TRAUMATIC

When a child lives with chronic abuse and/or incest, he often grows up having to live in a traumatic relationship or set of relationships. He surveys the world suspiciously and sees victimizers everywhere. This is actually a functional reaction when abuse is ongoing, a time when he may need to protect himself from further hurt and exploitation. However, this way of looking at the world often creates severe difficulties when he leaves the immediate world of his molesting environment.

For such a man, *relating itself* has become traumatic. The mechanism by which this happens was eloquently described by Julian who said, "We have a double whammy. We're vulnerable in two ways. First, we have families that make us yearn for contact so we're vulnerable to sexual predators. Then, we get abused by them, and we have nowhere to go back to for help, because we have those same families that can't give it."

Having lived with pervasive pathogenic family dynamics and dysfunctional systems of relating, a boy in this situation is likely to develop profound difficulties in interpersonal relating (see, for example, the cases of Patrick, pp. 141–144, 159–160, 186, and 248–250; and of Abe, pp. 190–191, 199–200, 221–228, 245–247, and 312–318). Through incest and abuse, he has developed severe disturbances about relating itself (Sands, 1994). Similar disturbances may also be the result of chronic familial boundary violations that do not involve physical incest.

Under such circumstances, relationships are experienced as fundamentally dishonest, dangerous, and mystifying. Abe addressed this problem when he plaintively said, "I need directness, or else I don't understand what's happening between me and other people."

Dishonesty in primary relationships leads a child to grow up distrusting *all* relationships. Cory communicated his anguish about this dishonesty by saying, "Our family motto was always, 'If you can't say anything nice, don't say anything at all.' But for me the best family motto would be 'If you can't say anything *honest,* say *nothing.*'"

DENIAL OF THE CHILD'S REALITY

A particularly damaging mystification occurs if an abuser is confronted about the abuse and denies the child's reality. In the movie *Spanking the Monkey,* a boy's mother denies having committed maternal incest after the boy tells his father about it. The father believes her denial, and the boy then tries to commit suicide. Such a denial may be overt, as in the movie, or covert, as when an abuser behaves blandly after the abuse is over, as though nothing untoward has happened.

In addition, when abuse is denied and secrecy is required of the child, whether because of overt warnings from the abuser or because of the child's inner sense that he must not talk about such things, the effect is more pernicious. As Uri put it, "Denial was our survival mechanism. My family lived on denial—air, water, and denial. That's how we got through." With gallows humor, he went on to say, "The cast had already died by the time I was born—my family was already dead and the die was cast for my abuse."

Victor reported a transferential dream related to having his reality denied:

"You were in it. We were having a session. I had had an epiphany about my abuse, about the way it has affected my life. I don't remember what it was, but it was very clear, everything suddenly made sense, and I was telling you about it. Suddenly, your pants were down around your ankles. I was confused, I asked you about it. You looked down as though to say 'Oh, no big deal,' and then they were up again and you continued as though nothing had happened. It was as though I had just noticed something of no consequence, like you had dropped a piece of paper, and I thought to myself, 'Why are you making such a big deal about it, thinking the one person in the world you should trust is trying to seduce you?' It made me feel bad that I would think such a thing about you. I woke up in a panic."

Later, Victor remembered that before my pants were down in the dream, I had been revealing about myself personally in a way I usually am not, and he had thought it was odd and wondered why I was using his therapy time to talk about myself.

"This dream shows how distrustful I am of everyone because of my abuse—even you."

I said, "In the dream I *did* do something inappropriate, and then I disowned it when you noticed. Having my pants down around my ankle *is* a big deal, it's not nothing. You realized that in the dream, but then I denied your reality. I said it wasn't important, and you accepted that and blamed yourself for having those thoughts. No wonder you woke in a panic."

His eyes gleamed as I said this, and he nodded, and said, "Yes, of course. No wonder I was confused."

"Sound familiar?"

"Yes—with my father—something was going on at night, but during the day it seemed like it was no big deal. I used to think I must be crazy."

"You had to dismiss what you knew to be real. That's a crazy way to have to live."

"Maybe that's the epiphany I was having about incest."

Brooke Hopkins (1993) eloquently recounts how he was affected by the secrecy surrounding his maternal abuse, abuse he still could not easily label as such: "But maybe the most damaging form of abuse (if that is the word to use) is silence, and the denial that is implicit in it. I mean the denial not only of what happened *but of the person it happened to*" (p. 51; emphasis added). Hopkins describes his need to confront and undo this silence: "I am writing this in order to break that silence, because the denial represented by it strikes me as something like a disease, a disease for which the only hope of a cure is in speaking, in making public what has been hidden for so long" (p. 37).

Similarly, Teo said at the end of his treatment, "What made me better is that through therapy and my group I was able *not* to keep this a secret any more—the more I could tell people, the better I got."

I will return in Chapter 8 to the effects of dishonest, secretive, and mystifying familial dynamics on adult relatedness.

COMPLIANCE WITH AUTHORITY

Children who are taught never to question their elders and to obey unquestioningly when adults tell them what to do are at particular risk for abuse. When a family expects unquestioning compliance with demands from adults, a child is primed to acquiesce in abusive situations.

Thus, families with authoritarian rules and structures tend to have children who do not know how to question abuse by someone in power. Whatever the inner cost, they are likely to accede to such abuse because they feel they have no choice. For example, Seth as an adult felt with growing fury that he had been programmed to comply passively with a family friend's molestation. And Cory recounted grimly how the stage was already set for his unquestioning acquiescence by the time his grandmother was raped when he was five. She had been walking with Cory outside his house, and when the rapist came up to her and grabbed her, she told Cory to go quietly into the house. "I was already programmed to comply—to not question or wonder. I was just a good boy and went into the house. I was quiet like she told me—I never said a word to anyone."

We also saw this dynamic in Bruno's reactions to abuse by a family doctor (see pp. 102–105). He had been taught by the actions of his physically abusive father and brother that peremptory, arbitrary, and near-random punishment was part of life, and he had been cautioned by his family to accept the derisive reactions of the nuns to what seems to have been his dyslexia. In this context, it is not surprising that he later also accepted molestations by the family doctor. Indeed, it is remarkable that he protested at all when the family kept bringing him back for further appointments with the doctor.

Another way for a young boy to deal with an authoritarian family is to learn how to outmaneuver and manipulate authorities covertly rather than to openly defy them. As adolescents, such boys may rebelliously break away completely from authority. We see both aspects of this in Yale's reactions to abuse by a nun:

Yale was an energetic gay man in his early forties with the grace and

compact body of the professional ice skater he had once been. In a committed relationship with a professional man, he was referred to me by
the therapist who had treated them as a couple a few years earlier. Yale
felt that he needed help dealing with his continuing fury over sexual
abuse throughout most of the second grade by the nun who was his
parochial school teacher. This nun would hug him and fondle his genitals, usually in the cloakroom while the class was doing an assignment
on the other side of the partition wall. With time, she encouraged him to
touch her body as well, including her breasts and, eventually, her vagina.

Yale tried to tell his parents that there was something wrong with
this teacher, but his mother berated him for being disrespectful about a
nun. He said the nun frightened all the children in his class and that he
always hated the sexual activity with her. She seems to have been psychotic at times in her own rampant expressions of anger in the class-
room. Yale claimed that he learned to manipulate her psychologically so
she could never be sure whether he would be willing to go with her into
the cloakroom again. He felt that as a result of these seductive manipula-
tions on his part she never got enraged at him, as she did with the other
children. Instead, she would murmur endearments to him during the
molestations, especially as he rubbed her to orgasm. Note, however, that
Yale's claims of mastery over the situation may well be an example of
how boys do not allow themselves to encode abuse as "feminizing" victimization but see it rather as something over which they had control.

As Yale grew up, he became a kind of terror in school. He was
bright and excelled academically, so there seems never to have been a
question of his being expelled. Yet his behavior, particularly after
puberty, was defiant toward teachers and sexually provocative with
other male students. In particular, student athletes and delinquents
would call him a faggot because of his interpersonal manner and his
interest in ice skating and dance. He said his method of dealing with
their derision was to seduce those who were most hostile to him. "After
I'd sucked them off a few times they'd leave me alone in public. We all
won! I enjoyed it. They enjoyed it. They stopped bothering me and I had
something to hold over them." He became increasingly contemptuous of
anyone who wielded power. His parents stopped trying to control him;
they did not know most of what was going on in his life and solaced
themselves with his continuing academic success.

At the time Yale saw me, he was starting a second career, one that
called on his intellectual prowess more than his successful skating career
had done. He expressed contempt for others who were further along in
his field though younger than he, particularly if he felt misused in some
way by them or felt that they had had success handed to them without
their earning it. On the other hand, he had difficulty maintaining bound-

aries when asked to do more than his share of work. In particular, he reviled female colleagues at his own junior level whom he said did not do their share of work and left it for him to do. He and his lover seemed to have a basically good relationship, though again Yale sometimes complained of feeling used and unappreciated by his lover.

In our initial two months of treatment Yale told the story I have just narrated. With withering scorn and sarcasm, he recounted stories about the nun, his parents, his high school classmates, and his colleagues and supervisors at work. He then decided to call the school where he had been molested to find out what had happened to his old teacher. He discovered that she had been replaced as a teacher, for "personality difficulties," not long after she had taught him, and that she had been dead for about ten years.

His fury continued to fill our sessions, and he began to drop his sarcastic tone and express more directly the anger and hurt beneath it. Eventually, he told me for the first time that he had initially consulted me with the idea that I could provide expert testimony in a suit he was contemplating against the Catholic Church. He had now given up on this idea, feeling that to start such a suit would keep him stuck in his anger and in his memories for at least the five or six years it would take to pursue such a court case.

I felt manipulated when I heard about his idea of suing and using me as a witness; I might not have been willing to accept him as a patient had I known about this motive for seeing me. We talked about his ability and willingness to exploit others without thinking about their wishes and needs. Further, we looked at how this old pattern that had served him well in second grade and thereafter was actually a product of some identification with his abusive teacher. This paradigm for his behavior greatly interested Yale. He had never seen it the way I was laying it out. It had simply been a survival mechanism for him, not something he had ever thought through.

This led us to consider how his exploitative stance kept him interpersonally isolated while he himself continued to feel misused. As we worked on this over a period of months, Yale began to be more direct at work about not taking on others' tasks. I suggested he think of his current interpersonal life as a kind of laboratory experiment for him in which he tried out new ways of approaching others' demands by setting limits with them rather than by manipulating them or seething inside as he satisfied their needs.

As he saw the success of these relational experiments, Yale began to talk more about the ways he felt ignored or exploited by his lover. The stakes in that relationship were higher for him, in that he was afraid he might lose his lover if he directly confronted him. To his surprise, however, his lover was receptive to him about these matters. Their relationship deepened and Yale became far more capable of emotional expressiveness as a result. His anger diminished and he was more likely to be compassionate about the people he had raged about, particularly his female colleagues and his mother. At that point, after eighteen months of once-weekly treatment, he felt ready to leave therapy. I agreed that we had done the work he most wanted and needed to accomplish. We both realized that there might be periods when further treatment would be helpful, but for the moment Yale felt he needed time to consolidate what he had done. If he ever returns to treatment, I believe the therapy will involve a much deeper and more difficult consideration of the exploitative and dismissive aspects of his transference.

TAKING CARE OF PARENTAL FIGURES' NEEDS

Obedience to authority also comes in subtle, covert forms. When a child learns he must please or take care of a parent, he is obeying an unspoken command to sacrifice his own needs for the wishes and desires of an adult. We will see how in Abe's case a father explicitly made it a child's job to care for an emotionally tempestuous and exacting mother. In Ira's case, his early experiences with his depressed and nonnurturing mother seem to have led him to accede to his sister's sexual demands. In turn, these experiences influenced his character, making him all too willing to acquiesce later to the wishes of a female authority who was simultaneously nurturing and demanding.

Ira came to me in his early forties because of a sense of failure in his career and a wish for intimacy and marriage with a woman. As he described it, he had allowed years to go by in which he had not made the necessary moves to turn a promising creative career into the success everyone had predicted for him. Instead, he worked at an unfulfilling job in an industry allied to his creative field. As an adult, he had not had a single relationship with a woman that had lasted more than a few months, and in the previous three years had not even attempted to meet a woman. He told himself there was no point in trying to establish a relationship anyway while he was such a failure in his career. Yet he saw life slipping by, and he was frightened by the prospect that he would grow old alone and would never have the children for whom he yearned.

As we talked about his history, he mentioned that he had left a prestigious university after two years, following the breakup of a relationship with a woman professor. He hastened to add that they had not begun to date until he was no longer her student. This relationship was one of many personal details he told me as we started to work together, and at first I did not register its possible significance. Some time later, however, Ira mentioned the relationship again in passing. I already knew that for two years after he left school he had made a few false starts in several directions before transferring to another university close to his parents' homes. He had also mentioned his regret at never again seeing his friends from the first college, and at losing the sense of belonging he felt for most of the two years he was there.

I asked what had happened with the teacher. Ten years Ira's senior, she had been his instructor in a grueling freshman course. She offered him special help with his work, as she did to other students. His grades rose from mediocre to excellent under her tutelage, and he received the highest grade among his classmates.

Ira's parents had announced to him during the summer between high school and college that they were getting divorced. This was not a total surprise to him, as their relationship had deteriorated badly in the years previous to his graduation, but it was still very disturbing. His father had a much younger girl friend, and told Ira far more about his sex life with her than Ira was comfortable hearing. His mother was depressed, and Ira felt responsible for taking care of her emotionally, a role he had played throughout his childhood despite her critical and nonnurturing nature. When he started college, he felt lonely and needy, and he gravitated to the teacher whose attentions felt so sustaining to him.

At the beginning of the semester following the course Ira took with this professor, they met informally once or twice, then she invited him for lunch in the faculty dining room, an unusual event at this school. Over lunch, she asked him to teach her some yoga exercises he knew, and suggested he drop by her apartment that evening. After they tried the exercises, she offered him something to drink and began to talk more personally to him.

In the course of this conversation, she asked him if he had ever thought of her as a woman rather than a teacher. "When she said that, I kind of froze. I knew what she meant. I actually *hadn't* ever thought of her as a woman. I was too embarrassed to say that to her. She was a teacher I liked a lot. She helped me, and I was grateful for that and wanted it to continue. But part of me knew I was at a crossroads—if I turned her down, I knew that would be the end of our special relationship. So I hesitated, and then went along with her. I never even put it into words this way at the time, but I was making some inner calculations. If I went to bed with her and made her my girlfriend, I wouldn't have to give up all this attention I craved—and, of course, I was young and the idea of sex with a woman was exciting, so it didn't seem like so bad a deal. We saw each other all semester, always privately, never in public. But it wasn't working for me—she was about twenty-nine then, certainly not old as I look at it now, but at the time I thought her breasts were droopy. I wasn't really attracted to her, and after a while I didn't even enjoy the sex. Eventually, I put an end to it, and the whole relationship went up in flames. I never quite said to myself that this was why I left school, but I guess it really was."

Ira did not know about my work with sexually abused men at the time we began our work together. When he started to talk about the relationship with his teacher, I was very careful not to lead him into thinking of it as abusive. I was at first unclear myself how to understand it. He had, after all, been of age, and he referred to her as his "girlfriend." The language in his initial descriptions of the liaison did not connote exploitation by his professor, but, to my surprise, he came in the session after describing what happened saying he sometimes wondered if the relationship would be considered abusive if it happened today. This was a word neither of us had used before. I asked what he meant, and he said he'd always thought he had exploited *her*, using her for sex and nurturance. "But, as I thought about it this time, I began to remember that she was a professor. *She* was the experienced one. She was needy, too—she had recently broken up with a boyfriend—and she used me to satisfy her need for attention from a man. She had the upper hand."

Ira was shaken by talking about this period of his life. He had never thought about how much pressure the relationship had put on him. At the time, the two friends he confided in about it thought he was "a very lucky guy." But, as he considered his subsequent relationships with women, he said, initially unconscious of the imagery he was using, "I decided not to thrust ahead any more in life, especially with women. I'd gotten too banged up."

In subsequent weeks, Ira told me about a period when he was about eleven that seems to have helped set the stage for his later sexual exploitation by his teacher. His parents used to leave him with his fifteen-year-old sister when they went out at night. "One time, we somehow wound up with all our clothes off. Then she started to kiss me, first on my body, then on my penis. I wasn't in puberty yet, I had no idea what was going on at first, but I got an erection and I had some kind of orgasm without ejaculating. It was exciting, and I kept giggling while it was going on. It was our secret, and after that we did it a lot. I never really touched her— I wouldn't have wanted to—she always started it and she was always all over me like that." I asked how their clothes "somehow" were taken off. "I don't know, really—I don't remember. But it must have been her idea, because I didn't think about those things yet. It was her need—she was overweight and unpopular—boys didn't like her and she wanted male attention. I enjoyed it, but I wouldn't have thought to do it. And somehow I knew I was making her feel better, too. We were very close and I felt sorry for her. I would never have turned her down for anything she really wanted." On the other hand, Ira continued, "She was a juggernaut. There would have been no stopping her. For her, I was no longer Ira. I became Boy, a symbol of all the boys who rejected her. At the same time that I felt excited, I felt very lonely—even invisible."

As we pieced together the disparate parts of his life, we saw a pattern of appeasing and taking care of women that started with Ira's depressed mother, accelerated with a premature and abusive sexual relationship with his unhappy sister, and continued into the disastrous affair with his needy college professor. He grew to see women as exciting and fascinating, on the one hand, but dangerous and exploitative, on the other. After the affair with the professor, he never again had a serious relationship with a woman, and he stopped himself from moving forward on all fronts. He had symbolically become an oedipal victor in the relationship with his teacher, achieving a conquest about which many men have conflicted and ambivalent feelings, despite the positive image such a relationship often has in the popular media (see Chapter 2). His problems with career success and intimate relatedness had multiple sources, of course, but they were closely bound up in this series of complicated relationships.

WHEN "BAD THINGS" CANNOT BE DISCUSSED

Many families have taboos about discussing highly charged questions and concerns such as incest and sexual aggression. Children learn and understand whether it is permissible to bring up such matters. If a child feels that it is unsafe to talk about abuse, he will not do so, and this is likely to lead to a more traumatic outcome because of his consequent ignorance, shame, and isolation.

Consider Seth:

Ironically, from an "objective," external point of view, Seth's molestation itself was less traumatic than that of many of the men I have treated. His trauma snowballed because of the familial circumstances already in place when he was molested. Seth never revealed to anyone his one-time molestation by an adult family friend till he began therapy in his late thirties. He said it had never occurred to him to do so, that he had totally incorporated his family's inability to consider or tolerate discussion of sexuality, psychological dynamics, emotions, and consequences of human behavior. The morning after the molestation itself, he pretended to his abuser that he had no idea that anything had happened. The pernicious effects of his silence, which further stunted his already-existing but suppressed need to have a forum for self-expression, led to an agonized adolescence and young adulthood.

Seth was aware that his molestation might seem minor to someone who had been chronically abused. He hesitated to join a group of sexually abused men because he felt that his own experience, while personally devastating to him, could not objectively compare to the persistent intrafamilial abuse he had read about in books, which he correctly surmised would be common in the group he joined. He felt he would be silenced by the experiences he would hear about, embarrassed that he had been so affected by what he thought should have been a relatively benign molestation.

Seth grew up in a small town, one of many brothers in a middle-class Catholic family. He went to parochial schools and attended church regularly. According to him, he learned in his family that obedience to authorities should be quick and unquestioned. This attitude was further enforced by his church and his school. In addition, he said, there was little tolerance in his family for discussing one's inner life. As a child, he took refuge in various artistic pursuits as a means of self-expression. His family did not actively discourage these activities. Indeed, in their characteristic style, they rarely mentioned them at all. Nevertheless, he felt they viewed him and his interests as odd and possibly distressing.

When Seth was about ten, Billy, a man in his thirties who served as handyman and assistant to a priest in another part of town, somehow attached himself to Seth's family. Seth did not recall how Billy first entered the family circle, but Billy quickly became a fixture there, coming to Sunday dinner after church, doing favors for the parents, babysitting at times, and generally making himself useful. Billy lived alone, and was viewed as limited in intelligence but harmless and pleasant.

Seth remembers Billy often coming in when he was playing or drawing, sometimes putting his hand on Seth's shoulder and leaving it there. In retrospect, Seth remembers Billy as a "creepy presence" in his life, but he is not positive that he experienced him that way till after Billy molested him.

When Seth was twelve, Billy offered to take him to New York City for his birthday, where they would see Seth's first Broadway show, go to museums, and stay overnight in a hotel. Seth was very excited about the trip, and his parents readily consented to it. All went smoothly until Seth and Billy were alone in the hotel room after the show. Billy began to massage Seth's back "to ease the exhaustion of the busy day," slowly undressing him and making the interaction more and more explicitly sexual. Seth cannot recall precisely what happened, but does know there was mutual touching of genitals. In the morning, Billy said to Seth, "I'm sorry about what happened last night. . . . " Seth interrupted him and professed ignorance, saying, "What do you mean? Nothing happened last night." Towering over Seth, Billy then said, "So you won't tell anyone about what happened last night?" Seth firmly answered, "Nothing happened last night!" Seth added that, perhaps because of his child's perspective, he experienced Billy as looming over him, large and threatening, when he asked Seth not to tell anyone. Seth's reaction was to close down, paralyzed, and enter into a self-induced denial of the events. Neither of them ever brought up the molestation again.

After they returned home, Seth avoided being alone with Billy, but did not tell anyone about what happened. He went over and over this fact as an adult, not forgiving himself for maintaining his silence. Yet he also believed that to do so, to talk about unpleasant, sexual, and aggressive feelings rather than deny them, would be breaking a central taboo in his family. As a boy, he never considered acting so contrary to the family's unwritten laws.

Billy maintained his relationship with Seth's family until his death twenty years later. Only then did Seth break his silence and enter therapy to talk about the feelings—about both his molestation and his constrained silence—that had malignantly intensified over the years.

In his mid-forties, seven years after he began individual therapy and three years after he joined a group for sexually abused men, Seth discovered, from a chance word said by the wife of one of his older brothers, that this brother had also been abused by Billy. Stunned, Seth got confirmation from his brother that he had been molested by Billy when he was twelve, the same age Seth had been at the time of his abuse, and in circumstances similar to Seth's molestation. The brother explained that at the time he had thought of himself as an adult who could take care of himself, and of Billy as a "homo" to be scorned. Only with time did he begin to realize that he had been a child who had been the target of a predatory adult, and that being in that situation had had long-term negative effects on his ability to trust or be intimately involved with others. He never told anyone about his abuse until he confided in his wife after they married.

Seth and his brother then asked their many other brothers about abuse, and discovered to their horror that a younger brother had also been abused by Billy, and that of their remaining brothers *all but one* had been molested by other men from outside the family. None had ever talked about their abuse as boys, and one brother had never told *anyone* about his abuse till he was asked by Seth. Each brother had considered the abuse a guilty secret that he carried with shame and suppressed rage. Each also now felt guiltily responsible for the abuse his younger brothers suffered, feeling that had he spoken up the younger ones would not have been molested. Characteristically, Seth's older brother said, "Of course,

Mom and Dad must never know about this." A sense of secrecy and shame continued to rule the brothers' way of dealing with their abuse, along with a continuing feeling that they must protect their parents from knowledge of "bad things."

When Seth told me about these revelations, I observed that each brother had lived in a private hell. He responded that his father had been severely traumatized during World War II, but had always refused to talk about his many battle experiences. I said quietly that he and his brothers had had a model for men living in private hells rather than revealing emotional anguish. He nodded, eyes filling with tears. The history of this family pattern was clear, but it had already begun to change. The brothers were talking to one another, with each opening up about his guilt, shame, and despair. This enlivened the emotional connections among them, which had been deadened over the years. With joy, Seth said that for the first time in thirty years he really had brothers again.

FAMILIES THAT CREATE EMOTIONAL NEEDINESS

Some family contexts create emotional neediness that make it nearly impossible for a child to resist the affection and tenderness that often appears to come along with abuse. Ezra's father was chronically depressed, and, as Ezra described it, he was emotionally inaccessible and even mean, a man who did little but go to work and do the other bare necessities required of him. If he felt provoked, he frequently lashed out emotionally or physically at Ezra and his sisters. Ezra was hungry for the attentions of a male authority figure, and was easy prey for the neighborhood teenager who enticed him into the woods and masturbated on his bare chest when he was ten. Afterward, Ezra said, "It didn't even cross my mind" to talk about the molestation to anyone in his family.

Thus, a needy and vulnerable child is more likely to accede to a molestation, especially if it comes in the guise of loving attention that has been heretofore absent in his life. That was Xavier's situation:

The seventh of ten children in a middle-class suburban family, Xavier felt that there was little emotional nurturance in his family at all, and almost none left for the youngest siblings. Both his parents had grown up in very large families, the father having been one of twenty-two siblings and half-siblings. Xavier idealized his mother, who died when he was about twenty, but felt her years of childbearing and the effects of a cold marriage had left her distracted and depressed. His father was hardworking, but inarticulate and emotionally distant. He derided his children's achievements and spent little time with them. The children, in turn, were derisive of one another, and there was little companionship among them.

Xavier described himself as having been a sensitive and lonely boy, intellectually curious but starving for affection. When he was six, his six-year-older brother invited him into a bedroom in an uncharacteristically tender manner. Murmuring what a sweet boy Xavier was, the brother caressed and held him, fondling Xavier's genitals and directing him to do the same for the brother until the brother reached orgasm. The sexual contact continued over time on an irregular basis, eventually including mutual fellatio and anal penetration by the brother. The brother's tone was always affectionate and tender during the molestations, but he remained brusque, derisive, and uncaring at other times.

When Xavier was eight, a second brother, this one four years older than he, approached him in a manner almost identical to the original approach of the first brother. In a seemingly loving fashion, he also held and fondled Xavier; sexual contact followed on a regular basis. Again, this brother was affectionate during the molestations but otherwise remained aloof.

Xavier believed neither brother knew that the other was molesting him, and Xavier himself never revealed the abuse to anyone until he entered a Catholic seminary, when he told his confessor. He felt deeply torn about the sexuality with his brothers, which recurred until Xavier went to boarding school at age sixteen. He felt what they were doing was wrong, physically ungratifying for him as a heterosexually oriented young man, and religiously immoral. Yet he desperately needed those moments of tenderness, whether or not the tenderness lasted beyond orgasm.

Xavier became a priest in his early twenties, having gone straight to seminary from his Catholic boarding school. He felt sure that the priesthood was his calling, rather than simply an escape from the legacy of sexual abuse by his two brothers throughout most of his childhood. On the other hand, he felt anxious in the company of other priests and was afraid of all intense emotional relationships.

In his mid-thirties, Xavier started what turned out to be a short but intense psychotherapy with me before being transferred by his order (for unrelated reasons) to another part of the country. In the three months we worked together on a three times per week basis, I came to feel that indeed Xavier had a calling to the priesthood; but it also became clear how his boyhood abuse had scarred him, affected his emotional well-being, and perhaps hurried him into seminary faster than he ever might have gone otherwise.

Whatever his suitability for the priesthood, Xavier's entry into a community of celibate brothers in Christ could also be viewed as an attempt to repair his childhood trauma by establishing safer loving relationships with new "brothers." Yet the new situation was also fraught with anxiety. Xavier was profoundly wary of relationships with fellow priests, loving the camaraderie but feeling that there was often a potential for a boundaryless melting into an overly intense relationship. He was not consciously afraid these relationships could become sexualized (though I believe that possibility might have emerged, perhaps along with some transferential sexual desire, had our treatment lasted longer). Rather, he said he feared they would arouse his emotional neediness and he would lose all sense of his own purpose. It was specifically because of such inner conflict about a potentially close friendship with a fellow priest that he sought treatment with me.

Because of the brevity of his therapy, we could do little more than lay out Xavier's history and start to make connections in it. The clarity of the narrative I have just related was not apparent to either of us immediately. Rather, it emerged as Xavier began to express the feelings and memories that had silently eaten away his insides for over twenty-five years. His bouts of anger in his family as an adult became more understandable to him, particularly his recurrent defiance of his father.

Interestingly, he was compassionate about his abusing brothers, at least during the time I treated him. He did not want to spend time with them, but he did note that their severe alcoholism and failed relationships were signs of how miserable their own childhoods had been. As he considered their lives, he realized he always assumed they had also been abused, and that there was probably a pattern of sexual abuse of young boys by older brothers or cousins throughout his extended family.

In the short time we worked together, I could do little more than provide a place for Xavier to tell his story, help him put its fragmented pieces together into the narrative I have recounted, and validate his anger. We agreed that this was very little in comparison to what he needed, yet he also noted what a huge accomplishment it was for him to have done that much.

THE INFLUENCE OF CULTURE

Cultural influences may create familial contexts in which behavior thought of as abusive by contemporary American mores are more acceptable for that particular family. It is not my intention to cover this vast ground here.[2] I do want to point out, however, that the meaning of sexuality in childhood, including same-sex sexuality and sexuality between adults and children, does change from culture to

---

[2] *Sexual Abuse in Nine North American Cultures*, edited by Lisa Aronson Fuentes (1995) is an example of a contemporary work that does treat this topic at length. See also Thompson (1988)

culture. These differences obviously affect how the child encodes his experience.

Writing in another context, Blechner (1998) develops precisely the point I am making here:

> [I]magine a man coming to you for . . . treatment. You discover that from age seven to twelve, he and many other boys were taken away from their families to a compound that was exclusively inhabited by men. It was a place where he was pushed to work, and, during leisure hours, he sucked the penises of the older males in the compound. They told him that it was good for him, that ingesting other men's semen would make him manly, so that the more penises he sucked, the manlier he would become. . . . Consider what effect . . . such an experience would have on this man's development, his adult personality, and the picture of his sexuality. . . . The scenario I have just described is the norm for adolescent boys in a tribe in New Guinea that has been studied by Gilbert Herdt (1981) and which he calls the Sambians. (p. 606)

Most people in our own society would describe this scenario as ritualized sexual abuse. For the Sambia, however, it is an initiation rite by which older men generously share semen, the quintessence of their treasured masculinity, with adolescent boys. For a Sambian boy, these experiences, which would be severely abusive in American society, are therefore unlikely to be traumatic. If anything, they would probably be thought of with pride as his entrance to manhood.

Particularly relevant for judging the degree of trauma involved in a particular set of sexual acts is whether the family, and therefore the child, feels the need to keep such sexual experiences secret. Generally, the more secretive the boy must be, the more the experience is deviant within his culture, and the more traumatic the sexual experience is likely to be.

An additional factor to be considered here is whether the child is growing up in the same culture in which his parents or grandparents grew up. This is an especially relevant consideration in families that are culturally transplanted, whether they emigrated voluntarily for economic reasons or fled their native culture because of war or other disasters.

Victor, for example, was born in the United States and thought of himself as completely assimilated to the American experience. His abuse and his reactions to it were embedded in two cultures, however, spanning the globe to the war-torn Asian society from which both his parents had fled. As I understand it, some of his childhood sexual experiences may have been culturally determined while most of them were not. But, growing up as he did in an urban area of the United States in the late twentieth century, his responses to all his experiences were refracted through the lens of American sensibilities. He therefore felt abused even by experiences that may have been culturally acceptable in his family and the country from which he came.

Victor's mother came from a prominent upper-class family in her native land. Her father had been a high government official, and he had moved the family from place to place during her childhood in order to ensure its safety during periods of danger, unrest, and war. Eventually, the entire family went into exile in another Asian country, where they lived comfortably, though on a far more modest scale than the lavish one to which they had previously been accustomed. In early adulthood, Victor's mother moved to the United States, where she met her husband. Victor described his father as "a kind of Asian Ricky Ricardo," a flashy dresser and suave dancer who swept his mother off her feet with his Americanized manners and seeming ability to make his way through society in the United States.

Though Victor's father came from the same country as his wife-to-be, he came from a class at the other end of its economic spectrum and grew up in a totally different milieu. The son of an elderly peasant man and his second wife, the father was seven years old when he, his mother, and his younger siblings were utterly impoverished by his father's death. They moved to a large city where a son from the father's first marriage reluctantly allowed them to live with his family. This half-brother did not otherwise support them, however, and they were reduced to begging on the streets to sustain themselves. Victor's father was clever, though totally without formal education. He seems to have developed a capacity to ingratiate himself quickly with those who might help him, and managed to beg or steal enough so that his family survived until he ran away at age sixteen. He then signed up as a sailor on a ship, eventually coming to the United States.

Using the skills he had perfected in childhood, he quickly constructed the Americanized public persona that so impressed Victor's mother when they met. He made decent money in a service job; however, he remained nearly illiterate in both his native tongue and English. Such deficits were not completely apparent to his educated wife until after they married. They were, however, central to the marital disputes that raged between them until they divorced when Victor was twenty following an incident in which the father physically attacked the mother. Victor never saw his father again.

From the time Victor was nine until he was about sixteen, his father regularly came to his bed at night, stroking Victor's torso, and, with time, his genitalia. As he did this, he would croon to Victor about how much he loved him, how handsome Victor was, and what a big strong man Victor would become. These, he said, were the reasons he was doing this to Victor, out of love and admiration of his beauty. Victor usually pretended to be asleep during these molestations; he rolled over if he was close to orgasm. He felt intense pleasure but also revulsion at what his father was doing.

Occasionally, Victor's father approached him during the day: "From the time I was twelve till I was fourteen or even fifteen, he'd beg me to take showers with him. He said he wanted to show me a secret way to keep my penis hard, but I never would do it. I'd say, 'I'm only fourteen— why do I need to learn that?'" Usually, however, his father tended to be gruff and verbally abusive to Victor in the daytime, as he was to Victor's mother and their other children. He particularly derided Victor's lack of scholastic achievement, and was punitive about the mediocre grades Victor often brought home.

In his late twenties, Victor started psychotherapy because he was depressed, had not been able to finish college, and, though presumably comfortable with his gay sexual orientation, had been unable to form an enduring intimate relationship with another man. In his work with a female therapist, he started to deal with his history of abuse by his father, which had never been forgotten. In doing so, however, he also began to remember an earlier series of incidents that he had never encoded as abuse.

These earlier incidents involved his maternal grandparents and occurred during visits to them in their Asian home-in-exile from about ages four to six. The grandparents played a game with him called "Where Are the Eggs?" In this game, either of them would chase him while he was naked to look for his testicles, which they playfully called eggs. When they caught him, they held him and mercilessly tickled him as they touched his scrotum and fingered his testicles. Victor remembered the game as exciting and accompanied by hysterical whoops of laughter on all sides. Sometimes his mother was present during the game, though she did not participate. When he began school, the game suddenly stopped, and his grandparents refused to engage in it even when he begged them to. He remembered feeling hurt and even depressed at the loss of this exciting connection to them.

Victor grew up with virtually no knowledge of the culture his family came from. Both parents tried to put their childhoods behind them and never spoke about their early life experiences. Victor stopped his visits to his grandparents in Asia at age six and had little memory of anything there beyond their home. As an adult, he had an aversion to learning anything further about the society of the country his parents fled, and shunned any cultural events related to it. He therefore had no knowledge of whether the "Where Are the Eggs?" game was traditional there. Nevertheless, he was deeply uncomfortable with the memory of it. He never discussed these experiences with his mother.

For Victor, then, there were two sequences of sexual betrayal. The recurring nighttime visits by his father were both abusive and traumatic. Victor instinctively knew to remain silent about them—both he and his abuser knew an incest taboo was being broken. The earlier games with his grandparents seem to have been culturally acceptable with a pre-school child. In any case, they were clearly considered appropriate in the specific milieu of his maternal extended family. The sexual play was openly acknowledged and was stopped when Victor was six. But whether the game was normative or abusive as far as his grandparents were concerned, it was eventually traumatic and shameful for Victor, who grew up assimilated to a Western society in which such play is not usually acceptable.

Victor's therapist referred him to me for further treatment when she left the city after he had been in therapy for four years. It was Victor's idea that he see a male therapist, although he was highly ambivalent about this decision. He was afraid he would fall in love with me and that this would make it impossible for us to work together. As we began treatment, however, he quickly moved beyond that fear, and our work focused on his distorted relatedness with various family members and how that affected his relationships with others as well. In particular, he reworked his relationships with his mother, father, stepfather, and siblings. We began to consider his distortions, based on those relationships, with people in work and social situations. In the first two years of our work together, he finally graduated from college at the age of thirty-four; developed a loving relationship with an older man (possibly a sublimation of erotic feelings he was afraid he would have about me, though he denied this); and changed jobs twice in his field, each being a clear step up in terms of both pay and responsibility.

In the next chapter, we will look more closely at families of sexually abused men, emphasizing the effects of chronic boundary violations on a boy as he matures.

CHAPTER 6

The Effect of Chronic
Boundary Violations

Boundaries are necessary in interpersonal relationships. Without them, people feel merged with one another, unable to act for themselves. But if boundaries are too rigid, people lose the flexibility that is necessary to navigate the vicissitudes of a relationship. An adaptive boundary, therefore, is one that is clear but not overly restrictive, permeable but not fragmented or too porous.

A meaningful measure of whether a family's functioning promotes health in its members is the way the family deals with its boundaries. This includes how the family respects personal space and whether it has appropriate expectations regarding the behavior of family members of various ages and generations. For example, parents are responsible for making rules and life decisions that affect their children. This responsibility requires a boundary that shifts in nature over time as the child appropriately is asked to give more input into how these rules and decisions are made. A very different kind of boundary is essential *between* parents, where, if things are going well, patterns of relating develop between adult equals who allow each other intimacy as well as independence. If a parent treats a child as a spouse, or if one spouse treats the other as a child, the boundaries have been inappropriately drawn, usually with negative effects. And when interpersonal boundaries are routinely violated in a family, its members may stop experiencing their identities as having real integrity.

Incest is an extreme form of boundary violation. Chronic incest becomes the familial grid on which a child's personality is formed. When incest has taken place, especially incest of a recurring nature, a boy is likely to have trouble with boundaries as he develops. He may define them overrigidly, not build them sufficiently, or otherwise relate to them in a distorted manner.

As we have seen, the violation of boundaries within a family can be incestuous in nature as well as in actual deed. A boy may feel psychological assaults on his personal boundaries in a sexualized relationship with an adult that does not include direct sexual activity. Like the boy who has experienced physically sexual activity, he is likely to have trouble with boundaries in adult relationships.

Sexually abused adults do indeed often have the refractory problems maintaining interpersonal boundaries that we might predict from their histories. Of course, boundary violations alone cannot account for these men's problems in living. But their histories highlight the importance for them of having boundaries that are clear, but flexible. They also emphasize the impact that violations and distortions have on psychic functioning. Most important, they affirm the need for a man who has suffered sexual abuse truly to define his own boundaries. In this chapter, I will look at both overt and covert familial boundary violations and explore their meaning for the men I have treated and their families of origin.

BOUNDARIES AND FAMILY THEORY

Among family therapists, Minuchin and his colleagues have particularly focused on the importance of maintaining appropriate generational boundaries in families. In their work with slum families (Minuchin, Montalvo, Guerney, Rosman, and Schumer, 1967) and, later, with families with psychosomatic illnesses (Minuchin, Rosman, and Baker, 1978), they demonstrate how boundary issues affect symptom formation and how therapeutic interventions that change inappropriate boundaries can lead to healthier family systems.

Particularly useful in understanding the effects of incest is their work describing inappropriate alliances and intergenerational boundaries in family systems with such pathology as *anorexia nervosa*. Aponte and Hoffman (1973) detail an initial consultation by Minuchin with a family in which an adolescent daughter is hospitalized with anorexia. As the consultation proceeds, it becomes clear that the father is overly close to all his children, but especially to this daughter, while the mother is isolated from the entire family. Using the metaphor of the open door to the

parental bedroom, a door through which all the children were inappropriately invited to enter, and thus invade the parental space, Minuchin
emphasizes the need for the parents *and* the children to have private time
and space separately behind closed doors. Once the boundaries were
changed and the alliances were redrawn, the girl was able to eat in front
of her parents.

Similarly, I and my colleagues (Gartner, Bass, and Wolbert, 1979)
have described a family that needed to establish a boundary between the
parents and their adolescent son. The son and the mother were in a fused
relationship that did not permit the son to develop appropriately and
make his way in the outside world. The father was an outsider to this
relationship, which disguised a psychological chasm between the parents. The son refused to speak to the father, apparently enacting the
mother's fury at her husband. The needed boundary was physically
inserted during the therapy by using a one-way mirror through which
the son watched his parents relate to one another. This forced the parents to settle their differences without using their son. Seeing his mother
fend for herself, the son became less fearful of leaving her. This shift in
boundaries was later perpetuated psychologically by the family.

I will now consider the stories of men whose boundary violations
were more explicitly eroticized than the cases just described. The three
men on whom I focus in this chapter represent the continuum of sexual
abuse histories from overt incest and abuse to covertly eroticized familial
relationships.

PATRICK

Patrick, a victim of frank and profound childhood incest, recovered
memories of his abuse during treatment and then graphically recalled
how he built defensive psychological walls, boundaries that enabled him
to survive his multiple violations. A charming and articulate thirty-eight-
year-old gay man working in a service industry, Patrick sought treatment
because of recurrent depression, night terrors about a stranger breaking
into his room, obsessive but impersonal sexual fantasies, long-term isolation, and difficulties in interpersonal relationships. While he had found
several previous therapies helpful, his overall symptomatic picture had
not changed. Initially flamboyant and seductive, during the first session
he nonchalantly remarked that for several years as a teenager he had had
sexual relations with his brother, who was three years younger than he;
that at age seventeen he had actively attempted (and failed) to seduce his
father; that he had later learned that his brother had also attempted
unsuccessfully to seduce his father during the same period; and that he

and this brother had once, as adults, had sex together with a third man. The brother had died of AIDS two years before I first met Patrick.

I will discuss Patrick's treatment from a variety of viewpoints in this chapter as well as elsewhere in this volume, particularly in Chapters 7 and 9. I saw him over a period of four and a half years for three or four sessions a week, using the couch. After the first year, we regularly had one double session each week, as we found this deepened his ability to express himself without feeling overwhelmed after our sessions (see Chapter 7). In addition, he participated in a group for sexually abused men for a year and a half toward the end of our work.

The necessarily foreshortened vignettes from Patrick's analysis that I recount here at least give a flavor of how his isolation, dissociation, and splitting developed and became the dominating defenses of his adult character. These defenses were all attempts to rebuild and bolster the boundaries his family had shattered. Furthermore, they make his initial symptoms of depression, isolation, night terrors of strangers, and obsessive impersonal sexual fantasizing all poignantly understandable as further attempts to secure his interpersonal boundaries.

The fifth of nine children in a middle-class family in which both parents were alcoholic, Patrick was himself a recovering alcoholic, as were several of his siblings. After he began psychoanalysis, his breezy, flip manner quickly disappeared as he expressed more of his deep depression, but throughout our work his seductive manner with me continued to resurface—as we shall see.

Over a period of months and years, previously dissociated memory fragments began to emerge of profound sexual abuse by Patrick's father that started when he was about age two or three and lasted for several years. As these memory fragments emerged, Patrick often was unable to articulate words clearly, making instead a strangled "Khh-khh-khh" sound as he reached for words. In his earliest terrified images he could only remember "the monster" coming into his room at night and fondling him. In later recollections, he recalled his father raping him orally, often banging his head against walls during the rape, then leading him crying back to bed after ejaculating in his mouth. Patrick also began to recall memories of repeated incidents of anal assault and penetration by a twelve-year-old brother when he was six. In the third year of psychoanalysis, Patrick suddenly remembered, though with much less clarity and certainty, that his mother was sometimes there afterward, wiping his mouth or anus clean but never saying anything about the molestations by either his father or his brother. He was never sure whether this was a memory or a fantasy. In either case, the image conveys how he experienced his mother's role in the abuse: she was complicit in the incest, either passively because she did not open her eyes to what was happening in her family, or actively because she did know but did not protect Patrick except by cleaning him afterward.

Shortly after talking about how his mother enabled the abuse to happen, he had the following dream: "I was with my mother, who was young. She had brown hair and I can barely remember her hair ever being brown. It's been gray for as long as I can remember. I had been very angry about something—I can't remember what—I had expressed a lot of anger. She was very nice, not angry at me. She gave me some colored pencils—a present—the kind of pencils I liked to draw with. I felt very guilty for being so angry—for being so bad—when she was being so nice." During our analysis of the dream, Patrick saw it as a reworking of a familiar theme. Symbolically, his mother was placating and soothing him after his father's abuse. The consequence of this was to make him feel guilty for having been angry about his molestations. In effect, he became the "bad one" rather than his father. The commonplace setting of the dream seemed to indicate that Patrick was confused about whether he had even suffered anything unusual in his abuse. In addition, the dream represented his question about whether he had any right to protest his boundary violations.

Patrick spoke about consciously building up walls to protect and isolate himself from his abusive environment. This was supported by two compelling fantasies from childhood, in which he did indeed build isolating walls:

In the first fantasy, Patrick was inside a construction site. Outside the construction walls, there were men he could not see, except for their penises, which were urinating though holes in the wall. He was excited but frightened, and had many questions about the fantasy. Did he want the men to break through the wall? Did he want to plug up the holes? Did he want to touch the penises? Did he want to be touched by the urine? Did he want to know who the men were? Did he already know who the men were? The answer to all these questions was both yes and no.

In the second fantasy, Patrick, with great hesitation, described a tower he had built to live in by himself, away from everybody else. This was a tower he still retreated to in fantasy as an adult, an intricately designed environment where food was delivered mechanically and Patrick never had to see another person. In the session after telling me about the tower, he said an alternate personality, Paddy, lived there with him and had been hiding behind a false wall while Patrick "showed me around." Patrick was terrified by the intensity with which Paddy swooped down on him after he left the analytic session, furious that he had allowed me into their private domain. (See Chapter 7 for further discussion of Patrick and Paddy in the context of a description of dissociation and multiple self-states.)

In this description of Patrick, we have a vivid, disquieting account of how a boy's boundaries were brutally violated and how he subsequently protected himself through fantasy and dissociation. We will see in further discussions of my work with him how these self-protective mechanisms perpetuated themselves by the time Patrick reached adulthood, severely limiting aspects of his psychological and interpersonal life.

KEITH

Keith's covert sexual betrayal by his mother and, to a lesser extent, his father involved boundary violations that were more subtle, at least on the surface, than Patrick's. But his reactions to them as an adolescent were severe and life-threatening. They carried over into his adulthood, when he carefully kept his distance from others while maintaining a friendly, well-related facade.

The most obvious manifestation of Keith's sexual betrayal occurred when he was six or seven. He heard about a movie being advertised that had naked women in it. He asked his parents if he could go to the movie, and when they asked him why, he told them he wanted to see these naked women. His father offered to show him his *Playboy* magazines instead, while his mother said, "If you want to see naked women, why don't I take my clothes off and you can look at me?"

When Keith came to treatment in his thirties he recounted this childhood memory, still feeling the confusion and repulsion he had felt as a boy. He said he had not wanted to look at *Playboy* with his father and he certainly had not wanted to see his mother naked, but he did not have the language available to explain any of this to them. Instead, he felt shamed by his request, though he was not sure why. He said he learned from the incident that it was wrong to want to see the movie, though he did not understand the reasons, and he never again directly discussed sexuality of any kind with either parent. Yet his relationships with both parents remained sexualized, dangerously so with his mother, herself a victim of childhood incest.

Keith's father was more openly inappropriate with Keith's sisters than with Keith. For example, he would wrestle them to the ground and lick their necks. When as adults they confronted him about such behavior, the father denied it had meant anything. Keith himself became his father's pawn in an affair that eventually split up his parents' marriage. "I would spend time with my Dad's girlfriend and her son. I didn't ask to spend time with him, but it was under the guise of this supposed friendship between their two sons that they got to spend time together." Later, his father stopped caring who knew about his affair: "My father would go out at all times of the night to spend time with his girlfriend—he was obsessed with her, as he has been with every girlfriend he's had since. I remember my mom saying 'Where are you going at ten thirty at night? Stay with your family!' But nothing could stop him."

Keith's mother was bitter about her relationships with both her own abusing father and her philandering husband. Only as he considered it in his adult psychotherapy did Keith begin to think about the implications for him of her aversion to men: "My mother hated men, really hated them. I wonder how that has affected me?"

His boundary violations and consequent inappropriate merging with his chronically depressed mother are illustrated by her picking him up at high school in her car, and bringing along a six pack of beer that she then shared with him. The mother was a near alcoholic at the time, shortly after divorcing Keith's father, and Keith became her drinking companion.

Keith's problems were compounded by severe dyslexia, which required constant tutoring and therapy as well as multiple changes of schools throughout his growing-up years. He felt himself to be bad and stupid, a problem child who would never be normal. He acted out in numerous angry and self-defeating ways, and eventually developed a profound drug and alcohol problem. He dropped out or flunked out of a string of special schools until returning to a regular public high school that had to accept him. Keith eventually attended college and distinguished himself in a field that did not rely on traditional reading skills.

As he recounted his descent into addiction, Keith said he had a "honeymoon period" from ages twelve to fourteen, during which he drank beer and used pot, LSD, and mescaline. He then began to "move on to hard liquor." From ages fifteen to eighteen, he was in his "crazy mode," during which he "took everything" but didn't think of himself as an addict. By age sixteen, he was drinking every day, often with his mother. "When I was sixteen, me and my mom were kicked out of a bar together—we were getting rowdy and they finally decided to ask me for my ID. Then my mom got mean and started hitting them. We were soon out on our asses." Finally, Keith was "completely addicted" for five years from age eighteen to twenty-three: "By eighteen I realized I was an alcoholic—I drank more and more viciously. I'd easily drink a quart of vodka at a time. I'd wake up in the morning and take speed to get rid of the DTs, then I'd drink continuously all day, then at night I'd take coke to prevent blackouts." At twenty-three, Keith entered a detoxification program and went through an extended rehabilitation. He had remained sober for over ten years when he began therapy.

While Keith was deeply ambivalent about his relationship with his mother, he only allowed the positive side into awareness in the years he was drinking and drugging. It was she, after all, with whom he felt he had the only nurturing relationship of his childhood. Two years into his analysis he said, "My mom was the only one who didn't expose the bad dyslexic me, so I accepted enmeshment with her. It seemed a small price to pay. But when she said I was 'special' I knew it meant I was stupid. I was never able to conceive of myself as unique in a positive way. Still, I was grateful that she wanted me and I didn't really care at the time about how totally inappropriate our relationship was." Two years later, Keith began to articulate the rage underlying his dependence on his mother. This rage had shown itself unconsciously in many ways throughout his life, however, ranging from the many ways he acted out in adolescence to his choice of a wife from an ethnic group he knew his mother despised. In Chapter 8, I will return to discussing Keith and the effects his merger with his mother had on his abilities to relate.

DAVID AND HIS PARENTS: A FAMILY INTERVENTION

Patrick's incest was obvious and extreme. Keith's was more subtle, though severely injurious to him. David and his parents, Mr. and Mrs. Jacoby, on the other hand, were a family in which physical contact occurred only rarely, and that contact was incestuous only in the loosest and most disguised definitions of the term. Yet boundary distortions and violations perpetrated by both of his seductive parents led David to a state of psychic paralysis.

I treated the Jacobys in family therapy after eighteen-year-old David, an only child, came home from a psychiatric hospitalization with a diagnosis of severe borderline personality and depression. David had a long history of unstable moods, impulsiveness with money, difficulty making long-term plans for his life, and chronic boredom and emptiness. He was spending most of his days at home in bed, rarely attending classes at junior college, going out most nights to clubs and discos, and returning home early in the morning, often intoxicated.

David's parents were both Holocaust survivors whose entire families had been murdered. They met and married in a displaced persons camp. Born in a small village in Eastern Europe, and with few cultural pretensions, Mr. Jacoby had nevertheless trained as a professional there, but he had to retrain in the United States in order to practice in his field. This required long years of night school while he worked at menial day jobs. When he did finish his degree, he worked for the civil service at a level much lower than he might have achieved elsewhere. Mrs. Jacoby originally came from a wealthy family in a large cultural center. A teen-ager at the beginning of World War II, she had attended a finishing school and been tutored in music and art. She worked as a translator until her husband finished his degree and then stayed at home with David.

The Jacobys had apparently been a mismatch from the beginning of their marriage. By the time they came into treatment, their relationship was characterized by mutual contempt, bitterness, and barely contained fury. Mrs. Jacoby was chronically depressed, while Mr. Jacoby was exceptionally controlling interpersonally. Each was in a rage at David for his passive–resistive inability to care for himself. Yet each was also inappropriately allied with David, and each felt the other was the cause of David's problems.

Despite his anger at David's irresponsibility about money and his own characteristic tightfistedness, Mr. Jacoby continued to supply his son with money for his nightly forays into the club scene and bought him a new car while simultaneously complaining that David's expenses would be his ruin. In addition, he often asked about David's experiences with girls, leering and winking at him so as to exclude Mrs. Jacoby. For her part, Mrs. Jacoby described chronic back pain and fatigue, yet she continued to make David's bed every day, cleaned his room, and mas-saged his bare legs and back. David himself seemed asocial and with-drawn in the presence of both parents together, but when alone with either of them he was livelier and shared private jokes, often about the other parent.

While the boundary violations in David's family were not flagrant, the overly close eroticized alliances between David and each of his par-ents, as well as the bitter distance between the parents, all represented severe boundary distortions. Eventually, I relabeled David's behavior as a self-sacrificing effort to force his parents to relate to one another, even at the cost of his own maturational progress. This intervention, a posi-tive reframing of David's symptoms and an implicit paradoxical injunc-tion that he continue to behave as he had been, was influenced by the schools of systemic and strategic family therapy (see Haley, 1973, 1976; Watzlawick, Weakland, and Fisch, 1974; Selvini Palazzoli, Boscolo, Cecchin, and Prata, 1978). Both the parents were shocked by what I said, and ignored it at first. They only began to react when I made the comment repeatedly, "congratulating" David on his skill at keeping his parents together. David himself began to laugh when I talked this way, the first time he showed any brightened affect when relating to me as opposed to either of his parents. He seemed to feel we shared a private joke, and began to ignore his parents' critical comments about him. I pointed out over and over how the parents and David continued to keep things as they were, and I even encouraged David's "indolence" and his parents' indulgence of it. Suddenly, the stalemate was broken. David started to get up early and attend classes. His mother stopped making his bed and rubbing his legs, while his father no longer showered him with cash. The Jacobys were by no means "cured" of their dysfunctional family dynamic, but David was loosened from its grip and began to join others his age in making a life for himself.

A TRANSFERENTIAL ENACTMENT
OF BOUNDARY VIOLATION

We will see in Chapters 9 and 10 how transferential enactments in the therapeutic relationship can help a patient communicate what has heretofore been unarticulated. When a dynamic is transmitted behaviorally like this, patient and therapist together can analyze the live interaction between them. In so doing, they have the opportunity to transform the message into a verbal one that is available to consciousness. In the following vignette, a man violated my boundaries, and our dialogue about this event helped us understand how he related to issues of privacy, separations, and personal space.

Isaac, who had endured twelve separate molestations or attempted molestations as a child, came into my office one day and, looking away from me, remained uncharacteristically quiet. When I asked what was going on, he flushed, then said in a seemingly offhand way that he hoped I did not mind, but he had gone into the kitchenette adjacent to my waiting room and gotten some milk for his coffee from my refrigerator. I remained quiet for a moment, then commented that he seemed to be having feelings about it. I asked what it had felt like to go in there.

"Well, I was pretty sure you wouldn't mind."

"You're having a reaction to going in there, though."

"Well, it's *your* kitchen, I guess it's your private space. And, of course, it's your milk. But it's not like I stole something of value."

"You're right—but since it *wasn't* something valuable, we can talk about what it meant without getting into thinking of it as a major theft. . . . What was it like going in to my private space?"

"I knew I should have asked you first. I felt a little guilty, but also curious."

"Curious?"

"It seems silly, but I wondered what might be in there." He laughed. "It's not like there were any surprises, though. There wasn't much in there."

"What if you *had* found something surprising?"

"You mean like a severed head in the refrigerator?" He laughed again.

I was taken aback and paused. "Well, that's an interesting thought."

"No, no, I knew there wouldn't be anything like that. But I see what you mean. It's a place where you could be storing something private, something that's none of my business. Maybe that's what I was hoping for."

"To see something private of mine?"

"Well, yeah. I don't know what. I'm just curious about you, I guess."

"What are you curious about?"

"Lots of things."

"How come you never ask?"

"Oh! I didn't think of that. I didn't think I was supposed to. I guess I could have asked for some milk, too."

"What would that have been like?"

"Strange. I'm not used to asking for things. I expect you'd say no, and I didn't want you to say no. Then, too, I expect you'd say no about answering my questions about you."

"Why is that?"

"Isn't it supposed to be unethical for a therapist to answer a personal question?"

"Even if I didn't answer *all* your questions, if you asked them, got them out there between us, at least we'd both know about your curiosity—that might be more interesting than my answer would have been."

"But I already know about my curiosity. Maybe I didn't want *you* to know about it."

"So you didn't want *your* privacy invaded!"

He laughed. "That's right."

"Have you ever had the experience of someone invading your privacy?"

"Not really. . . . Well, now that I think of it, I suppose that's been my whole life."

From here, we went on to a discussion of his abuse situations, and his sense that people could touch him physically or get close to him psychologically without caring whether he wanted them to or not. He said he didn't expect his privacy to be respected, and he often did not respect others' privacy, either, though he had never thought of it that way before. In subsequent weeks, Isaac brought up occasions when he had sneaked looks at his employer's private papers, and he began to experiment with deliberately keeping within interpersonal boundaries, both with me and outside the therapy room. This led him to set boundaries with others more easily. For example, he began to say no to a fellow employee who often asked him to trade shifts and work at an inconvenient time.

In this anecdote, we see how a man's feelings about invasions of boundaries and privacy emerge through a thorough investigation of a seemingly small live behavior in the therapeutic relationship. These were issues Isaac had never addressed directly before. His fantasy about a severed head hidden in my refrigerator revealed the extent of his fears about what I (or, presumably, any authority) might hide under my apparently normal exterior. It also revealed the primitiveness of his own unconscious aggression. With expectations like this, it is not surprising that he would feel the need to protect himself by invading my boundaries and discovering for himself what secrets I might be hiding from him. Boundaries for Isaac were permeable and amorphous. This is how he related to others and what he expected from them.

WORKING WITH BOUNDARY CONFUSION AND DISTORTION

The specific problems raised by chronic boundary violations were voiced by Cory, who said, "People were intimate with me without my permission—and very early. You'd think that would make me used to being intimate—but, no, it means I haven't let anyone get close again. I'm only learning now why anyone would even *want* to be intimate."

Thus, an abused man may carry into adulthood a fear of all interpersonal contact, a fear that was realistic when he was being abused but now is inhibiting and disabling. Struve illustrates this (Morris et al., 1997) when he describes a man who experienced a touch on the shoulder as a punch in the stomach. Similarly, when Max had the collar on his coat straightened by another man in his group, he considered the act a major abusive violation. The concept of "nurturing touch" was alien to both Max and the man who touched him.

Thinking about sexually abused men in terms of boundary violations provides intriguing clues about how to work with them in treatment. Remembering that a man with such a history may not experience having real interpersonal boundaries, it is important to reinforce his ability to form them. I have found it useful to empathize with his need to create a defined sense of where he stops and another person begins. For example, with Patrick I accepted his need for a fantasy tower. I then asked questions about what he was protecting himself from, without directly challenging his judgments. After all, he knew better than I did what monsters could threaten his survival. Only after many months of my supporting his need for isolating and protective boundaries could he decide on his own to question them. He then, in fantasy, made a hole in the tower wall, took his child-self Paddy by the hand, and hesitantly turned to others for help.

Similarly, when Keith spoke in flat tones about the essential aridity and lifelessness of his adult relationships, I remarked on how his need to establish rigid boundaries and an inflexible separation from his mother had been a necessary and life-sustaining prerequisite to his attaining sobriety. He had required their boundaries to be overly restrictive at that time to emphasize the absolute change he was attempting to make in a relational pattern where boundaries had barely existed before. He accepted my comments about the adaptive aspects of his isolation from his mother when he originally attempted to gain sobriety. We could then talk about whether such draconian measures were still needed in his other relationships. He began to make efforts toward intimacy, first with his wife, then slowly with others.

In a parallel manner, when I reframed David's behavior as an effort to reform family boundaries and alliances, I implied that this effort was healthy under the circumstances. Hearing that their need to fuse with one another was understandable in the context of how they had constructed their lives eventually helped David's family to deal with one another in a more functional manner.

Other men have also talked during treatment about their boundary problems, which were demonstrated in a variety of ways. For example, Abe, who could not maintain boundaries, said "I always spill the beans too much, and always regret it." Seth, who, like Keith, maintained rigid boundaries internally while externally seeming to be friendly and related, remarked that the only place in the world he felt truly safe was in his canoe, "alone and with lots of water between me and the next nearest person." Beau, who had been raped and severely abused both sexually and psychologically by numerous people, pointed out that he never had his disabling anxiety attacks when he was alone in his room, "just me and the four walls," weekend after weekend. But he was terrified that having to go to these lengths to preserve his boundaries meant he was destined to be alone for the rest of his life. Andreas, who functioned superbly at work but at great inner cost because of the severe dissociation required to do so, recounted a conversation with his supervisor: "My boss said to me, 'Why do you think you keep getting the employee of the month award? You *never* say no!' After he said that I fell apart." He saw how he unconsciously acceded to requests that were often inappropriate, and how this was a psychological repetition of his acceding to his multiple abusers' demands that he return to them weekly for further abuse. Musing on his tendency to lose himself in others' demands and needs, he said, "I do what others want and do what others want, and then when I look in the mirror there's no one there."

Finally, Quinn illustrates how a man can create interpersonal boundaries within his own flesh. After seven years of individual treatment and five years of group therapy, Quinn wanted to face his weight problem, and began to attend a weight loss group. There, he came to the realization that his weight was literally an armor he had built up for two purposes: First, his massiveness made him a man no one would be likely to confront or abuse. Second, the weight protected him from being an object of desire. In his early adulthood, he had been athletic and muscular, and he often found himself in what were to him bewildering situations where women made clear their attraction to him. Unable to navigate the complicated waters of such relationships, he built up a wall of fat that saved him from such situations by rendering him both unattractive and unapproachable.

In the next chapter, I will consider the later dissociative consequences when a boy needs to distance himself psychologically from the trauma and the intense emotions he would otherwise experience during and after sexual abuse.

CHAPTER 7

Dissociation and Multiple Self-States

Recent literature on sexual abuse has increasingly emphasized the role of dissociation, rather than repression, as a protective defense against the terrifying, inchoate, and disorganizing feelings that accompany childhood trauma. Repression, first hypothesized by Freud (1900), has historically been considered a primary defense mechanism by psychoanalysts. But the roots of dissociation as a construct go back earlier, to the nineteenth century (Charcot, 1887; Janet, 1887, 1889, 1898, 1907; Prince, 1890, 1907). In the history of psychoanalytic theory, Freud, Ferenczi, Balint, Sullivan, Fairbairn, Bion, and Kohut all wrote about dissociation as a response to early experience of psychological trauma (Bromberg, 1991). In recent years, dissociation has received more attention than repression in the literature, and, indeed, J. Singer (1990) has gone so far as to argue that repression has lost its usefulness as a concept.

The history of the concepts of dissociation and repression have been well documented elsewhere (for example, Putnam, 1992; Davies and Frawley, 1994). Rather than fully recount that history again here, I will focus selectively in this chapter on the aspects of theories of dissociation and multiple self-states that have proved most helpful to me in my own work. I will describe dissociative models for personality organization as well as for dealing with trauma. I will also cite literature, most of it written about women, that conveys how dissociation works for sexually abused adults and suggests how to deal with it in treatment. In addition, using case material, I will demonstrate throughout the chapter how dissociative processes have affected the lives and psychotherapies of the sexually abused men I have treated.[1]

DISSOCIATIVE PROCESSES

"Dissociation" refers to an unconscious severing of connections between one set of mental contents and another, often before they enter awareness. "Repression," by contrast, refers to the mastering of conflictual material by actively pushing it out of awareness.

By "mental contents," we refer to several types of dissociated material. Most often, we are talking about dissociated affect, but we can also speak of dissociated behavior, dissociated knowledge of facts, and dissociated sensation, as well as dissociated interpersonal patterns (Pearlman and Saakvitne, 1995). Dissociation is accomplished through self-induced hypnoid states that protect the individual from psychic disorientation and pain. In dissociated mental states, the now-separated mental contents dwell side by side without reference to one another. In such states, good and bad feelings about the same object can thus coexist without conflict, for there are no connections between them that would alert the individual to the incongruities involved. This is how dissociation allows an individual to be conscious of the *fact* of a traumatic event in his history while dissociating and therefore not experiencing the overwhelming *feelings* about it that would otherwise disorient him.

In their most extreme form, dissociative phenomena result in what in the past has been called "multiple personality disorder" (see Putnam, 1989, and Ross, 1989), but is referred to in current diagnostic manuals as "dissociative identity disorder." More frequently, dissociative disorders of a milder nature are seen in adults with histories of child sexual trauma.

Dissociated experience has never been allowed into awareness, and therefore has never been encoded into language. Indeed, much of what we are exposed to in life is never verbally symbolized. Donnel Stern (1983, 1987, 1989, 1997) refers to this as "unformulated experience." Many such experiences remain unformulated for benign, nondefensive reasons. They may, for example, be unimportant or irrelevant at the time. Stern (1997) says that these experiences are dissociated in the

---

[1] In general, I focus in this chapter on the psychoanalytic literature about dissociation. The trauma, psychobiology, and dissociation literatures have also influenced my thinking, but I do not discuss them in a comprehensive way. For integrations of those literatures, see Hopenwasser (1998a, 1998b).

"weak sense" (p. 113). Drawing on the work of Harry Stack Sullivan (1956), he points out that the ability to dissociate is an important component in the development of personality. Every individual must dissociate "not me" experiences as he evolves psychologically in order to gain and maintain a reasonably consistent sense of self. Thus, experiences that, if integrated, would challenge that sense of self are dissociated, or, to use Sullivan's term, "selectively inattended." They are not verbally encoded and never enter awareness. These experiences, Stern (1997) says, are dissociated in the "strong sense" (p. 113).

Briere (1995), whose work I discuss later in this chapter, sees dissociation intrinsically as an adaptational *talent* rather than as a pathological *defense*. Price (1994) speaks to this issue when she notes that in incestuous situations a child is totally dependent on those directly and indirectly involved and responsible for the child's abuse and exploitation. Dissociation, as she points out, is one of the defensive and adaptive strategies the child develops to deal with this untenable situation.

The adaptive aspects of dissociation are highlighted in another way by Hegeman (1997). She emphasizes that in Western culture trauma is usually thought to cause dissociation, but that dissociation is a culturally patterned phenomenon. She notes that culturally patterned altered states of consciousness have been found in 90 percent of a sample of 488 societies. In these cultures, dissociated states may be both accepted and valued, as in trance states induced during shamanistic practices. By contrast, in our culture such states tend to be pathologized or marginalized, as in charismatic religions.

Philip Bromberg (1991, 1993, 1994, 1995a, 1995b, 1995c, 1996a, 1996b, 1998), an interpersonal theorist like Sullivan and Stern, has written extensively about dissociation, both as a response to trauma and as a central organizing aspect of personality. Like Briere, he considers dissociation adaptational (Bromberg, 1994). He also posits it as a universal process that helps all human minds become systems of discontinuous and shifting states of consciousness. He believes dissociation is as basic to personality organization as repression (Bromberg, 1994, 1995a, 1995b; see also Goldberg, 1995), and that every well-functioning individual has been shaped as much by trauma and dissociation as by inner conflict and repression. We will return to Bromberg's conception of dissociation later in this chapter.

TRAUMATIC DISSOCIATION

Everyone has an ability to dissociate to greater or lesser degrees. Ordinary dissociation often results in daydreaming or other benign mental activities. By contrast, traumatic dissociation, a response to overwhelming life experience, has both numbing and intrusive features. It is a means for the self to maintain some fragile sense of functioning.

Traumatic dissociation has usually been thought to be the far end of a dissociative continuum that starts with everyday dissociation, although some (for example, Stern, 1997) suggest these may actually be two different kinds of dissociation. Because it is easy to get the concepts of traumatic and everyday dissociation confused, Hirsch (1997) has suggested reserving the term "dissociation" for traumatic dissociation and calling everyday or developmentally normative dissociation by Stern's (1983, 1997) term, "unformulated experience."

From where do pervasive dissociative states emanate? For Price (1997), dissociation results from cultural bans that determine and define acceptable speech, thereby preventing the symbolization and linguistic encoding of events that the culture will not allow into consciousness. For Bromberg (1991), dissociation arises when early object relationships have not allowed the normal development of tension-reducing mental structures. Because of this, presymbolized experience that is too intense to be cognitively processed is instead retained as raw data in unbearable mental states that are then dissociated in order to preserve other areas of functioning. Thus, dissociation is a protection against being incapacitated by the shock of "aspects of reality that cannot be processed . . . without doing violence to one's experience of selfhood and sometimes to sanity itself" (Bromberg, 1993, p. 165).

Davies and Frawley (1992, 1994) describe the dissociative process in more detail as a means to avoid ego dissolution when trauma presents the individual with too many disturbing stimuli. They describe how such material is split off from awareness before it has been symbolized, as well as how it emerges eventually in disguised forms. The ego is split, resulting in two or more self-states. These ego states, organized and functioning independently, enter consciousness separately, thinking, remembering, behaving, and feeling differently from one another. Not available to the rest of an individual's personality, "[t]hey are likely to make their presence felt via the emergence of recurrent intrusive images, violent or symbolic enactments, inexplicable somatic sensations, recurrent nightmares, anxiety reactions, and psychosomatic conditions" (Davies and Frawley, 1992, p. 31).

Traumatic dissociation thus exists to protect the individual from the full shock of trauma. The ability to dissociate allows people to act as they must in order to save themselves from the overwhelming emotions that they would otherwise experience. Thus, a child who is raped nightly may learn to dissociate his unformulated terror and proceed in the daytime as though he lives an ordinary existence. This enables him to build up areas of competence while encapsulating his traumatized reactions to his abuse. If he has little capacity to dissociate, he might be so paralyzed by his feelings that he is totally unable to learn in school, relate to others, or develop other skills he needs in life. (I am talking here about *relative* competence. Many abused children do indeed have deficits in these areas despite their attempts to dissociate their trauma.)

As a reaction to trauma, dissociation protects against personality fragmentation (Bromberg, 1994). It is a way of shutting down the information-processing mechanism so that pain is neither registered nor experienced (Madison, 1995). Its goal is "to maintain personal continuity, coherence, and integrity of the sense of self and to avoid the traumatic dissolution of selfhood" (Bromberg, 1993, p. 162). Thus, paradoxically, *it is through fragmentation that dissociation restores a unified sense of self.* This is accomplished by using hypnoid processes to separate out and unlink disorienting self-states of consciousness. These separate states of consciousness then become discontinuous, disparate, and unrelated experiences that coexist in multiple self-states. I will discuss the concepts of "unified sense of self" and "multiple self-states" later in this chapter.

One of the protagonists in Scott Heim's novel *Mysterious Skin* (1995) illustrates this process. Molested twice by his baseball coach at age eight, he "loses time," and becomes amnesic for the periods when the abuse occurred. As he grows older, he comes to believe that during the lost time he was abducted by aliens. In a way, this is a creative reinterpretation of his alien experience as a molested child. He experiences himself as a relatively unified individual who must have had a unique experience that accounted for his loss of memory; he thus manages to maintain a cohesive sense of self through his dissociation. For years, he reads everything he can about UFOs and claims of alien sightings and abductions, until the dissociation finally begins to break down in his late adolescence.

Brooke Hopkins (1993) is a layman who writes about his childhood maternal incest. Without using professional language or jargon, he finds poignant words to articulate his inner experience of traumatic dissociation:

> There must be a form of trauma that produces what can only be described as an out-of-body experience, a trauma so total that one is *forced*, in order to preserve oneself, to view what is going on around one as if one were a detached spectator. . . . I seemed to experience all this as if I were somehow outside myself as well as in, as if I were viewing it all from some position two or three feet above my body as well as experiencing what was going on from within. (p. 45)

In this description, Hopkins is simultaneously conveying the experiences of the child he was in the past and the adult he is now, an adult looking back on his childhood trauma and finally finding grown-up words to describe it.

The immediate effects of dissociated reactions to early childhood trauma were conveyed to me even more directly by Patrick. In Chapter 6, I described how Patrick split off at least one child part, a furious, protective, and frightened child whom he named Paddy. I will return to that split shortly, but I note now that Patrick had already showed me a different frightened child-self who did not have Paddy's fury. I experienced this terrified and traumatized child in Patrick when he first began to recall fragments of his dissociated childhood abuse by his father. The language he used was the language of a preschool child. He talked about "the monster" coming into his room at night long before he attached that monster's presence to any particular person or event. At another point, he started to cry as he said he wanted to keep his pajamas on. The words he used were those of a very young child, simple words of one or two syllables, often without complete sentences.

Patrick's dissociative defenses were the vehicle by which he initially recalled his abuse. His very first memories about his molestations did not seem to be related to abuse at all, but rather were about "yellow roses all around me." He was very anxious as he described the roses, but could not elaborate on his panic. He and I were both confused about why he was frightened by the flashing image of these yellow roses, an image that recurred over many weeks. He eventually remembered that the roses were in a pattern that corresponded to the wallpaper in the living room of the house he lived in as a child, a room where some of the earliest abuse had occurred. It was a long time before we understood that he concentrated on the wallpaper while he was being abused as a means of self-hypnosis in order to "not be in my body" and therefore not experience the abuse. In other words, this was his way of dissociating his abuse experience as it occurred. In doing so, he learned the self-hypnotic techniques that he later used pervasively.

With time, Patrick was flooded by many fragmented memories of abuse by his father. As he described these incidents, Patrick talked in a singsong, childlike voice, speaking of himself in the third person as "the little towheaded boy in his pajamas." It was as though Patrick himself were on the ceiling, watching a child being abused, much as Hopkins describes in the passage about his maternal abuse quoted above. This seemed to be a latter-day demonstration of how Patrick's adult dissociative defenses began. These dissociative defenses were formidable in his case, so formidable that they had kept Patrick amnesic about his sexual abuse throughout his life. Indeed, it seems likely to me that the ability to dissociate his experiences so completely saved Patrick from psychosis and enabled him to develop psychologically without needing, for example, a delusional system to deal with the abuse. Instead, Patrick developed rigid and suffused dissociative defenses that enabled him to maintain an amnesia that continued over the course of several otherwise helpful psychotherapies. This amnesia only receded in the context of an intense psychoanalytic relationship with me.

By contrast with dissociated experiences, repressed memories are considered to have already had a previous shape in consciousness. They were somewhat integrated before being pushed out of consciousness, and are therefore experienced by the individual as familiar if they reemerge. If dissociated traumatic material comes into awareness, on the other hand, as Patrick's did, it breaks through as nearly the same terrifying experience it was before the disintegrating self severed the experience's ties to consciousness. Unverbalized, unsymbolized, fragmented, and undigested, this dissociated experience emerges exactly as it was in its original traumatizing context.

GENERALIZED DISSOCIATIVE PATTERNS

The chronicity of Patrick's abuse led him to resort to dissociation as a commonplace way of warding off anxiety in almost any uncomfortable situation. What had started out as a useful, perhaps even lifesaving, way of dealing with his trauma ended up as his principal mode of being-in-the-world. He developed compulsive behaviors like alcoholism, incessant masturbation, and anonymous, unpleasurable sexual activity as a means to hypnotize himself and return to a dissociated state. While behaving compulsively, Patrick entered trances, self-induced hypnotic states that replicated essential elements of his original dissociative reaction to trauma. These trance states provided Patrick with a speedy reentry to the protected dissociated state he had created while being abused.

For example, rather than experience anxiety and unhappiness when he returned from holiday visits with his abusive family, he went directly to gay bars and fellated dozens of men in the back rooms (this happened in the years before the AIDS epidemic). Concentrating on the penis in his mouth was like concentrating on the yellow roses of the wallpaper in his living room as a child. It protected him from his emotional experience—in this case, the reemergence of his many conflicts about being with his family. After a night of compulsive and ultimately unsatisfying anonymous sex, Patrick was numb, exhausted, and could barely remember what had happened either at his family's home or in the back rooms of the bars to which he fled.

Indeed, Patrick's dissociative tendencies were so well ingrained that they also took over in much less conflicted situations. He had not developed other ways to cope with anxiety, nor could he differentiate between states of minor versus overwhelming anxiety. Instead, he went through life on automatic pilot. When his unconscious radar signaled him that danger *might* be near, he began to dissociate. This happened once, for example, when he thought a waiter in a restaurant was being over-friendly. Momentarily anxious about the meaning of this approach, Patrick suddenly found himself out on the sidewalk, not remembering the act of leaving his meal on the table and walking out to escape the possible attentions of the waiter.

But the dissociation did not always work completely, as witness his recurring night terrors of a stranger breaking into his room while he slept. In that case, danger was signaled by the "simple" act of going to bed at night. Going to bed, in his early experience, had meant that a "monster" might well come into his dark room and molest him. At times, he could fend off his anxiety about this. At other times, the anxiety broke through and he experienced a terror similar to what he must have felt as a small boy. In these states, he could not sleep, and constantly checked the locks on his doors and windows to assure himself that he was safe.

As Patrick's patterns demonstrate, then, dissociation, though not in itself necessarily pathological, can become so. Individuals who have lived with chronic trauma like incest are likely to dissociate as their first reaction to *all* anxiety. But dissociation may or may not be an objectively appropriate reaction to every anxiety-arousing stimulus. Bromberg (1994) points out how the dissociative cure for anxiety can itself become the problem. By always mobilizing for disaster, the individual unwittingly contributes to its likelihood. In discussing Freud's case of Emmy von N, for example, Bromberg (1996a) writes that her "need to maintain the dissociative structure of her mind was her way of protecting herself against trauma that had already occurred—a protection against the future by plundering her life as if it were nothing but a replica of the past" (p. 70). Patients who have endured trauma can never be "cured" of what they have lived through—it will always be part of their history—but therapy can help them stop what they *still* do to themselves and others as a result of that traumatic past.

People who dissociate chronically have large portions of their emotional life unavailable to them, and may have deficits of memory for many external events as well. Their ability to see the world realistically may thus be seriously compromised (Silber, 1979). Indeed, Rivera (1989) maintains that it is not multiplicity that gives problems to an individual with a multiple personality disorder (now called dissociative identity disorder), but rather the accompanying defensive dissociation and consequent inability to be fully cognizant of the world and even of the self. Through this distorted reality, caused by "dissociative virtuosity" (Herman, 1992, p. 102) in dealing with overwhelming and traumatic psychic hurt, traumatized individuals "learn to ignore severe pain, to hide their memories in complex amnesia, to alter their sense of time, place, or person" (Herman, 1992, p. 102).

Most abusers were themselves abused (although, as I noted in Chapter 1, most abused children do not grow up to become abusive). They are likely to have learned to use trance and are often in dissociative states while committing sexual abuse. This helps explain why abusers often disown and disavow the enormity of their acts, or even have no memory of the events. They dissociate their guilt and thus feel a subjective sense of innocence (Grand, 1997). Victims may identify with the disavowed shame of their abusers, thus setting the stage for their own shame about the abuse (see the discussion of Lorenzo in Chapter 8). Acknowledging and remembering the abuser's dissociation can affect how both sexually abused adult and therapist think about the abuse situation, since it reminds them of the likely inner state and history of the perpetrator. This in no way excuses an abusive act, but it does sometimes make it more understandable.

ANDREAS

Consider Andreas, a man whose pervasive dissociation suffused every aspect of the life he constructed, distorting his perceptions, confusing his relatedness, and compromising his sexuality:

Andreas's deeply dissociated states led him at times to lose co-consciousness among them, and the nature of these multiple self-states might qualify him as having a dissociative identity disorder. Even after years of intensive individual and group therapy, Andreas often maintained that he had no feelings at all other than anger, fear, and occasionally anxiety. When in his initial consultation with me Andreas said flatly that he had no feelings other than these, I answered that I did not believe him, although I understood he was not aware of them. He later told me he almost got up and left my office when I said that; he was angry because he felt that I was calling him a liar, but he was also afraid that I would make him feel emotions other than anger and fear.

An example of Andreas's rigid dissociation was his claim that his physically and emotionally abusive father had no effect on his life, since the father had been missing through most of Andreas's childhood and had neglected Andreas or punished him when he was present. As

Andreas described it to his group for sexually abused men, he had erased his father's presence from his mind and therefore was unaffected by him. When over many weeks group member after group member disputed this assertion, he finally said that he understood intellectually the arguments they made that the lack of a father must have affected him powerfully. "But," he contended, "if I truly acknowledge that my father affects my life, and of course he does, then my life is no longer in a neat little bottle that I can put on the shelf and just forget about. I'd get worried, I'd get anxious. I don't know if I can live like that."

Andreas remembered his sexual abuse history over the course of a lengthy treatment with another male analyst before he was referred to my group. He recalled several men who, having initially snatched him off the street when he was eight, periodically abused him for about six years. The abusers seem to have been a ring of child molesters. Membership in the ring changed from time to time, and there were always several other boys being simultaneously victimized. Sometimes Andreas was forced to have sex with the other boys; this was particularly traumatic to him, and it left him with the irrational feeling that he was these boys' abuser.

Andreas could not forgive himself for having obeyed these men when they ordered him to be in a certain place every week so they could come get him and continue their sessions of sexual abuse. He continued to ask himself, when he did not dissociate the entire experience, why he went to meet them weekly, never doubting their authority over him even though he did not know them and never even learned their names. He insisted, "By going back week after week, I became my own perpetrator." Only after several years of working with me did he tell me his abusers warned him that they would kill his mother if he did not come back to them as ordered. He believed them and returned because he was terrified that they could and would murder her. Despite this, he continued to blame himself for going back and for "not stopping the abuse."

He never told anyone about his molestations. His parents finally found out about them when he was seriously injured one night by multiple anal rapes. He returned home bleeding profusely from the rectum. As he recounts it, his mother took him to the hospital but never asked for details about the abuse. His father sneered and said Andreas deserved whatever had happened to him. When memories of his sexual abuse returned shortly after his own son was born, Andreas was not sure whether to believe them. His recollections were finally confirmed, however, when he searched hospital records and discovered that his rectum had been surgically rebuilt during his childhood.

Andreas also recalled repeated physical mistreatment and neglect by his father and an incestuous relationship with his mother that he could only allude to momentarily because it so sickened him. Both parents and all of his siblings were or had been substance abusers. In addition, his father was contemptuous and abusive toward his mother, who was of a different race than he. Isolated and depressed, living in an ethnically homogeneous community from her husband's background that refused to relate to her, the mother appears to have led a miserable existence throughout her marriage. Andreas thus had many repeated emotional traumata within his family to dissociate along with his sexual abuse by outsiders. This family context left him unprotected and vulnerable to abuse by strangers.

Andreas's dissociative patterns helped him succeed in establishing an external life that was remarkable given how little support he had available to him during childhood. His story illustrates the positive, adaptational aspects of dissociative defenses. He graduated from college; married and raised a large family; was a pillar in his church; held a substantial and remunerative position with considerable authority over other workers; and maintained interesting side businesses as well. But his thoughts and feelings were rigidly and dissociatively separated. He constantly and consciously surveyed himself to make sure he did not allow himself to experience any emotions except anger. Not knowing how to feel anything in moderation, he made sure he felt nothing. He called this "living topside," meaning living solely in his head. On the rare occasions when emotion slipped through, he fell apart. If he allowed himself to feel, he always returned in fantasy to the occasion of his first molestation, and then could easily become flooded, crying incessantly. When this happened, he ruthlessly made himself furious at everything in his life: "After four or five days of being enraged, I'm back in control."

Andreas maintained that he had no feelings about anyone except his children, and that he had only had intense feelings about them at the time of their birth. He forced himself to play with them "because it's good for them developmentally that I do so," but never felt playful or joyous around them. Sex with his wife had on the surface seemed successful in the first few years of his marriage, but he finally admitted to her that he felt nothing during sex. He could maintain an erection almost indefinitely, but he experienced no sensation and had no erotic fantasy life. He continued sexual relations with her because it was the "right thing to do morally," but he maintained that he had absolutely no other reason to want to have sex. He consciously dissociated so he could perform sexually: his wife would give him advance notice that she was interested in sex, and he would then get himself into a dissociated state, sometimes using marijuana and at other times creating a trance state. He was then able to perform sexually and satisfy her while "not present." Experiments with men had confirmed his belief that he was not gay, but rather that he had made himself virtually nonsexual. Later on in his treatment, as his dissociation began to break down, Andreas reported experiencing glimmers of sexual desire, but said he initially felt instantly nauseated whenever his sexual feelings were aroused.

Andreas approached my group for sexually abused men with a curious mixture of indifference and terror. These existed in him side by side, with no reference to one another—exactly what happens during a dissociative episode. In group he initially disliked "checking in," the process in which every group member tells the group as it begins about his current emotional state (see Chapter 11). He hated how this made him immediately visible to the group, although he simultaneously knew instinctively that the group experience had great potential to help him. He felt exposed by the expectation that he would be self-revealing, and he also was reluctant to disclose the paucity of his emotional center. He often arrived late to avoid the check-in, even though this usually meant he stayed silent for the rest of the group. At first, he was unable to have a real verbal interchange with other group members; instead, he lengthily spoke *at* them. His competence in the work aspects of his life was very clear to all, but the near-void in his interpersonal relating was totally at odds with that competence.

Over the first few months that he was in the group, Andreas gradually became slightly more comfortable, though he maintained his basic unrelated stance toward other group members. His first crisis came the first time a new man, Seth, entered the group. Already enormously apprehensive about a new man joining the group before ever meeting Seth, Andreas called me five days later and asked to see me individually. He was gray and glassy-eyed; his terror had broken through his dissociation. He told me that he had been unable to sleep since the night Seth entered the group, because he was sure Seth was an abuser. He asked me whether I knew if Seth had molested anyone, and I reiterated my policy of not allowing men in the group who had been abusers as adults. Since this was my general policy, I could say without compromising Seth's confidentiality that to the best of my knowledge Seth did not have such a history. I added that I could not guarantee this, of course, but that I thought it was important to explore why Andreas was so sure Seth was an abuser.

It took a long time for Andreas finally to identify the specific reason for his terror, which was that Seth's hands seemed to him to be exactly like the hands of one of the men he remembered abusing him. Seeing Seth's hands had plunged Andreas back into the panic state he had endured as a boy. Never having allowed this dissociated panic into awareness before, he was now terrified in exactly the same ways he had been at age eight.

Articulating this enabled Andreas to return to the group and tell them, and Seth, about his panic reaction. This was a breakthrough on several levels: Andreas had to relate to other group members more authentically in order to communicate his internal perceptions; he forced himself to relate his feelings and part of his history; and he began to identify some of the distorting mechanisms that suffused his experience.

As his therapy continued, Andreas started a medication regime that helped him avoid the extreme bottoms of his occasional emotional breakthroughs. Only after many months of being on medication did he volunteer the information that the medication also helped him in his efforts to feel nothing at all. Fearfully, he acknowledged that he wanted to try having feelings and asked to take lower dosages of medication. Titrating his medication dosages allowed him to experiment with having feelings without the extremes he had always feared. He later said, "I've learned that when I feel nothing—*that's* when something's happening that's very important to me." These were, of course, only a few steps on his long and arduous path toward a less dissociated mode of being.

DISSOCIATED SEXUAL COMPULSIVITY

Compulsive sexual activity can be a compelling way to soothe the unregulated affect that emerges when dissociation breaks down. In common with other compulsive dissociative adaptations to trauma, such as gambling, overeating, and various addictions, sexually compulsive behavior is a dissociative solution to the problem of managing anxiety. Addictions can help a man experience highs that prove to him he is still alive when he begins to feel depersonalized, numb, and empty (Schwartz, Galperin, and Masters, 1995b). But they are also tools for numbing out when he is starting to feel and think in uncomfortable ways. Paradoxically, addictive behaviors, which themselves often seem to be examples of poor impulse control, are ways of controlling *other* impulses that are even more dangerous, like harming oneself or others.

When the body is hyperaroused, it releases chemicals called opioids to tranquilize itself. The biological underpinning of how sexual compulsivity soothes anxiety involves the stress-induced analgesia that results when these chemical opioids are released to assuage pain during and after trauma (van der Kolk and Greenberg, 1987; van der Kolk, 1996). This analgesia is compellingly seductive. The bodily change is powerfully reinforcing, and the individual is moved to experience it again and again. A man is thus motivated to repeat the sexual behavior that first induced these self-soothing chemical opioids to be released. Since the secretion of the opioids was a reaction to traumatic sexual activity, the victim may become compulsively sexual as a means of recapturing those tranquilizing effects. Engaging in compulsive sex thus allows a man to reexperience directly the biochemical means his body used to calm his anxiety when the abuse first occurred. Also, in addition to offering some degree of physical discharge in itself, sexual compulsivity has the added force for a sexually abused individual of being very close to the original traumatizing behavior. The behavior itself becomes the central focus of his attention, allowing a self-hypnotic dissociative trance to take over his consciousness (see Spiegel, 1990).

Both these self-soothing aspects of compulsive sexual behavior—the releasing of the opioids and the hypnotic focusing on the sexual behavior—serve to help the man regulate unmanageable affect that is triggered by seemingly innocuous reminders of his abuse (Briere, 1995; M. Schwartz, 1998, Cassese, in press). However, unpredictable situations may contain triggers that suddenly lead to unmanageably high levels of sexual arousal. In turn, this may lead both to greater dissociation and an inability to monitor the safety of his sexual activity (Cassese, in press). Dissociation thus puts him at risk for harm. For example, a dissociated individual has a reduced capacity to judge the danger of a sexual behavior like unprotected sex. Sexually abused individuals for this reason may be at greater risk of HIV infection (Cassese, in press).

A man in this situation may also be less capable of saying no to a potential sex partner. This is certainly true when there appears to be no clear risk to the encounter, but may also be the case if danger is recognized. Lorenzo was a gay man who had been abused by a number of presumably heterosexual men in the small town in which he grew up. While he practiced safe sex when in dissociated states, he repeatedly put himself in potentially dangerous situations like picking up strangers in parks. As he began to recognize and intervene in this process, he described what he went through trying to say no when a man he disliked unceremoniously demanded to have sex with him: "I have this neighbor who claims to be straight but always comes to me for sex. I don't really like him, and I don't like sex with him. But yesterday he met me in the hall again and said, 'Wait for me, I'll come by.' I got panicky. I didn't know if he would really come by—sometimes he doesn't when he says he will—but I knew that if he did come I *couldn't say no*. I go into some other state about it. I like it that someone wants me, and I feel so bad about myself that if he wants me—*even if I don't want him*—I have to say yes. So I left my own apartment, which is better than I've done in the past, when I've waited and had sex with him, or waited and he never arrived. Still, I had to leave my own home in order to not submit when a man told me it was time to be sexual with him."

Earlier in this chapter, we saw how Patrick's dissociative sexual compulsivity soothed him when his anxiety was triggered. Such dissociative compulsions became Devin's principle approach to his life. Devin was originally referred to me for an evaluation related to serious legal charges resulting from compulsive sexual behavior. I cannot be specific here about the nature of those charges. Although I usually do not do evaluations for legal matters, I made an exception in Devin's case because I believed that he had committed a victimless crime, and that he had possibly been set up to be arrested for behavior in which he did not usually engage, although it seemed related to his history of sexual abuse. Sometime after that evaluation, while still waiting for a resolution of his court case, Devin sought treatment with me.

In our first evaluative sessions, Devin revealed his involvement in an extraordinary number of compulsive behaviors, most of which were self-destructive either directly or indirectly. No longer actively drinking, chain-smoking, or doing drugs, his current compulsions included gambling, looking at pornography, overeating sweets, and maniacally collecting baseball cards. He followed sports scores doggedly, laboriously making endless lists that duplicated information he could otherwise have obtained easily and instantly in computerized form. He spent many hours in sex-oriented Internet chat rooms, and ran up immense phone bills on phone-sex lines. He shopped far beyond his means, incurring huge charge bills for items he never used. "When I have to buy something, I don't care about anything except the high I feel when I'm getting it. I have to have it! Then I get home, and I feel dirty and foolish. It's never stuff I really need, and I get embarrassed about buying it so I never use it. It just sits there in my house—I'd feel too embarrassed to take it back to the store." He went to peep shows and allowed men to fellate him there, sometimes vomiting afterward because of his conflicts about participating in homosexual acts. (He claimed that if he had the money he would compulsively go to female prostitutes instead.) Even when building a shelf in a closet, a positive activity in his own mind, he spent hours making exhaustive measurements and calculations, and could not rest till every closet in his house had shelves. "I didn't eat till it was done. I stayed home from work to do it. And I *hate* doing home repairs, I don't really know what I'm doing. But once I decided to make a shelf, it was like someone else was in my body, making shelf after shelf after shelf."

Devin told me about his history of sexual abuse calmly, reciting the facts of his abuse history as though they had happened to someone he knew very distantly. In a way, they had, so detached was he from his own experience. His compulsions served to keep Devin out of touch with his inner life. Although occasionally emotion did break through his compulsive defenses, as when he noted that he was nauseated all the way to my office the first few times he saw me, usually he did not experience any disturbing feelings.

For example, after being found guilty of the crime that had led to our initial consultation and failing to get a reversal after a lengthy appeal, Devin seemed indifferent to his fate. While awaiting sentencing, he said blandly that he knew he should be worried but wasn't. He added that anything could happen between now and the time he was sentenced, so he did not let himself think much about what he had done or what might happen in the future. Once sentence was passed and he was awaiting the start of a jail term, his mood remained similarly bland and even cheerful, though he did note the inappropriateness of his affect.

Devin's father began to abuse him when he was about five years old. In the beginning, his father fondled him in the bath, but soon he was coming to Devin's room at night, groping and fellating Devin and asking him to touch the father's penis and squeeze it. Later, his father took Devin on business trips where the sex sessions were more extensive, and the father also took photographs of Devin in explicit pornographic poses. The abuse ended when Devin was about fourteen.

Devin described his father as brilliant, a talented athlete whom Devin adored. "Everyone loved him—I always felt he was a good father—I never thought about all the other stuff. It was like some other person did those dirty things at night." The father was a dry alcoholic, nondrinking from the time Devin was three, and active in AA. He continued to smoke marijuana daily, however, and also sometimes did "other weird drugs." He bought a gun for no apparent reason, and would go off by himself for days on end without explanation—a habit Devin repeated in his own marriage. In addition, the father had a long-term girlfriend while still living with Devin's mother, and raised a child with her.

Both paternal grandparents died from active alcoholism, and one paternal aunt died of a combined drug and alcohol overdose. None of Devin's siblings was alcoholic, but Devin had had severe alcohol and cocaine addictions. His driver's license had been revoked for repeated drunken driving offenses. At the time I first saw him, he had been alcohol- and drug-free for over two years following four attempts at rehab programs, and he attended AA meetings daily. But his life remained chaotic, pulled together loosely by his compulsions and his continuing capacity to function at his job. He was divorced, though he maintained a relatively positive relationship with his ex-wife, who knew about his history and his compulsions, and with his children.

Devin never confronted his father about the abuse. He said he would have been far too embarrassed ever to raise the issue. "While it was happening, I'd get disgusted. Usually it felt bad—then I would pretend to be asleep. But I never told him to stop—it was not at all terrifying. And sometimes I wanted him to do it. It felt good and bad at the same time. When I heard him coming up the stairs, I'd get excited—it became pleasurable." Devin turned red as he said this, saying he was afraid I would think he was gay. Turning away from me, he added, "I knew there was something wrong with what we were doing, but it made me feel special. I loved my father so much, and I loved having this special secret with him. He never said to keep it a secret, but I knew I should. At the same time that I felt disgusted, I also felt special." Asked how he felt talking about the abuse, Devin said, "I know I should feel rage, but I don't. I don't actually miss him but I also don't hate him—I'm emotionless. I guess I make sure I have no feelings about him."

When Devin was in his early twenties, his father was indicted for molesting a neighborhood boy. He asked Devin to testify on his behalf, and Devin did so, swearing in court that he could not imagine his father doing such a thing to anyone. The father was acquitted, but Devin was positive his father had committed the crime of which he was accused. He felt terribly guilty about the boy whose charges had been judged to be unsubstantiated. "I did a terrible thing to him. I'm not as bitter now, but I hated myself for what I did. Why did my father ask me to testify? I perjured myself when I was still young and idealistic about the law. Since then, I've been bitter and cynical about everything."

His father died five years before my first meeting with Devin, and on his deathbed he apologized to Devin for what he had done. "Even then, I hated having to talk to him about it. It made me uncomfortable, very embarrassed. I told him it was okay, even though it wasn't." The father also told Devin's mother about the abuse before he died.

Devin married in his early twenties, and could not say why he married his wife except that she wanted him. "I liked her but I never really thought I loved her, and within weeks I was fooling around with other women." His sexual problems with his wife included humiliating difficulties maintaining an erection and ejaculating. Although she seems to have been supportive about this, he avoided sex with her whenever he could. He had similar sexual difficulties with any woman with whom he had a relationship, but not with pickups or prostitutes. Apparently, with women he did not know there was less overwhelming emotion that had to be dissociated during sexual intimacy.

His sexual problems with women made him wonder whether he was homosexual, as did the childhood abuse itself, especially in light of his sexual arousal during the molestations. He insisted, however, that he had no conscious erotic desire for men. Indeed, he got highly anxious in response to interpersonal approaches of any kind from a man, and was phobic about saying or doing something that might make him appear gay or, by extension, appear interested in men for anything at all. This seemed to be an aftermath of his conflicted pleasure when his father abused him. We also explored the alternate possibility of his having unconscious homosexual desires, whether related to the abuse or not, as represented by his allowing men to fellate him in the heterosexually oriented peep shows he frequented. These homosexual concerns affected his relationship with his son. While he had claimed to have no fantasies or impulses about molesting boys, he was worried that somehow he would abuse his son anyway. He had always refused to bathe the boy, and obsessively worried that he was spending too much time with him or looking at him too much.

Devin's chronic homosexual panic was a constant in our work together. He sat miserably in his chair at the beginning of every session, afraid to make eye contact, warily surveying any slight behavior on my part that might possibly be construed as a sexual advance. He was unable to dissociate these feelings successfully. Yet he never missed a session and, indeed, the most hopeful aspect of our early work was his expressed wish to learn to sit with me without these interfering apprehensions. With time, he acknowledged shamefacedly that he looked forward to seeing me. Characteristically, this "confession" was accompanied by further alarm about its possible sexual implications. In this manner, in fits and starts our work proceeded slowly from, and returned frequently to, Devin's basic need to reestablish human relatedness through his slowly growing alliance with me (see Chapter 9 for a further discussion of this concept). Gradually, as our interpersonal connection grew, there was some diminishment of his dissociative compulsive behaviors.

DISSOCIATED REENACTMENTS OF ABUSE

Dissociated experience, unsymbolized in thought and language, exists as a separate entity outside self-expression, cut off from human relatedness, deadened to full participation in the psychic life of the rest of the personality. Price (1997) observes that trauma lies not just in traumatic events but in their unassimilated nature. Its effects cannot be healed until the wound from the trauma has been reopened in a new situation where it can be linguistically encoded. It has not been symbolized, and it is not amenable to verbal interpretation before encoding occurs. This is a crucial process in work with sexually abused patients because in most cases they cannot heal from dissociated trauma until they can think about it and experience it (Madison, 1995). For some severely dissociated individuals, however, traumatic experience may be linguistically encoded but the dissociation, while pervasive, is not powerful enough to protect them from feeling recurrently overwhelmed by their feelings.

The effect of not symbolizing sexual abuse linguistically is far reaching. Recall the work of Conte (1985) and Gilgun (1990, 1991), who found that abused boys who had a confidant as they were growing up were less prone to develop symptoms. In particular, Gilgun found that boys with confidants were not as likely to become rapists, molesters of children, or violent criminals. These boys had verbally encoded their abuse experiences by talking about them to their confidants. Conte's and Gilgun's work demonstrates that dissociating traumatic experience rather than verbally symbolizing it makes the boy more likely to reenact his abuse unconsciously, often through acts of violence and criminality that occur in manhood when he is in a dissociated state. Those who have linguistically encoded their abuse experience are much less likely to need to reenact it in these ways.

Of course, unconscious reenactments of abuse do not always take the form of criminal acts. They can occur in the course of everyday life, as when Abe gave gifts to emotionally abusive colleagues, repeating an unconscious pattern of placating his abusive mother. In addition, patients often reenact dissociated trauma in a therapeutic relationship. In such cases, the reenactments can create challenging and difficult therapeutic impasses, as we shall see in Chapters 9 and 10.

BREAKING THROUGH DISSOCIATION

As Sullivan (1956) notes, people are programmed to resist any breakthrough in their dissociative patterns: "[T]he dissociated personality has to prepare for almost any conceivable emergency that would startle one into becoming aware of the dissociated system" (p. 203). Hegeman (1995a) discusses the consequent difficulties of using traditional treatment strategies in working with dissociated individuals, since the object of such work is to help patients confront material that dissociation has held at bay. Cognitive–behavioral approaches (see Ross, 1989; Putnam, 1992) suggest ways to restructure cognition about trauma as a means of resolving symptomatic responses to it later in life. While these approaches are certainly helpful, they do not address the damage that has been done to an individual's core ability to live in relationship with others.

Transference cues play a crucial role in helping both patient and therapist gain access to dissociated material (Davies and Frawley, 1992, 1994; Hegeman, 1995a; see also Chapter 9 in this book). Treatment must change internal accommodations made to avoid awareness of the original trauma because such accommodations also interfere with the self's development. Most important is the need to focus on a dissociated individual's relatedness: "[The] very fragmented, doubting self . . . must be mobilized to engage with and negotiate the dissociated material. Therefore maximum attention must be paid early in treatment to restoring the patient's capacity for relationship" (Hegeman, 1995a, p. 187).

This is a particularly apt way of considering what occurs when a traumatic *relationship* must be dissociated, as in chronic incest. In such cases, there may be a severe disturbance about having relationships at all because relating to others is itself linked to terrifying dissociated experiences (Sands, 1994). I will discuss the ramifications of this problem in Chapter 8.

A sexually abused individual is likely to be very conflicted about allowing dissociated experience into awareness. Each step presents new strains and reasons to put brakes on the process. Saying he was afraid to open doors in his life and move beyond the plateau he had reached, Abe once recounted the story of Bluebeard, which had been a favorite of his in childhood. In that story, as he remembered it, Bluebeard told his wife she was free to go anywhere in the house that she wanted, but she was not to open a certain door or she would be punished. Eventually, curiosity got the better of her and she opened the door. Behind it she discovered the dead bodies of the previous wives that Bluebeard had killed. Abe said he was frightened about what dead bodies he would find if he opened more doors to his experience. I pointed out that opening up these doors had saved the woman's life, since she then knew what she was up against and could flee her husband. Abe had not thought about this aspect of the story before. Taking it as his cue, he went on with his difficult interior self-exposure.

Numerous accounts have been written about how dissociated memories of traumatic sexual abuse can come rushing back in adulthood. Without entering here into the controversy about the validity of such recovered memories, a controversy I have written about elsewhere (Gartner, 1997b), I will cite one of these reports:

Brooke Hopkins (1993) discusses how one night during his twenties he was suddenly inundated with memories of his sexual abuse by his mother:

> I vividly recall how more or less involuntarily they came back . . . how dumbstruck I was as I watched those memories come out, almost perfectly intact, after what seemed at the time like so many years, the almost physical excitement I felt as that whole portion of my childhood continued, with just a little renewed pressure, to unfold. (pp. 35–36)

He tries to describe how these memories had remained inside himself. Struggling with the inadequacy of language to convey his experience, he uses the term "repression" to describe what sounds like dissociation as defined in the opening sections of this chapter. He acknowledges how "recall" is a misleading term for how his memories of abuse suddenly consumed his awareness. After describing his mother's physicality in sensuous detail as he remembered it from his nights embracing her in bed, he writes:

> [S]uch closeness was utterly engulfing in its immediacy, engulfing and fantastically exciting. That's why, once the repression is lifted, it is not difficult to recall (if "recall" is even the right word); like Proust's involuntary memory, *there are no intellectual structures to mediate the sensations.* They are simply, overwhelmingly there, and they remain part of your body forever, a burden as well as a blessing. (p. 41; emphasis added)

REGULATING AFFECT
AS DISSOCIATION BREAKS DOWN

John Briere (1988, 1989, 1991, 1992, 1995; Briere and Runtz, 1987, 1988) discusses the problems that occur when dissociated material is finally experienced during psychotherapy. He notes that in general the sexually abused man is likely to be hypervigilant—extremely sensitized to possible danger signals like noise or sudden movements—as well as easily put into the hyperaroused states that are triggered when these danger signals are perceived. He has a reduced capacity to tolerate such hyperaroused states or to modulate his affective response to such danger signals. Thus, emotional reactions of fear and rage easily get amplified to devastating levels that can interfere with his cognitive abilities. Because of this, he learns to avoid intense feelings rather than try to tolerate them. This may be especially true for men who were traumatized before the age of five, because at the time of their abuse they had not yet identified sufficiently with their parents' capacity to handle and tolerate strong affect (Huizenga, 1990).

Such a man may then become phobic about all emotions. Keith summed up his need not to feel: "When I feel emotion, I'm all consumed and lost and hurt—that's what it was like when I lived with my mother—I was either alone or consumed with her and by her. I was so emotional as a teenager, so sad, so unhappy. I had to do drugs to numb it out, but they can't numb it out completely. I equate emotion with pain—I'd like to feel emotion without all that pain but I'm not sure if it's possible."

Briere emphasizes the traumatized individual's reduced capacity to recover from the heightened emotional states likely to result from experiencing dissociated terror. Ordinary self-soothing mechanisms such as deep breathing are unlikely to alleviate the intense and disorienting feelings he has at such times. Instead, to distract himself he may try to alleviate his stress by resorting to self-soothing but self-destructive behaviors like substance abuse, overeating, self-mutilation, and compulsive sex. We saw this in Patrick's response to visiting his family by becoming compulsively sexual and in Devin's pan-dissociated way of dealing with the world, both described earlier in this chapter.

Briere (1995) argues that dissociative defenses exist for a purpose and are helpful because they keep toxic emotional states at bay. Dissociative defenses must therefore be honored in the treatment because they helped the individual survive unbearable situations. For this reason, Briere prefers the term "dissociative solution" to "dissociative disorder." This solution got the victim through his childhood experience. It did not, however, permit him to accomplish the necessary task of habituating the stressors of the abuse. This would have made them less toxic because they would have been allowed to enter the realm of ordinary experience and become familiar (see Breuer and Freud, 1893–1895, for an early discussion of a similar process). Effective psychotherapy reduces the need for this dissociative solution.

We saw the dramatic defense against being overwhelmed emotionally in Andreas's rigid maintenance of barriers between his emotional life and his consciousness, described earlier in this chapter. Aware that he was not equipped to deal with strong affect, Andreas tried not to allow himself to experience any emotion at all. On the other hand, if a traumatized man never reexperiences any of his dissociated affect, he will continue to be ruled by it (Madison, 1995).

It is important to remember that if trauma occurs very early, the man may, like Andreas, have *only* learned to dissociate in response to strong feelings. For this reason, Briere warns against helping an individual recover dissociated affect too quickly. If he does, he will lack the necessary psychological container for his distress and may have to self-medicate or plunge into self-destructive methods of defusing his pain. The cycle has been interrupted and he no longer soothes himself in the same ways, but he is allowing more emotional danger signals into awareness than he previously did. This is because when an individual who tends to dissociate changes and starts to integrate his experience, the dissociation breaks down. When this occurs, he will initially experience a *higher degree of distress* until he finds new ways to cope with these emotions.

For example, Harris reported that at certain stages of his psychotherapy he began to experience severe headaches and backaches from tension; he had never experienced either when he had operated "on automatic" during his young adulthood. Harris's memories of sexual abuse by his father returned to him after many years of therapy. He and his therapist had never focused on this issue, and both were surprised when with a rush he suddenly recalled that over a period of years his father had taken him to the park and molested him. He said he was thankful he had not recalled the abuse earlier because he did not believe he could have borne the psychic pain, panic, and turmoil brought on by these recollections without the years of preparation in his individual psychotherapy.

While Harris had altogether dissociated conscious knowledge of his abuse experience, Seth never forgot the facts of his molestation. He did, however, dissociate the emotions that accompanied it. This affect suddenly inundated him when as an adult he endured another trauma, this one related to a serious accidental injury on the job. As he put it, "It was always there, but my mind just skipped over it till I was seriously injured in that accident. Then, as I was reacting to that trauma the emotions from the abuse flooded me. I couldn't function at all."

Abe, on the other hand, framed in a more positive light the increased anxiety he felt as his dissociation broke down. He noted with wonder that the uncontrollable shaking of his leg during therapy sessions was a sign that he was no longer emotionally deadened. This led him to consider how pervasive his dissociation of feeling had become.

Similarly, as Patrick and I worked to understand his dissociation, it began to work less well, and for an extended period he felt more anxious much of the time. But, during this period, while Patrick did feel far more emotional pain than previously, he was simultaneously able to consider in a less dissociated way how he had chosen a job he derided because doing it fulfilled his need to serve others in a self-demeaning manner. This recognition enabled him to embark on an ambitious and arduous course of study for a career he cared about. I don't believe he could have made such a decision while in the dissociated state he had lived in for years.

Dissociation, then, exists for a self-protective purpose, and it is crucial that the dissociating individual not get flooded by toxic emotions as he begins to experience what had been dissociated; he has no way of dealing with such states. Briere emphasizes that you are retraumatizing the man if you explore his abuse prematurely, giving him access to overwhelming feelings without strengthening his capacity to cope with them. The therapist must therefore titrate as much as possible the degree to which dissociated feeling emerges.

How does this titration occur? Some writers emphasize the need to address pacing and containing affect when working with dissociative states (see, for example, Kluft, 1989b; Dolan, 1991; Fine, 1991; Grame, 1993). Dolan (1991) suggests how to use a patient's ability to dissociate as a creative resource by making the unconscious tendency to dissociate into a conscious capacity to do so. If he learns to dissociate at will, he will be able, for example, to hypnotize himself if he feels too intensely, or to use such techniques as locating the trauma in a specific part of his body. Grame (1993) suggests internal containment strategies like teaching benign self-soothing techniques and internal visualization, using spiritual support, and utilizing time-outs to maintain impulse control. She also advises employing such external containment strategies as adhering to the agreed-upon length of therapy sessions, maintaining boundaries about touching, and limiting telephone calls.

This issue of maintaining traditional rules is a controversial one, however. Such writers as Davies and Frawley (1994) have commented on the impossibility of always maintaining conventional therapeutic frames and boundaries with this population. Some patients require extended sessions in order to feel safe enough to explore traumatic memories. Or they may need to be allowed phone contact if they are experiencing disorienting object constancy problems between scheduled sessions. The decision to break with tradition under these circumstances needs to be made carefully and judiciously.

For myself, while I feel it is best to err on the side of caution and not deviate from established therapeutic practices unnecessarily, it is clear that extending myself beyond the usual therapeutic boundaries can be helpful and necessary at times. For example, at one point I actively encouraged Abe to call me and leave a message on my answering machine at any time of the day or night when he felt he was getting "lost" and allowing abuse to occur. Hearing my voice and speaking to me, albeit on tape, helped center him psychologically and allowed him to reexperience the moments of relative autonomy he felt during therapy sessions. Our agreement was that I would call back only if he asked me to, and that such a response might not be immediate, though it was likely to come within the day. Abe never misused my invitation. In addition to the technique helping him directly in the moment, he experienced my offer as a sign of caring and empathy that he usually had trouble believing was possible.

Similarly, when Patrick was inundated by affect as he began to recall his early sexual abuse, it became clear to me that our usual forty-five-minute sessions were not adequate for his needs. He often did not allow himself intense emotions until thirty or even forty minutes into our sessions. I became concerned that in the time we had left in the session he was not able to recover from these feelings so that he could leave my office and continue with his outside life. He became frustrated and frightened, often backing off from affect just as he started to feel it. Aware that this pattern of experiencing strong affect so late in the session might also reflect a resistance to having such feelings, I nevertheless felt it was important to see if longer therapy sessions would help him sustain and digest what he was going through. We experimented with having one double session and one or two single sessions each week, and this worked well. In the longer sessions, he felt safer to allow his terror into awareness, and he often used single sessions to articulate, and thus encode, what he had been going through in the double sessions. Accommodations like these are commonly used by many clinicians accustomed to treating traumatized patients.

To encapsulate the process of allowing dissociated material into awareness without overwhelming the patient, Briere (1995) conceptualizes a "therapeutic window" that gives the therapist and the sexually abused adult a psychological space in which to process abuse. In this space, anxiety-arousing feelings are experienced, but the individual does not feel he is drowning in them and so does not resort to processes like dissociation that help him escape from them. If material emerges from dissociation too quickly, however, he develops intrusive symptoms, like panic or anxiety. When these intrusive symptoms get overwhelming, he uses avoidant strategies, like self-destructive self-soothing behaviors, to deal with them. As long as the dialogue between therapist and patient remains in the therapeutic window, however, neither symptoms nor avoidant strategies interfere with the patient's functioning.

The therapist's job in this situation, then, is to access a window of opportunity in which the man is allowed to experience more traumatic material than had been previously possible, but is not overwhelmed by it. This requires the therapist to keep interventions gentle enough so the patient will not feel overcome by anxiety, but also deep enough for him to experience his trauma more fully than previously. As the therapeutic process moves forward, at every step the therapist needs to monitor the patient's ability to stay in this window. If he gets overwhelmed by his feelings, the therapist must either help him reduce his psychic pain or enable him to raise his capacity to deal with it (see Krystal, 1975, for a related discussion of helping addicted patients learn to tolerate intense affect). Thus, the parameters of the therapeutic window are constantly shifting.

The therapeutic window can exist, according to Briere, because people defend themselves somewhat more than they have to. This creates a psychological place where dissociation is not necessarily used or needed but is still available, and therefore the psychic material does not overwhelm. Therapist and patient can do their work in this space. But the therapist can easily undershoot the window, say, by only nodding and giving support, thus not helping dissociated material to emerge. Alternatively, the therapist can overshoot the window, for example, by asking intrusive questions too early in the process.

The therapist must therefore work to process emotional material with the patient at an appropriate level (Briere, 1995). Abstract questions about the trauma feel safest to the sexually abused man and are therefore least likely to push him into becoming symptomatic. An example of such a question might be, "Did you feel you could talk to adults about upsetting events?" Questions like this are helpful when a man is just beginning to talk about his experiences and cannot yet describe them with any specificity. A man with a somewhat greater capacity to reexperience the trauma might be asked narrative questions to help him reconstruct the story of the abuse. An example of questions like this would be, "What was the sleeping arrangement in the bedroom you shared with your brothers, and where were they when your father came into your bed?" This kind of question helps the patient develop a symbolized, verbal conception of what he went through. The questions most likely to overwhelm the man involve sensory aspects of the abuse, which ask him to verbalize his physical sensations. A question like this is, "What did you feel inside when your mother was rubbing your belly and penis that way in the tub?" Hearing this might push a man to start feeling boundaryless or panicky. On the other hand, if questions like this are never broached, he cannot extend the limits of what is tolerable to him. Questions like this last one are most likely to be helpful to a man who has already succeeded in bringing some of his dissociated experience into awareness.

Briere warns that there is danger in pushing the parameters of the therapeutic window too fast. For example, some clinicians believe that delving directly into the content of traumatic material during the first year or so of sobriety of a patient who has been addicted to drugs or alcohol may push him back into the addiction (Robertshaw, 1997). It is important, however, eventually to expand the therapeutic window and allow the man to begin to feel his traumatic emotions. The trauma cannot be resolved without both reexperiencing the memories and experiencing, in the context of a therapeutic relationship and often for the first time, the feelings that accompanied the abusive event. This allows the man to become desensitized and habituated to the overwhelming affect surrounding his molestation and thereby allow it into his everyday experience. Anxiety that cannot be felt cannot be habituated (Briere, 1995). This is why desensitization has not worked for him in the past: he can't get habituated to dissociated feelings he does not experience. And if he did begin to experience them, he was likely to avoid them through such means as drugs, alcohol, or compulsive sex, all of which serve to soothe and distract him from the affect he was unable to regulate in any other way.

Unless habituation occurs, the abuse will continue to organize his personality on an unconscious level, forcing him to continue to be unthinkingly suspicious or untrusting, to develop somatic symptoms, or to maintain any of the other sequelae of sexual betrayal we see. For these reasons, simply doing supportive psychotherapy with a sexually abused man is not enough. It is essential also to address the trauma and push his limits so that he processes his previously dissociated traumatic affect. At the same time, however, it is important to remember that most trauma therapists have given up the idea that every traumatic memory must return for health to be regained (Hegeman, 1998).

MULTIPLE SELF-STATES

Classical psychoanalytic approaches have generally considered the goal of treatment to be the resolution of internal conflicts. Contemporary psychoanalytic literature written by those who consider themselves relational, interpersonal, and poststructural (for example, Rivera, 1989; Mitchell, 1992, 1993; Bromberg, 1993, 1994, 1995a, 1996b; Harris, 1994; Davies, 1996a, 1996b, 1997), rather than classical, has instead posited that understanding self organization, states of consciousness, and dissociation is central to psychoanalytic work. In particular, the ability to dissociate is thought to be key to the development of personality for all individuals. Most important, personality is thought never to be organized to produce a unified self, but instead is *normally* a set of *multiple self-states*, disunified and decentered, evolving out of the individual's *normative dissociative tendencies* (Pizer, 1996a). The concept of a single, unified self is considered a social construction, a "largely nonexistent unity of consciousness" (Bloom, 1997, p. 33).

Davies (1996a, 1996b, 1997) likens personality organization to a kaleidoscope that makes "intricate patterns, varied but finite, conflating and refiguring themselves from moment to moment . . . whose patterns become recognizable over time, yet whose parts will come to light in different constellations of prominence and obfuscation" (1996b, p. 562). Each self-state embodies a particular position according to the role that self-state learned to play as part of the individual's overall survival strategy in childhood (Rivera, 1989). For these writers, we all exist in multiple self-states, states that are usually interconnected although separate. No one self-state represents the "real" self. Bromberg (1994) conveys this idea when he adapts Polonius's famous advice to Laertes in *Hamlet*:

"To thine own *selves* be true" (p. 518; emphasis added). In this section, I will lay out the theoretical ideas behind the concept of multiple self-states, and in the next section I will illustrate the concept with two case examples.

For traumatized individuals, the content of an idea may be dissociated from the affect surrounding it, as when an individual knows he was abused but experiences no feelings about it, or when an internalized concept of a parent as an abuser may be dissociated from the internalized good and nurturing parent. But it is not only discontinuous and conflicting affective states that lead to the organization of multiple self-states. Rather, according to this line of thinking, *all* individuals are organized this way. Psyches are nonunitary, a series of separate self-states that with time "attain a *feeling* of coherence which overrides the awareness of discontinuity. This leads to the experience of a cohesive sense of personal identity and the necessary *illusion* of being 'one self'" (Bromberg, 1994, p. 521; emphasis added).

Different self-states are created in the different relational matrices through which we all move in our lives. Sullivan (1953) speaks of individuals having different personifications of personality in different interpersonal contexts, depending on the relationship with the significant other person. Laing and Esterson (1964) capture the flavor of such relational matrices in their discussion of families of schizophrenics:

> Each person does not occupy a single definable position in relation to other members of his or her own family.
> The one person may be a daughter and a sister, a wife and a mother. There is no means of knowing *a priori* the relationship between: the dyadic set of reciprocals she has with her father, the dyadic set with her mother, and the triadic set she has in the trio of them all together, and by the same token, she may be a sister to her brother, and to her sister, and, in addition she may be married with a son or daughter.
> Let us suppose that Jill has a father and mother and brother, who all live together. If one wishes to form a complete picture of her as a family person, let alone as a person outside the family, it will be necessary to see how she experiences and acts in all the following situations:
>
> Jill alone
> Jill with mother
> Jill with father
> Jill with brother
> Jill with mother and father
> Jill with mother and brother
> Jill with father and brother
> Jill with mother, father, and brother. (p. 6)

While Laing and Esterson did not intend what contemporary writers have called multiple self-states in this description, they did lay the groundwork for understanding how an individual comes to feel like and *be* a different person in different interpersonal configurations. In essence, this is the concept that is used in contemporary theories of personality to challenge the idea of a single integrated self.

Traditionally, treatment goals have included the unification of different self-states when they are thought to exist so that they are replaced by a stable, central self. But for theorists like Rivera (1989), concepts like "unity of the self" and "defined individual identity" are no longer therapeutic goals but rather are thought to be dangerous fictions that erase differences among self-states and between human beings while fostering conformity to cultural norms. Yet Rivera believes that the concepts of self integration and the essential decenteredness of personality can be reconciled. She suggests that the general treatment goal in relation to multiple self-states be that the individual is *simultaneously able to hold contradictory emotional states and points of view*, as represented by different self-states, in a "central consciousness" (p. 28). Pizer (1996b; see Pizer, 1998) calls this the "capacity to tolerate paradox." This, Rivera says, can be accomplished if, rather than silencing the multiple voices, the individual develops an increased capacity "to call all those voices 'I,' to disidentify with any of them as the whole story, and to recognize that the construction of personal identity is a complex continuing affair" (p. 28). Or, as Price (1997) puts it, one must listen to the voices of these multiple self-states "not as a unified choir, but as singular voices begging to be heard and recognized and simultaneously fearing such recognition" (p. 133).[2]

In this theoretical perspective, then, personality is not unitary, but is instead a mental structure consisting of a group of multiple self-states that become *relatively* cohesive as maturation occurs. There is actually no such thing as an integrated self, though there may be the illusion of it because the individual usually *experiences* the cohering self-states as a continuous, unitary selfhood.

Within this "acquired, developmentally adaptive illusion" (Bromberg, 1996b, p. 515), however, there are dissociated gaps between self-states. These gaps are masked and are not usually experienced by most normatively organized individuals who take for granted a unified sense

---

[2] Some writers, including both classical analysts and self psychologists (see Paul, 1994; H. Schwartz, 1994; Lachmann, 1996), have criticized this conception of multiplicity on a number of grounds. In particular, they have warned about the danger of reifying and furthering the separations among multiple self-states by treating them as totally separate from one another.

of self (Bromberg 1993, 1995a). For other people, however, the experience of continuity of self is never assumed, and they have lifelong struggles dealing with a variety of relatively or entirely dissociated states. To differentiate between these two, the personality organized normatively by dissociation and the personality organized by traumatic dissociation, Pizer (1996a) suggests calling the former the "distributed multiple self" and the latter the "dissociated multiple self" (p. 504).

Unbridged spaces between multiple self-states exist side by side without knowledge of one another. A sign of psychic health is the ability to negotiate and cross with relative ease such gaps between dissociative states. As Bromberg (1993) puts it, "Health is the ability to *stand in the spaces* between realities without losing any of them" (p. 166; emphasis added). A traumatized individual may, however, through dissociative processes, lose the capacity to make interconnections among the selves that live in his various unique relational configurations. Or he may be prevented from ever forming these primary connections. To the extent that the spaces between the selves cannot be bridged (Pizer, 1998), the individual is living with a diminished ability to deal with his world.

Thus an essential goal of psychotherapy is to form linkages among the multiple realities of different self-states to make it easier for the individual to negotiate these spaces with relative fluidity (Bromberg, 1994). Working this way requires a focus on relational restructuring in addition to the cognitive reconstruction advocated by cognitive–behavioral therapists. I will discuss relational restructuring via the therapeutic relationship in Chapter 9.

MULTIPLE SELF-STATES: TEO AND PATRICK

If dissociation is a normal and inevitable aspect of personality organization, dissociative identity disorder is the most severe of the many organizational possibilities that may ensue. Let us consider first Teo, a man who exhibited a relatively minor disorder of dissociation and multiplicity, and then Patrick, whose multiplicity was complex, rigid, pervasive, and appropriately termed a dissociative identity disorder.

The lack of connectedness between his multiple self-states was all too apparent to Teo when he was first referred to my group for sexually abused men. Indeed, the main object of our work was to allow him to move easily among those states. This could only be accomplished after his mute child-self learned to speak to others about his sexual abuse.

Teo had worked his way out of the gang-ridden streets he grew up in and became a globe-trotting businessman whose skills and abilities kept him in demand all over the world as a consultant. The father of six children from three marriages, he found in his third wife a woman who supported his need finally to face the demons from childhood sexual abuse by his godfather, Arnie. His abuse memories were vague, but he had no doubt that there had been a sequence of sexual activity, probably including mutual fellatio and masturbation, while Arnie baby-sat for him when he was seven and eight. In his late forties, Teo began an individual psychotherapy that forced him to confront the effects of this abuse. In doing so, he temporarily had to undo much of what he achieved as "Ted," the accomplished executive and entrepreneur, in order to find again the frightened child, "Teo," whom he had silenced four decades earlier.

In our initial consultation for group therapy, Teo asked me to call him by that name, noting that to all his colleagues, friends, and relatives he was known as Ted. A veteran by that time of five years of individual therapy with a woman analyst, he had come to view Ted as the protector of Teo. He said he wanted at last to allow Teo, the child-self in whom all his dissociated fear and anger resided, to be known to his adult self and to others.

Likeable and highly articulate when he chose to be, Teo took a mostly silent role in the group. Unusually, other group members allowed him this silence, accepting his statement that he had spent too much of his life being overly glib, and that for him talking was a way of hiding his pain and fear. His essential warmth and supportiveness to other group members came through in the brief remarks he did make and in the expressions on his face as others spoke.

Teo was devoted to the group for the two years he attended it. He arranged his international business trips around the night the group met so that he rarely had to miss the group because of them. If he did miss a meeting, he often called from wherever he was to say hello at the hour we met. When he spoke in the group, it was often to offer support to other group members based on his own life experiences about whatever they were addressing at the moment. If he talked about himself, it was usually about how tired he was of being capable "Ted" in the business world; or about problems he might be having with one of his children; or, eventually, about his rage toward his godfather, Arnie, and toward the parents who did not protect him from molestation.

A year after entering the group, Teo announced that he had sent a letter to all his clients worldwide, saying that for the present he would continue to work for them via fax and electronic mail, but would only rarely accept phone calls or be willing to travel for his work. He explained in the letter that this was due to personal stresses and needs. His clients were remarkably accepting of these terms, and he lost relatively little business, though he said he had been determined to go through with his plan no matter what the consequences were. He had decided to give Ted a rest and allow Teo out into the world.

If anything, Teo was now quieter than before. He was not able, and no longer tried, to voice what was happening inside. His Teo child-self was available to him, though he did not yet have the language to give it a voice. He bided his time, and neither the group nor I ever criticized him for this.

After some months of near-muteness, Teo began to emerge as though from a cocoon. He began to tell some of his clients about his abuse history and his reasons for withdrawing into himself. He gave voice to his corrosive and alienated anger and cynicism, telling the group how he had bitterly divided the world into victims and victimizers: "The world is full of either victims or Arnies—or, at best, victims-in-training or Arnies-in-training."

A few months later, Teo felt ready to leave the group. He was immensely grateful to it and his therapists. As he put it, "What made me better was that through individual therapy and my group *I was able not to keep this abuse a secret any more*—the more I could tell people, the better I got. It seems so simple, but I would never have believed it on my own." Here again is a demonstration of the need to symbolize trauma verbally in order to ameliorate its effects.

Looking back at his dissociated mode of relating to the world, he was able to describe how he had coped with this world, and the price he had paid: "I learned a tape to say. I could handle any situation by turning it on and hiding while my mouth talked. It was only by learning that it was OK to be quiet—not to be on top of everything—that I found *my* voice. That was the paradox—I had to be quiet to find my voice." In the language of the theorists who posit multiple self-states, this voice was actually a group of several voices, those of Teo and Ted as well as other self-states that had never been as clearly delineated to me as these two. They constituted a chorus in which each voice was heard. Teo had learned to negotiate the gaps between these self-states.

I return now to Patrick, the man whose child-self, "Paddy," was furious at the adult "Patrick" for allowing me into their private domain. Patrick was always clear that he and Paddy were different aspects of himself, and that there was always co-consciousness between the two. Yet Patrick and Paddy seemed like distinct entities, and I began to see them as separate personalities. Over the course of treatment, other personas emerged, unnamed but clearly different from these two. Patrick never completely gained an ability to move fluidly between his self-states, but he did learn to bridge the spaces between them more of the time.

I have described (see p. 143) how Patrick developed the alternative persona of Paddy, the furious and frightened child he had been while he was being abused. As Patrick, he ambivalently wanted me to enter his world. He invited me to share his childhood fantasy of living in a walled-off, protected tower. As Paddy, he was furious and frightened; he felt invaded by me and was in a rage at his own adult self for having allowed me to transgress into this protected, private space. Therefore, Paddy attacked Patrick after the session when Patrick allowed me, in fantasy, into their private tower.

As we talked about Patrick and Paddy, it became clear that "Patrick" represented the part of him that had to interface with the world—charming and placating, though brittle—while "Paddy" represented the terrified, furious, and traumatized child who could not bear to be near another person. In a subsequent session, Patrick recalled that his abusive father had called him "Paddy" as a child.

"Paddy" and "Patrick" exemplify Davies and Frawley's (1994) compelling description of the child and adult selves in the sexually abused women they write about: "The child self may be condemned to a world of unrelenting paranoia, but the adult persona, having ejected these toxic experiences, attempts a rudimentary integration" (p. 72). Davies and Frawley describe at length the vicissitudes of treating an adult like Patrick who has such bifurcated self-states, noting that such an individual often develops in treatment to a point where it is possible to articulate "the ongoing struggle between that aspect of personality that wants to function independently and successfully, and those more child-like aspects that feel such an adaptation to represent a 'sellout' and betrayal of the child who suffered so unmercifully" (p. 73). They then emphasize the critical importance of reaching some integration of the experience of the adult and child personas.

Patrick displayed other prominent self-states besides Patrick and Paddy, such as the toddler I described earlier in this chapter who was afraid of the monster who came into his bed at night. I often felt I was dealing with a different person in one session from the man I had treated the session before. Indeed, he sometimes seemed to switch suddenly before my eyes. For example, in one session he described with pain how in all seasons and all weather his father, while supposedly doing childcare for him and his siblings, took them to the edge of what Patrick now knew to be a gay beach, then disappeared for hours. He got very quiet, clearly close to tears. Then he startled me as he suddenly laughed harshly and mockingly: "This is silly! I don't know why I'm talking like this. What I really want to tell you is how much I want to suck you off and have you as my lover!" In a flash, he had again become the seductive, bold, and brittle man who in our first session had told me with a smile how he had had sex with his brother for several years and tried to

seduce his father at age seventeen. Because of the emergence of such separate personas, the rapid oscillation among them, and Patrick's seeming
inability to bridge the spaces between them, I came to see Patrick as suffering from a moderate dissociative identity disorder.

By the fourth year of treatment, we had finally progressed sufficiently to talk about Patrick's sexual relationship with his three-year-
younger brother during adolescence and even once in adulthood. Doing
so forced him to reconsider the implications of that relationship and his
need to dissociate many aspects of it. He remembered that he and his
brother were always so furious at each other during the day in the years
they were sexually involved at night that they seemed truly to hate each
other. They never spoke to one other during sex or about the sexuality in
their relationship. With time, Patrick acknowledged that his brother, the
"bottom" in their sex acts, never seemed to enjoy the sex, and never
achieved orgasm with Patrick. On the other hand, Patrick, the "top" and
the consistent initiator of the sexual activity, was nearly always orgas-
mic. Another self-state, that of a predatory teenager, thus gained prominence, and one day Patrick said, with horror, "I guess I was his abuser. I
never realized that, I never thought of it that way." He began to wonder
about his brother's life trajectory: Had he also been abused by their
father? Had he led a promiscuous life in part because of his abuse experiences, whether with Patrick or with their father? Had that led him to
contract HIV and die? When he verbalized these unanswerable, previously dissociated questions, we sat together in silence, allowing their
implications to sink in. These implications were as unbearable to us both
as the memories of his own abuse.

An individual whose personality is organized by dissociation, then,
is likely to have a lowered capacity to link his multiple self-states to one
another. Whether the result is a relatively minor dissociative tendency, as
in Teo's case, or a pervasive dissociative identity disorder, as in Patrick's,
it influences his ability to manage interpersonal relationships. In the next
chapter, we will focus more specifically on sexually abused men's relatedness.

CHAPTER 8

Intimate Relatedness

Sexually abused men often have flawed or distorted concepts about relating to other people. Chronic disturbances in relationships have been detailed throughout the clinical literature on incest (for example, Gelinas, 1983; Courtois, 1988; Ehrenberg, 1992; Davies and Frawley, 1994). We saw in Chapter 5 that relating itself can be traumatic for men with histories of abuse. In Chapter 7, we further saw that this trauma becomes especially pernicious when terrifying early dissociated experiences are linked to the very fact that one is in a relationship. Sexually abused men may not understand what involvement with others entails and what they risk or, alternatively, do not have to risk when they are intimate with others. Distortions about intimacy are a logical extension of having had faulty, corrupt early relationships with abusers and, often, other adults. Their understanding of interpersonal relating was often valid in those early destructive relationships, but such perceptions interfere with their ability to create nonabusing intimate relationships in adulthood.

Situations involving trust, sexuality, intimacy, power, and authority may pose particular problems to an abused man. Abuse is likely to have occurred when he was especially receptive to interpersonal approaches as a boy (Briere, 1995). If he was undermined at this vulnerable developmental stage, when he was especially needy for contact with others, he may be starved for intimacy while simultaneously remaining phobic about it. He will have potent fears for his safety in human relationships, and these will affect the extent to which he can accept the interpersonal closeness he often desires.

Many men ignore such intimacy disorders in young adulthood, only coming to acknowledge any deficits in their relationships later in life. In early middle age, when many abused men seek therapy, they may feel more secure psychologically. By that time in their lives they also may be forced to relate to others more intimately. If they encounter problems relating to partners, making career changes, or having children, they may finally be moved to face developmental impasses about trust and intimate relating that were impossible to address in childhood or early adulthood (Horsley, 1997).

In this chapter, I will discuss how sexually abused men's adult intimate relationships are affected by their histories. Themes that have recurred in my patients' lives and treatments relate particularly to the areas of abuse, trust, and sexuality. I will therefore focus on interpersonal problems stemming from distrust, anxiety, and rage; from men's difficulty differentiating abuse from other interpersonal dynamics; from their frequent ambivalence about themselves as sexual beings; from the emotional and sexual distance characteristic of their relationships; from the ways they relate to others through their sexuality; from the ambivalence some of them feel about their abusers; and from the propensity many of them have to develop relationships that are predatory and abusive, on the one hand, or masochistic and victimized, on the other.

DISTRUST OF POWER AND AUTHORITY

A child who has been fundamentally betrayed in a relationship with a parent, caretaker, or other parent substitute often expects similar betrayal in future relationships, especially from those he perceives as authorities. His ability to form attachments is seriously compromised by his internalization of authority figures as treacherous and undependable. He consequently develops the sense that he will be betrayed by those he cares about and trusts. Wariness and anxiety about interpersonal encounters influence all relationships for such a man.

Isaac described feeling endangered when he was singled out by an authority. He had returned to college in his forties, and he became so alarmed when a professor openly praised his work that he left the class. Anxious and intimidated by this attention from someone with power, unsure whether it had some sexual implications, he never returned to the course, taking an incomplete grade instead.

For Lorenzo, distrust stemming from molestations by men in his small town was compounded by the reactions of a trusted priest to whom he confided information about the abuse and his own growing sense that he was gay. By the time he was fifteen, Lorenzo had had numerous exploitative sexual encounters in which he sexually serviced older boys and men, all of whom were publicly identified as heterosexual, and many of whom were married. Confused about the meaning of his own behavior, and only vaguely knowledgeable about sexual orientation, he did nevertheless begin to wonder if he were gay. He had no idea who to talk to about this in the working-class mill town in which he grew up. Then he remembered a priest who had once served in the town for two years before being transferred to a large city three hundred miles away. He'd always thought this priest was "cool," and so he called him and said he needed to talk to him. The priest came to Lorenzo's town for a visit, and Lorenzo first told him about his abuse experiences and then said he thought he was gay. "He looked at me and said, 'I knew you were gay the minute I laid eyes on you!' So, I said, 'Why didn't you tell me?' and he said, 'Some things are better to discover on your own.' So, at first he was good about it—he invited me to visit him, and when I did he took me around the city and showed me gay neighborhoods, gay bars, gay shops. That part was good, but then we went back to the house he lived in with other priests, and I wanted to get high—I was a crazy kid in those days, and I asked him where to get grass. He said, 'No problem, just go upstairs and ask Father Donald.' So I went upstairs, and there was nice Father Donald, and we got high together, and then he made a pass at me." Lorenzo laughed. "It was the first time anyone serviced *me*, and I really liked it. When I went downstairs and told the first priest about it, he said, 'Oh, sure, Father Donald does that with everyone.' Can you believe this? He *knew* what was going to happen when he sent me up there! Later, I found out he was gay too, and had sex with other boys, though never with me." Lorenzo was talking faster and faster, and I asked him to slow down and tell me what he felt about all this. "I thought it was funny. And exciting." Then he paused. "But, you know, I'm thirty-five now, about the age Father Donald was then. I have no interest in fifteen-year-olds! My nephews are that age! I'd never go near them for sex." I asked again how he felt about what happened with the two priests. For the first time, he seemed reflective. "It was a terrible thing to do. They knew how fucked up I was about sex with all those men, and how unsure I was about being gay. I went to them for sanctuary! And they just helped me party with them." Lorenzo began to look sad. "In those days I really believed in the Catholic Church. No more."

The anticipation of betrayal may take the form of fears, fantasies, or even outright expectations of inappropriate sexual advances. Thus, in our initial meetings Seth focused on the facts that my office is situated in a hotel and that I have a couch in it that he felt could serve as a bed. Reminded of the circumstances of his molestation in a hotel room by a family friend, his anxiety overwhelmed him and interfered with his ability to form a relationship with me. In order to continue our consultation, he had to remind himself that he rationally understood my professional status and believed I must be ethical since I was recommended by a therapist he had grown to trust over many years. Greg had a comparable phobic response when he first met me, which I will discuss in Chapter 11. Being the stimulus for these men's panic was difficult for me. I felt compassion and empathy for each of them, yet they both instantly experienced me as toxic and dangerous. While on one level I understood this as a transference reaction, I was viscerally unsettled by the contrast between their reactions and my usual sense of myself as a relatively warm and calming presence in my consulting room. When they started group therapy, these feelings were reactivated for both Seth and Greg, and they became intensely anxious and distrustful about being in a group of men whom they felt could overpower and control them.

The power differential between child and abuser can dramatically affect the boy in later life (Dimock, 1988). This may emerge as a need to control the partner in a relationship. Power has been eroticized during sexual abuse. It was through power and control that a boy was introduced to sexuality, so his adult sexual relationships are often driven by attempts to regain and maintain control and power over an intimate other. Thus, love relationships cannot be shared partnerships. Instead, they become arenas for power plays about who is in charge and in control. Lewis, for example, had such a need for control in intimate relationships that he had thrown partners across the room if he even momentarily felt they were physically taking charge during lovemaking.

To an abused boy, vulnerability often becomes associated with powerlessness. In adult relationships, he either needs complete control, as Lewis did, or when feeling vulnerable he anxiously reacts as if he were still powerless and needed to pacify authorities. Consider, for example, Abe, whom I discuss more fully later in this chapter. He was explicitly told by his father that it was his job in life to take care of his capricious, imperious, and narcissistic mother. Abe both adored and hated her, and tried hard to please her. He usually failed, however, and would then be subject to ferocious lambastings by her, and then again by his father when the father had to deal with the mother's subsequent viciousness. Abe expressed his anger about his burden by being antisocial in other relationships. Then he became afraid his antisocial behavior would infuriate his mother. He recalled once bringing home a report card that listed excellent academic grades but contained highly negative comments about his interpersonal skills. He wrote his mother an elaborate and distraught letter of apology, which he placed next to the report card, strewing the table around them with rose petals in a futile attempt to appease her. As an adult, he anxiously gave presents to people he felt he had displeased, as well as to those who were abusive to him. He felt powerless and vulnerable in relation to them, and hoped that these presents could somehow placate them and keep them from attacking him. It simply never occurred to him that he could be directly confrontative or survive their disapproval.

Abe's sexual betrayal by his mother involved mostly covert seductive excitation and overstimulation. Hypervigilant anxiety like Abe's, bordering on paranoia, has been especially noted in the literature on men who were incestuously involved on an overt level with their mothers (Margolis, 1977, 1984; Rothstein, 1979; Shengold, 1980, 1989; Gabbard and Twemlow, 1994). Rothstein believes this anxiety originates in a feeling that their mothers will ridicule them if they do not perform adequately. Gabbard and Twemlow (1994) elaborate on this idea, writing that this anxiety relates to a "feeling that one's role as the narcissistic extension of mother is a precarious one contingent on doing her bidding. These men often feel they are walking on a tightrope that could lead to catastrophe if they make one misstep that displeases mother" (p. 184). Should this happen, the boy may experience himself as his mother's inadequate lover. If he has internalized male gender expectations, this can be a source of further shame and despair, since men expect themselves to be sexually skilled and potent. Dread of failing his mother may exist dissociatively, side by side with the sense of specialness and entitlement also common in men who were sexually betrayed by their mothers (see my discussion of maternal sexual betrayal in Chapter 2, as well as Sue Shapiro's description in Chapter 10 of sexually abused men's inflated sense of their seductive powers).

MAINTAINING EMOTIONAL
AND SEXUAL DISTANCE

A common way to fend off the anxiety that accompanies a sexually abused man's interpersonal relationships is to keep them as distant, formal, and emotionless as possible. When relating is traumatic and he is phobic about emotional attachment, he can only allow himself to be emotionally cool and removed. Whether consciously or unconsciously, Andreas, Beau, Devin, and Patrick all attempted, with varying degrees of success, to keep their interpersonal relationships as distant and free of feeling as possible. In this section I will describe how this process worked for Keith and Willem.

Although Keith seemed friendly and well-related, there was an inner wall that kept him removed from others. Consider his relationships with his wife and with me:

Keith's roller-coaster, incestuously tinged relationship with his mother, coupled with his emotional and later physical abandonment by his father, left him guarded and vigilant in his adult relationships. He married his wife at a time when she suffered from a very serious illness that seemed likely to cause her early death. He was universally admired by their friends for his loyalty to her, but privately he himself felt he had only been able to commit to her because he was convinced the marriage would be brief. When she did not die, he was fatalistic about the chances of their relationship lasting, saying he did not believe any relationship could endure over time. He continued to keep himself removed from her emotionally, consciously reasoning that he needed to protect himself in anticipation of their inevitable breakup. This logic seemed sound to him in light of his experiences with his seductive mother and his parents' inability to achieve good relationships with one another or with subsequent spouses.

The emotional distance from his wife extended to their sexual relationship. Keith described his ambivalence about intimate sexuality with his wife: "She isn't satisfied with her sex life. She says she wants to be 'engulfed by my masculinity.' But I don't want to engulf her, to merge with her like I did with my mother." Instead, Keith held back from her both emotionally and sexually, despite his own and his wife's longing at times for greater intimacy.

Our work together evoked Keith's intimacy problems again and again. Keith frequently tested me, both to see if I would abandon him and to monitor whether I would get suffocatingly close. Would I call back if he had an emergency? Would I allow him to reschedule an appointment at the last minute? Would I accept his going on a quickly arranged vacation without becoming punitive? He explored his own hopelessness about relationships, and his growing commitment to treatment bespoke a wish to come to terms with it. He noticed small shifts toward trust in his outside relationships. Yet such a transformation must perforce be very slow, and neither he nor I could know how far he would ultimately change as he continued to face his history.

In contrast to Keith, Willem was openly distant in his interpersonal relationships. He maintained such a coolness in relation to others that he believed he had no relationships whatsoever, nor did he acknowledge or remember a history of relating closely to others in his earlier life.

Willem grew up in a European country, the son of an alcoholic mother who had a series of husbands, boyfriends, and one-night sex partners. He had no doubt about the veracity of his vague and disturbing memories of direct abuse, apparently by one or more of these men. He also believed he witnessed his mother's sexual relations with them at times. His own father left the family when he was about three, and Willem had no memories of him, except for a visceral feeling of fright and danger when his name was mentioned. The one time he visited his paternal grandparents, they also scared him. At the time we first met, he did not know if his father was still alive.

Willem felt rootless because of his mother's unstable relationships. This feeling was magnified when she married her third husband. He was a man whose career took the family to live abroad in other cultures for a year or so at a time, so any friendships Willem made ended after a brief time. Yet this was the only period of his childhood during which he had a sense of a cohesive family.

Shortly after his mother and her third husband divorced, the mother died suddenly. He was never told the cause of her death. Willem was twelve, and went with his ten-year-old sister to live with his maternal grandparents. He recalled this household as gloomy, grim, and filled with bickering. He was glad to be sent away to boarding school after a year and a half, although he felt guilty about the sister he sexually abused during this period (see my discussion of this abuse later in this chapter).

As an adult, Willem had great success in a career that required keen intellectual prowess and analytic ability. He maintained that he had no feelings, and indeed his emotional life was sparse, barren, and brittle. He had acquaintances, but no friends, and on the surface he had no capacity to bond to others. He had married in his mid-twenties, and when his wife divorced him five years later he precipitously tried to commit suicide in a particularly lethal way. His life was saved, and he entered an inpatient psychiatric facility from which he emerged more openly vulnerable, needy, and dependent. He quit his career, and was convinced to start outpatient psychotherapy.

Willem called me for a referral, saying he could only work with a woman, and I referred him to a female colleague. About eight months later, she referred him back to me for group therapy. His decision to see me and join the group was in essence a decision to face his internal demons about men. Willem's deep suspicion of men originated both in his shadowy memories of sexual abuse by his mother's boyfriends and/or husbands, and in the fear surrounding his internal image of his own father. These feelings made it very difficult for him to consider seeing a male therapist or to enter a group of men. Intellectually, however, he realized that he was desperately in need of a supportive network, such as the one he had found during his inpatient hospitalization. Additionally, he said he wanted to face his fears of men and their ramifications in his life.

For a period of time, his other therapist and I devised, at his request, an unusual joint treatment in which he attended the group and saw both his female therapist and me for individual work. This diluted the intensity of his bond to each of us. Paradoxically, however, by engaging in attenuated relationships with us, he was able to further attach to us both, since he felt less threatened by the intimacy of each situation.

In sessions with me, Willem was wary, seemingly waiting for me to make a false move. Over the course of our work together, he repeatedly demanded more connection to me than he felt he had. Each time we addressed this issue, however, he seemed to disappear. He either canceled appointments because of other commitments or came to sessions and just sat there, impassive and impermeable.

Nevertheless, we made progress. In our early contacts, we went over Willem's history and saw how little he knew about his early life or family origins. He then decided to try to find out about his mother's death. He made international calls, wrote to the appropriate authorities, and eventually received copies of his mother's death certificate and the transcript of the inquest that followed her sudden death. He was shocked, and yet not totally surprised, to discover that she had committed suicide. He tried to integrate the little information he had about her depression and alcoholism with his memories of her dour parents and his frightening picture of his own father and paternal grandparents. The court records reported on Willem's depressed emotional state before and after his mother's death, and he found it comforting to realize that someone had tried to understand him when he was a child. As he considered his mother's death, his own suicide attempt became more understandable as an unconscious repetition of her suicide. His need not to rely on other people or to create bonds with them also seemed reasonable in this context. As he confronted these themes, he gained a clearer sense of wanting to live and accomplish something important in his own life. He eventually decided to pursue a career in which he could advocate for abuse victims.

After a few months, his other therapist and I consulted with one another, with Willem's permission, and decided that to continue to allow him to see us simultaneously would reinforce Willem's problems in committing himself to either of us. He agreed in principle that it was a good idea to see only one of us individually, but he wanted us to decide for him which of us he should see. We refused to make the decision for him, and he struggled between preferring to see her or me. He told me he experienced her as nurturing and comforting, but vague and nondirective. At the same time, he said he found me impenetrable and uninvolved, although incisive and able to stir him up in frightening ways that might ultimately be positive for him. I told him I did not think it mattered which of us he chose, since he had some positive feelings about each of us, but that it was very important that he make a commitment to one person and stick with it. Willem eventually chose to work with his female therapist.

Willem's commitment problem remained a constant. He periodically dropped out of one therapy or the other, ostensibly for financial reasons, often without informing the other therapist about what he had done. Despite this, he made remarkable strides in the rest of his life. Having originally stated that he had "no history," meaning virtually no early memories and no relationships with anyone from his childhood, he eventually contacted the sister he had abused, who was very glad to hear from him. He learned from her that he had a maternal uncle who was interested in seeing him. She even told him that his father had resurfaced, and that his stories about the parents' marriage made him a far more sympathetic figure than he had seemed during their childhood. He recontacted former friends in his native country, and began to observe with some emotion that his pattern in adult life of moving from city to city, job to job, and girlfriend to girlfriend reflected an understandable but devastating incapacity to connect to others. Progress in these areas was slow, but when he left the group after two years, again giving financial reasons, he had partially healed in the area of relating to men, and he was no longer a man without a history.

RAGE: ONE EMOTION ALLOWED TO MEN

We saw in Chapter 3 that masculine gender norms endorse anger as one of the few emotions open to men (Bruckner and Johnson, 1987; Lew, 1988; Sepler, 1990; Struve, 1990; Isely, 1992), and that rage is the only affect many sexually traumatized men can express (Dimock, 1988; Sepler, 1990). As Crowder (1995) puts it, "Anger is powerful and energy-filled and it is an affective state that is egosyntonic with masculine cultural roles. Anger and rage can become a 'catchall' emotion for male victims. Because it is a powerful and active emotion, expressing anger is more acceptable than displaying more vulnerable emotions" (p. 24). In many cases, underlying sadness, loss, and desolation are hidden beneath this rage. But Crowder notes that "male survivors tend to be able to contact their anger and rage at having been abused long before they can feel their grief. They often display active and violent revenge fantasies. Women survivors, on the other hand, are initially more in touch with their sadness and depression" (p. 38).

The consequences of a furious mode of living in the world are obvious in men who become sexually or emotionally predatory or abusive as adults. Many nonabusive men, however, also live with an unbridled rage that affects their capacity for intimacy and the quality of their relationships. In Quinn's case, discussed later in this chapter, his anger stayed front and center for years as he confronted his abuse by his grandfather. While he never acted out his rage antisocially, it frequently broke through, affecting his ability to work with supervisors and clients, and influencing his more personal relationships as well.

Quinn's considerable rage was easy to recognize, but consider the monumental fury underneath Beau's seemingly quiet, passive, and polite exterior. This fury flowed unchecked and periodically overwhelmed him, nearly drowning him in its intensity. Beau, having had emotionally unsupportive and victimizing parents, was raped by three student athletes and a coach in high school, and then was further victimized by many other students. During his college years, he continued to be sneered at and derided by classmates. He was hospitalized for psychiatric reasons three times between the ages of eighteen and twenty-six. Each hospitalization was precipitated by an explosion of temper following a dissociative episode in which he felt the ground or furniture moving. During the hospitalizations, his feelings emerged about the rape and its aftermath, about being gay, and about his extreme sense of being ostracized and not belonging anywhere.

In the meantime, Beau put his energies into doing well academically. He remained emotionally isolated, telling himself there were good reasons to distrust every group he encountered: gays and straights, men and women, every racial and ethnic group. He had superficial relationships with one or two gay men and had two brief love affairs. Neither relationship lasted long, and together they further embittered him. When the second affair ended, he moved to New York City. There, he met older men who took him away for weekends and bought him expensive gifts. While ambivalent about the mercenary character of these relationships, he rationalized that he had the right to take what he could from these wealthy men, since his expectation was that they would exploit him and then desert him.

Beau took a job that kept him in contact with teenage boys. This was highly conflictual for him. He was attracted to the boys, and they presented a temptation he had to be careful not to act on. Yet he also seemed to communicate to them his vulnerability to being manipulated or abused by them, and he was apparently the frequent butt of homophobic jokes and derision. Even though he was nominally the adult authority in these relationships, he reexperienced with the boys the helplessness he had felt with the student athletes who had raped him. He considered himself these boys' victim while also being attracted to them and feeling seduced by them. The combination of feeling seduction, arousal, fear, and rage in these interpersonal situations periodically plunged him into dissociative episodes on the job. On one such occasion, he left his workplace and traveled to another part of the city while in a fugue state.

Because of these problems on the job, Beau, then in his late twenties, sought individual psychotherapy, and a few months later was referred to my group for sexually abused men. Seemingly gentle and soft-spoken, for the first few weeks after entering the group he was quiet, hardly appearing to attend to what others said. Eventually, he started to talk about his trouble relating to the teenage boys at work. In particular, he focused on his susceptibility to being sexually aroused by them and his fury at them. At this point, group members asked more about his internal experience. As he described his feelings, he suddenly erupted in a frenzy I have seldom seen outside an inpatient unit. With his face distorted by rage and his body moving half out of his chair, he railed inchoately about his rapes and his fury at abusive men and cruel women. After ten minutes of near-psychotic fury, he collapsed, weeping and gasping for air. The group was hushed as he exploded, but afterward most of the men talked about identifying with his rage, some in fear they might similarly erupt, others in envy that they were unable to do so. Each understood Beau's rage from firsthand experience, and seemed not to be afraid during his outburst.

RESPONSIBILITY FOR OTHERS' FEELINGS

We have seen that boys often feel responsible for their abuse. This feeling has several sources. Being responsible for one's fate is part of the socialized masculine gender ideals every boy internalizes to some extent. In addition, boys often attribute their abuse to having given off a message saying they were interested in sex with their abuser or were vulnerable to predators in general. This may be compounded by an abuser telling the boy that this is happening because the boy is so handsome and desirable, or because the victimizer loves him so much, or because the abuser knows this is what the boy "really" wants. The abuser thus confirms that it is the boy's fault that he is being molested. In addition, abused boys may have been told implicitly or explicitly that they are responsible for their family's well-being, or for the mental health of one of their parents.

The boy's sense of responsibility for his abuse may build to a generalized sense of responsibility for everything that happens to him and for the emotional health of those around him. Abe, Andreas, and Owen all provide examples of this dynamic. Its pervasiveness for Victor came to light in the following incident:

One day Victor arrived back at his office from our session and found that his supervisor had forgotten to cover for him, although this was a standing arrangement they had made for his therapy appointment. He called me anxiously and explained that we had to change our appointment time so that this would not happen again. The next day he called again and said he would be able to keep the usual time. When he came to his session, he began to talk about his reactions to tension in the air at work. He said he had assumed that the anxiety in the office when he returned was about his absence, that he had gotten panicky about his job, and so he had called to change our appointment. Upon reflection, however, he realized that his bosses were stressed about something unrelated to anything that had happened when he was gone. "When I feel tension in the air, I assume it's about me, and I have to give in or submit to whatever is demanded, whether it's at work or with my family or with my lover." By the time he got to my office, he seemed both resentful of his supervisors and of me because he assumed I was put out by his call and I had not wanted to accommodate his wish to change the appointment time. I pointed this out and he agreed, "Yes, after I give in or submit, I get very angry at whoever it is I give in to, and I create scenarios about their being disagreeable or uncaring about my needs."

Recall that, while molesting Victor, his father would tell him the abuse was happening because he loved him and because Victor was so handsome. Victor's sense of being responsible for the abuse was compounded by the sexual pleasure he felt simultaneously with his disgust and shame. In addition, he felt that the nightly molestations calmed his father down and kept the family somewhat more peaceful than it otherwise would have been. He remembered how he felt when his father got tense or angry. The father would cry out, "If it weren't for all of you I wouldn't have to be here—I'd be free!" Victor said he accepted the blame for his father's moods. He added, however, that his current reactions of feeling responsible for others were also colored by his history with his mother. She would tell Victor he was perfect and worth all the sacrifices she made: the job she hated, the marriage she was stuck in. Feeling responsible for his mother's disappointments, Victor again reacted with anxiety. He felt as trapped as each of his parents felt in their marriage. The reactions to the incident at work were influenced, then, by the guilt and fear he felt in relation to both parents, the responsibility he felt for their unhappiness and for easing their pain, and the resentment he ultimately felt about this dynamic.

DIFFERENTIATING ABUSE FROM OTHER
INTERPERSONAL DYNAMICS

Men with sexual abuse histories may have little real sense of the differences among sex, love, nurturance, affection, and abuse. For them, these concepts are roughly equivalent. As Price (1994) notes, "Intimacy becomes identified with abuse, exploitation, sexuality, engulfment, and enmeshment" (p. 213). The origins of this confusion are chillingly described by the protagonist of Heim's *Mysterious Skin* (1995) ten years after he was abused by the baseball coach he idolized at age eight:

> "He had chosen me, you know? Out of all the boys on the team, he'd picked me. Like I'd been blessed or something. He taught me things no other boy on the team or at school could know. I was *his.* . . . Coach took me to the movies, told me I was his star player. He stuffed me full of candy and let me win a trillion video games. And then he was there, on top of me on the kitchen floor, rubbing his dick against my bare belly." (p. 285; emphasis added)

For this lonely boy, the affection, nurturance, and love he felt from and for his coach became indelibly identified with sexuality, abuse, and exploitation.

Misidentifying relational experiences is an adult sequel to the sexually abused child's "confusion of tongues" between the languages of tenderness and passion described by Ferenczi in 1933 (see also Gelinas, 1983; Johanek, 1988; Ganzarain and Buchele, 1990). Explaining his near-phobia about emotion-laden experiences, Keith said, "For me, violation means intimacy, and intimacy means violation. Someone has an emotional flareup and I want to dive into it. I *fuck* it, I become one with it, I feel those raw emotions again, like I did with my mother. Then I wind up being the caretaker of the person with all the emotions."

For me, the best illustration of how sexuality, love, nurturance, affection, and abuse get confused for sexually abused men lies in the words of Abe, whom I describe later in this chapter. A man who suffered from exceptionally inappropriate seductive overstimulation as well as verbal abuse, Abe said one day in despair: "No one will ever love me unless I'm completely their servant. So I bring gifts to people who have abused me, I allow sadistic sex. I don't yet know to what lengths I'll go to feel loved. I keep returning to that wonderful cozy nest of abuse and incest. It's a sewer and yet it's my spiritual home. Why do I continue to allow abuse as an adult? Because when I'm being abused, someone's attention is completely focused on me. I know that's not love, but it really feels like love." Abe summed up his family's confusion of love and abuse in a motto often repeated to him by both parents: "It's better that we shit on you than that someone else kisses you." In other words, their abuse was the best love he could hope for in life.

In a psychology where emotions are blurred this way, affection is highly suspect and is experienced as both sexual and abusive, erotic and violating. Abe, for example, at one point acknowledged that any interpersonal movement toward him, even a dinner invitation, could be experienced as hurtful and abusive. This distorted view of positive relatedness was poignantly highlighted by a verbal slip made by Xavier, who once said, "I was depraved [sic] of love by my family."

Long-term, arduous work is required in psychotherapy before a man can begin to allow himself to embrace more freely his own loving feelings. Cory inadvertently discovered he had begun to make this shift after his wife suffered a miscarriage. In wonderment, he said, "I had let myself love it. I didn't even worry about the pain I feel now. And even though I cried all this week, I know now that I've opened up a big wonderful space in my heart where there had been a void—and I can love my child—I can love my child when I have *me*."

AMBIVALENCE ABOUT BEING SEXUAL

The difficulty differentiating sexuality, love, nurturance, affection, and abuse has many consequences for relationships involving intimacy, sexuality, and/or love. It also affects a sexually abused man's relationship to himself as a sexual being. Having experienced his first sexual arousal in an abusive context, he links sexuality to "coercion, nonmutual exchange, and sometimes violence. . . . The pairing of secrecy and sexual arousal often leaves a victim feeling very ashamed of his sexuality, especially if he senses that his sexual expression is deviant. Some survivors are unaware that their sexual behavior has been shaped by abuse processes and they believe that they are misfits or weird or crazy because of the nature of their sexual desires and expression" (Crowder, 1995, p. 32).

"Although incest is an abuse of power, it is also an abuse of sexuality" (Price, 1994, p. 224); this abuse causes distortions about all sexual situations. Experiencing erotic excitement becomes negatively charged. As Victor succinctly put it, "All pleasure is bad. Do you know why? It's bad that my father is touching my penis. His touching my penis gives me pleasure. Therefore, it's bad to have pleasure." Victor elaborated on the ambivalence he developed about sexual arousal with his father: "I hated when my father talked to me while he touched me. He'd say, 'You're so big, you're so hard, you know Daddy loves you and that's why he does this.' But I don't think I ever believed him. I felt like a hooker when he said that. I'd rather he would have just touched me, and kept quiet. At least it felt good and I didn't have to think about it being my father who was doing it. When he touched me, he'd open my pajamas and by the time I woke up he'd have fished my dick out and it would be hard. I'd let him touch it for a while—then I'd get upset and I'd turn over. He'd beg me to turn back. Sometimes he'd sigh and say 'OK, if that's how you want it,' and I'd feel guilty. I felt I wasn't doing what a good son would do. So I'd turn around again and let him continue, and he'd be so grateful." Noting one Pyrrhic victory in his struggle about sexuality and abuse, Victor forlornly concluded, "At least I never came with him—I always made him stop before I came."

Lorenzo, a gay man who had numerous presumably heterosexual male abusers as a boy, said one day that he felt shame whenever he experienced sexual desire. "I realized one day that I was in the gym, looking around, admiring men's bodies, not coming on to them, but feeling attracted and yet terribly ashamed of my desires. It was crazy—I felt like a pedophile, even though these men were my own age and I have no interest in children. I couldn't understand it, but then all of a sudden it hit me. The men who abused me had no shame about what they did. They invited me to come give them blow jobs when I was as young as eight and nine, and then I'd see them in church with their wives or on the street, and they were totally casual, pillars of the community. Sometimes it was as though they hardly knew who I was. *So I took on their shame!* I took it in. They couldn't own it, so I did—*and I still do!* I walk around feeling my desire, and feeling I'm terrible for having desire, that desire itself is abusive. I feel the shame they should have felt but never did!"

Not surprisingly, many sexually abused men feel ambivalent about being sexual at all. They have learned to be extremely wary both about their own sexual feelings and about sexual approaches from others. (In this, they resemble sexually abused women.) Sexual situations, or situations interpreted by the man as including sexual elements, tend to bring up the dissociative defenses he learned as a boy while being abused. Sexual dysfunctions are common among these men, including lowered or excessive sexual desire, sexual aversion, erectile disorder, inhibited orgasm, and premature ejaculation (Glaser, 1998).

Hugo, a gay man in his forties, was seventeen when he went through the last of a series of molestations by older male cousins. "I was trying to express my anger at the way I was being treated, so I willed myself not to have an erection, and I succeeded. I only meant for *that* night! But the result was I could never again have a spontaneous erection with anyone I cared about." As a result, he spent years trying to negotiate satisfying relationships, knowing all the time how "defective" he was in comparison with the men to whom he was attracted and whom he tried to engage intimately. Not until the drug Viagra came on the market was he able to achieve erections regularly when he felt aroused. Only at that point did Hugo realize the extent to which his sense of masculinity and power had been compromised by his impotence. He had to mourn the losses to his self-concept from twenty years of battling paralyzing shame, self-doubt, and feelings of inadequacy whenever he tried to be sexual in a related, intimate way.

An additional problem about being sexual involves the shame a sexually abused man attaches to having been abused. This shame often becomes associated with all sexual arousal (Rusinoff and Gerber, 1990; also see Hastings, 1998), so that arousal itself becomes shameful. Also, if a man restimulates memories and fantasies about his abuse experience, he may confuse these with sexual desire (Briere, 1995), which may add to his shamed and phobic response to sexuality. One goal of treatment in such cases is to separate out and attempt to repair these feelings.

In the course of their psychotherapies, both Andreas and Cory became aware of severe dissociation during the sex act. Andreas "functioned" sexually with his wife but felt physically and psychically numb. Cory had felt physically paralyzed as a nineteen-year-old when a male college dorm counselor tried to seduce him. In adulthood, he continued to dissociate during sex: "Once I get things going in sex, I can just turn the machine on automatic and leave."

Some sexually abused men avoid interpersonal sexuality altogether. Others may attempt to manage sexual relationships while suffering from the ambiguous intensity they experience during intimacy. The pain of this situation was summed up by Cory when on various occasions he said, laughing but only half-humorous, "The trouble with sex is there's always someone in your face," and "I don't want any spontaneity in sex unless I know what's going to happen," and "If you really think about sex and all that happens in it, who would ever want it?"

SEXUALITY AS INTERPERSONAL CURRENCY

On the other hand, a child whose sexuality has been compromised by early abuse and eroticized relationships learns that sexuality and seduction constitute his interpersonal currency. Having learned that his sexuality is valuable to others, he may make it the basis for his self-esteem. If that happens, sexuality permeates all his interpersonal encounters. In addition, interpersonal closeness often becomes eroticized because sex is the only way for the man to feel intimate (or seemingly intimate).

Hungry for interpersonal contact but phobic about it, believing that sexual closeness is his chief opportunity to feel loved but experiencing love as abuse, a sexually abused man who allows himself to be sexual at all often solves his dilemma by engaging in frequent, indiscriminate, and dissociated sexual encounters. These are not free or joyous expressions of hedonistic, lusty sensuality. Rather, they represent a man's imprisonment in an empty behavioral circuit from which he feels there is no exit. Incessantly pursuing sex, he nevertheless achieves very little intimacy. Nonmonogamous sex is not necessarily bad, but it is often not fully intimate (Glaser, 1998), especially when it involves compulsive seeking after partners. In these situations, a man usually looks for sexual release to allay his anxiety rather than because he feels sexually interested in or aroused by another person. He is momentarily soothed by impersonal expressions of sexuality, much as he might be by other compulsive or addictive behaviors like drinking, taking drugs, or overeating. Yet he does not feel loved once the sex act is concluded. These incidents leave him feeling empty and lonely, while the idea of fully pursuing interpersonal relatedness fills him with a dread of repeating his abuse history.

While it is not uncommon for men who have been sexually abused to become sexually abusive as adults (see below), these men, like their female counterparts, often enough find adult relationships in which they themselves are sexually abused or otherwise exploited. Such relationships often include boundaryless merging with the loved one, so that the man is eternally anxious about being left, never feels capable of having independent thoughts or feelings, and increasingly wants to devour and be devoured by his mate. Sometimes a man alternates impersonal compulsive sexuality with a drivenness to merge with a partner, with each tendency balancing and saving him from the excesses of the other. Either way, he ends up continuing to feel unloved while striving to regain a momentary sense of being loveable.

Examples of how sexually abused men express these conflicts include Chet and Patrick. Chet, a straight man who became an icon of the underground counterculture, went to bed with countless groupies while simultaneously drowning in intense, boundaryless love affairs. Patrick was a gay man who would return to the city from holiday visits to his abusive family and go directly to the back rooms of gay bars, where he would fellate dozens of men.

Some men use their sexuality to get what they need, to bond to authorities, and to manipulate others if necessary. What may have started as a desperate means of keeping some sense of power in a relationship where he is outmatched becomes a man's characteristic way of relating. This can create considerable grandiosity about his sexual prowess and unrealistic expectations about his influence over others. This grandiosity is an attempt to transform trauma and helplessness into omnipotence and control. In adulthood, it can turn into a general sense of unrealistic entitlement that is in line with a child's developmental level, both cognitively and psychologically (Price, 1994).

Victor was forced to confront his inflated view of his seductive powers when he heard Gene, a married man in his therapy group, talk about experimenting with bisexuality. Victor realized that he was angry at Gene. At first he thought his anger resulted from his feeling that Gene was ignoring his wife and children when he had liaisons with men. Then, as he spoke, he suddenly blushed, saying that he had just realized that deep down he was jealous because he himself was not the object of Gene's desire. Victor was very surprised by this insight. He had not thought that he was even attracted to Gene, and observed that he had only become interested as he began to think of Gene as bisexual. He then confessed that he was often attracted to bisexual men. This led him to acknowledge a previously disowned adolescent fantasy that his father would take him away from the family and they would live together with Victor as his father's lover. In this fantasy, Victor's passion and love for his father would transform the father into a loving man capable of supporting Victor emotionally. His father would then be consistently warm with Victor, as he often seemed to be during the abuse, when he would praise Victor's looks and abilities, in marked contrast to the competitive and jeering attitude he evinced toward Victor during the day. Victor then began to think about his relationship with his much older male lover, and how he often fantasized about transforming the lover through his passion. During this fantasy, he made his lover into a far colder, angrier, and more punishing man than the lover actually was. Victor came to realize that in the fantasy about Gene, Victor's great passion for him would transform Gene from the cold, automaton-like person he sometimes seemed to be into a passionate and emotional human being. From here, we were able to consider how Victor's abuse led him to become grandiose about his expectations of power over men, expectations that often led him to confusion and disappointment.

Like Victor, Ramon had a sense of himself as someone whose worth and power were defined by his sexuality. For Ramon, however, such distortions were far more pervasive and damaging. While his psychological dysfunction arose from a number of sources, his childhood sexual abuse was a central part of his personality organization.

When he first came to see me, Ramon was a forty-year-old man who for the first time in his life was about to start formal training for a career, following years of drug addiction, drug dealing, jail, psychiatric hospitalizations, and rehab. At the time I first met him, he had been drug-free for two years. He had been diagnosed as schizoaffective, with both bipolar and paranoid symptomatology, but a combination of antipsychotic and mood-stabilizing medications had helped him achieve relative psychological balance. He was deeply disturbed, however, about memories of child sexual abuse that were breaking through his thoughts at all times of the day, and he was afraid that these thoughts would make it impossible for him to study. Nevertheless, he could not bring himself to seek help and find a therapist. Instead, his girlfriend made calls all over the country, located me, and made the initial call and appointment for him. She accompanied him to that consultation and stayed in the waiting room while he hesitantly followed me into my office.

A likeable man with remnants of the Latin good looks that had made him the object of many adults' desire as a child and teenager, Ramon stuttered, cried, and seemed to be falling apart before my eyes as he tried to tell me about his first molestation. I stopped him gently and said he did not have to go into it quite yet, that perhaps we should get to know each other first. I asked him about the rest of his life.

Breathing a sigh of relief, Ramon began to tell me about his years of drug dependence and small-time drug dealing, and then of his decision "to be decent" and get sober after nine failed attempts in various rehab programs. His girlfriend, a high-achieving professional woman, had been a major steadying and supportive influence on him, and had stayed with him throughout the rough period while he was getting sober. He now had several friends who were "productive and made contributions to society," as he wanted to, but he was afraid he could not manage the training ahead of him because he had had academic difficulties throughout school. In addition, he feared his childhood memories would engulf him and prevent him from concentrating on anything else in his life. These memories were already ravaging him. He had never talked about them to anyone, afraid they might consume him even more if he did, but he had begun to realize that he had no choice: not talking about them no longer worked to keep them out of his consciousness.

Ramon's father, a merchant seaman who was rarely home, was physically abusive to his wife when he did appear. He deserted the family, and the parents divorced when Ramon was six. Ramon did not see his father again for fifteen years. After his father left, Ramon seems to have been left to shift for himself while his mother worked. When he was eight, he was invited to the house of Sam, a well-known neighborhood "character" who delighted children with his impromptu sidewalk puppet shows. Once there, Sam amused Ramon with his puppetry, then began to caress him. Sam cajoled Ramon into letting Sam undress him, then he lubricated Ramon and penetrated him anally. That night, Ramon bled profusely, and for several days he stuffed tissues inside his shorts to stanch the blood. This was the first of many similar visits to

Sam, who always treated Ramon in a loving manner while molesting him. With time, Ramon yearned to spend more and more time with Sam, the only seemingly caring and kindhearted adult in his life. Ramon therefore often greeted Sam affectionately when they met in the street. The abuse went on for two years. Ramon cannot remember how or why it stopped, though he knows Sam moved out of the neighborhood. Ramon described his relationship with Sam in conflicted terms. Continuing yearning, desire, and regret alternated with shame and depression. He reported, however, that when at age thirty he saw Sam on the street one day he got so enraged that he tried, unsuccessfully, to buy a gun to kill him.

After Sam moved away, Ramon regularly met another man who originally approached him in his schoolyard. They went on car rides together and the man molested Ramon in the car. Ramon would also go to the park from age ten to twelve, often allowing himself to be picked up by both men and women who would engage in sex with him. Money or expensive gifts were often exchanged for the sex.

During this period, Ramon frequently accompanied his mother to bars, where she would meet men and go out with them. He tried to dictate the men to whom she could talk. She didn't always listen to him, and they fought when he became insistent. Eventually, finding him unmanageable, she sent Ramon to a military boarding school in her native city.

After his return to New York City at about age fifteen, Ramon met an older, wealthy gay man who invited Ramon to live with him. While the two never directly engaged in sex with one another, this man often gave Ramon body rubs with oil and on numerous occasions watched Ramon have sex with women and men whom he would procure for Ramon. Ramon lived with this man until the man lost interest in him. Ramon assumed he was no longer enticing to this man because he was getting too old to be physically attractive and was too stupid to be appealing on any other level. At age nineteen, Ramon married a somewhat older woman who seemed willing to take care of him. The marriage lasted a year.

Ramon was afraid that being in therapy would make him discover he was gay or bisexual. He had not had sex with a man since he was eighteen and had no sexual fantasies about men in general; but he was aware of intense excitement when he remembered being molested by the puppeteer. He did not have these feelings when thinking about any other men, but the excitement he felt when remembering his original abuse haunted and confused him. He had no way of understanding it except to think he was gay or bisexual. This perplexed him because he said he liked sex with women and claimed not have any sexual interest in men.

On the other hand, Ramon said he sometimes did not care whether he was with a man or a woman, that his strongest motivation was to make sure his partner did not leave him. "They always left, even though they seemed to care so much about being with me. Every time I was with someone, I figured, I've got this one, they're really attracted, they'll stay. But they always left." Interpersonally, his need was for nurture and kindness rather than for mature genital relating. While he worried about the stigma of being seen by others as bisexual or gay, and indeed as an adult had always chosen female partners, he sometimes acknowledged that the sex of his partner was not as important to him as a sense of being cared about and supported. His desperation about being abandoned, as he had been by his father physically and by his mother in many other ways, was the motor that ran his psychological machine. As he left the session during which he laid this out, he poignantly whispered as he passed me at the door, "I hope you don't get tired of me."

Ramon's early experiences left him confused about his value. "There was something wonderful about knowing I was blessed with good looks and my body produced this liquid that felt so good and could make other people so happy too." He then confessed, however, that he had never felt he was good for anything else, that he did not feel he had anything else to offer the world besides his body. "I know how to make men or women happy in bed, but that's all I know." It was therefore a major step to embark on the educational program he was about to start.

Ramon related a fantasy he had during sex: that he could crawl up into the woman's vagina and "just stay there." When I asked him about this fantasy, he hesitated, then said he imagined being reborn and having a second chance to be innocent. "I never had that innocent time a child has." I said it did indeed sound like he had been robbed of his childhood. There was a moment of silence and then Ramon began to cry.

AMBIVALENCE ABOUT THE ABUSER

The ambiguity and complexity of feelings concerning their abusers tend to influence sexually abused men as adults so that all close relationships become suffused with suspicion and irresolvable ambivalence. This is especially likely if the abuse occurred in the context of a seemingly loving relationship, particularly a familial one. Intense intermingling of love and hate for an abuser leads to highly charged, fluctuating feelings about loved ones in adult life. Cruelty can be eroticized as sadism; being violated can be sexualized as masochism. We will see examples of both of these in later sections of this chapter. The ambiguity may itself be paralyzing, as with David, who eventually was hospitalized when he could not deal with his conflicted and eroticized relationships with both parents.

Julian was deeply ambivalent about the man who simultaneously mentored, loved, and molested him. He was abused for three years by Father Scott, a parish priest who when Julian was twelve required that he come for special counseling sessions in order to get confirmed. Father Scott made Julian his special altar boy, invited him to visit him in his rooms, and undertook to educate him in classical texts, languages, and music. Julian came from a psychologically and physically invasive family in which emotions and boundaries were ignored. Although he flunked out of school after Father Scott began to abuse him, once the abuse stopped he became an A student, largely, he said, because of the earlier influence of the priest. He eventually went on to get an advanced degree.

Father Scott taught Julian to idealize the male relationships described in classical Greek texts. These included intellectual mentoring, deep interpersonal commitment and intimacy, and physical sexuality, which began between them a few months after Julian started being counseled by Father Scott. Father Scott led up to the initial seduction by encouraging Julian to talk about the pain he felt about his physically abusive but otherwise unresponsive family. After these sessions, Father Scott would hug Julian. These hugs were precious to the boy, who was starved for physical affection, or, indeed, any kind of positive regard from an adult. With time, the hugs got longer, and then one day Father Scott kissed Julian, putting his tongue in the boy's mouth and making the kiss last for minutes. Julian was startled and confused, unsure of what was happening and what it meant. After the kiss, Father Scott said with a meaningful look, "*I know you want more,* but that's all for now." Julian was bewildered at the time, but as an adult he said, "So right from the beginning he made it that the abuse was my idea, so I felt responsible and guilty that it was happening even though I had no concept of men kissing at the time, and certainly no interest in it." Shortly thereafter, Father Scott introduced Julian to anal sex, and for two years they had regular sexual encounters that included anal sex and mutual masturbation. Father Scott also encouraged Julian to have sex with an older boy whom Father Scott was trying to seduce. The two boys would engage in sexual activity, and then Father Scott had sex with each of them.

The priest maintained that their relationship existed on the highest plane possible for two human beings, that they had attained the ideal glorified by the greatest poets and philosophers of the ancient world. He reiterated that they experienced all forms of love together: love of beauty, love of thought, love of logic, love of art, and love of one another that was intellectual, sensual, and emotional. Julian did love Father Scott, and he craved the companionship and deep interest the priest offered him. Nevertheless, he was confused and conflicted about the sex that accompanied it. "He did so much for me! Anyone would think he was the best mentor a boy could ever have, and, except for the sex, he was." He said the activity with Father Scott was never what he really wanted sexually, yet shamefacedly acknowledged that it was satisfying in some ways as well. As Julian started to go out with girls, he would often sneak out of his house after dates and go to Father Scott's rooms, where he would find physical release for the sexual arousal he felt with his girlfriends, and emotional comfort that never existed at home. Likewise, when he was beaten by his parents for flunking out of school he went to Father Scott for comfort. He only realized years later that the relationship with the priest had contributed to his depression, anger, and inability to concentrate in school.

Almost as an afterthought, Julian mentioned that when he was about fifteen he was once offered $25 by a woman on the street if he would allow her to fellate him. He went back to her apartment, where she locked the door, told him to undress, then took off her own clothes, revealing herself to be a male transvestite. "I didn't know what to do—the door was locked with a key, and he was about 200 pounds while I must have weighed 140. He wanted to fuck me, and finally I said to myself, 'Oh, what the hell, you've done it before, and you'll get hurt if you don't do it now. It's not a big deal, and you know it'll be over in ten minutes if you cooperate.'" Afterward, he was allowed to leave and given $25, which he immediately contributed to a church charity. "It makes me realize I felt like damaged goods—it hardly mattered any more what anyone did to me."

At age fifteen, Julian entered a new school, where he did well, having put a stop to the sexuality in the relationship with Father Scott. After he left for college, his family moved away from the parish where Father Scott served, and Julian rarely returned to his old neighborhood. He excelled in school and eventually married, but remained ashamed, conflicted, and secretive about his relationship with the priest. He remained grateful for the intellectual and emotional expansion the relationship with Father Scott afforded him. Simultaneous with this, however, he was covertly enraged about the exploitation and mystification involved in their sexual activity. As an adult, he was a compulsive masturbator driven to furtively view peep shows; he seemed consumed by female pornography when he was anxious. He felt out of control, in the grip of the sexual impulses that flooded him at such times.

At age thirty, Julian attended a funeral in his old neighborhood, and there saw Father Scott, who came over and introduced himself to Julian's wife. Julian was furious that the priest could approach him with such nonchalance and could speak to Julian's wife as though he were simply an old friend of Julian's. But he also felt paralyzed, wanting to shame and hurt Father Scott but barely able to speak to him. The priest drew him into a corner and whispered, "You may feel better than the rest of us now that you've left town, but you and I know that all I have to do is rub your belly and you'll squeal like a puppy!" Feeling helpless and shamed once again, Julian finally got in touch with the full extent of his rage at his former mentor.

Ambivalence toward the abuser may be resolved through denial of one or the other side of it. A boy may then either experience *only* the abusive or *only* the loving aspects of his molestation. Such a denial keeps a man stuck in an untenable psychological position, and he may swing abruptly from one side of his ambivalence to the other.

Keith, for example, initially held on to a positive image of his covertly seductive mother, the only person he could cling to in a hostile and denigrating world. He developed life-threatening substance addictions that allowed him to stay merged with her, and later had to virtually cut off contact with her, rejecting her almost completely, in order to attain sobriety and build a life separate from her.

As Keith explored all the reasons he held himself back from having intimate relationships, especially with women, he focused at first on his fear of merging with the mother who had overwhelmed him emotionally and whose companion he had been in her descent into alcoholism. Eventually, though, our work revealed another side to his isolation: by maintaining his fear of relationships, Keith was actually *holding on* to his relationship with his mother. Isolating himself kept him fixed in the push–pull of the romance he had experienced with her, and, ironically, this served to keep her psychologically close to him.

By not allowing himself to recognize his mother's covert sexual abuse, Keith doomed himself to years of very serious substance abuse and other acting-out behaviors, as well as to a lifelong inability to commit to relationships despite the initial impression he conveyed of being warm and friendly. After three years of psychotherapy, he said in hindsight, "I had an emotional orgy with my mother. I could explode my emotions. I see now that I'd be exhausted by all this emotional give-and-take with her, and when I was exhausted my emotions wouldn't get in my way so much. I'd create situations with her—I'd act out, I'd get caught doing something awful by someone's parent and it would get back to her—then I'd be thrown back to her and again we'd have this orgy of emotion. It was sexual in some way I didn't understand. She had not come to terms with her own childhood incest at that time—and we'd cling to each other emotionally until we were both drained and worn down. We'd keep repeating that process over and over—she must have needed to exhaust herself emotionally too."

The ambivalence can extend toward the nonabusing parent as well. Victor described how his abuse history affected his relationship with his mother, making him unable to tolerate the ambivalence caused by his perception of her passive role in his abuse: "I don't know how to feel about my mother. She should have protected me from my father. But I'm a hypocrite if, even though I'm angry with her because she didn't stop him, I still want to go home to have her dinners and get her approval."

Victor also acknowledged ambivalence about the sexual "play" he engaged in with his grandparents from ages four till six. They stopped their sexual games when he began school, and Victor recalled trying to get them to play them again, and becoming depressed and lonely when they would not. Having been overstimulated by them at an age when he had no capacity to regulate his emotional response, he grew to crave the internal high that accompanied the games and thereby became linked to interpersonal closeness with his grandparents.

Quinn and Isaac provide further examples of how ambivalence about an abuser gets expressed in later life.

Quinn: Oscillating Feelings about a Beloved but Abusive Grandfather

Quinn was able to experience only one side of his ambivalence toward his abuser at a time. He did not permit his fury at his grandfather to enter consciousness until after he remembered his sexual abuse at his grandfather's hands. Once he recalled the abuse, however, he could no longer allow himself also to remember the loving, affectionate aspects of his relationship with his abusing grandfather. His healing did not truly begin until he gained the capacity to simultaneously feel both sides of this ambivalence.

Quinn began to remember sexual abuse by his maternal grandfather when he was twenty. He never spoke to anyone about it until after his grandfather's death three years later. At that point, Quinn got depressed, and eventually sought treatment from a woman therapist. When he was referred by her to my group for sexually abused men at the age of twenty-eight, he was in a constant rage. Overweight, temporarily disabled because of a severe injury, at odds with the woman he had lived with for three years, Quinn was barely able to talk about anything in treatment except his outrage at his grandfather and the parents who had not protected Quinn from him. While he proclaimed that he had worked through his victimization, and that he now considered himself a "survivor" rather than a "victim," these claims were hollow indeed. He could not talk about anything but his victimization, and was angry if anyone suggested he "let go of it."

Quinn's grandfather molested Quinn for a period of four years starting at about age four. The molestations, which occurred approximately on a weekly basis, took place in the grandfather's basement workshop when Quinn was visiting his grandparents. His grandfather fondled Quinn, performed mutual fellatio on him, and penetrated him anally with fingers and, at times, his penis. The interpersonal context of the abuse was one in which the grandfather was very affectionate to Quinn, telling him this was something they did because the grandfather loved Quinn so much. The grandfather took many photos of Quinn, some with Quinn partially undressed and in semiseductive poses. Although Quinn does not recall being told to keep their activities a secret, he instinctively felt he should not tell anyone.

The youngest of several siblings, Quinn grew up in a working-class suburban family. His mother had "married down," according to her own family, which had been of a different ethnic background and higher economic status than his father's large immigrant family. Over the years, however, the mother's family lost their money, while Quinn's father was successful in his blue-collar field.

Quinn's father was a martinet at home, and seems to have been threatened by any sign of competence from Quinn. For example, at age eleven Quinn designed and built a remarkably elaborate treehouse in the backyard, installing electricity and running water in it. His father decided the treehouse had to come down because he thought that if it were discovered his property taxes would be raised. There was never any discussion regarding Quinn's ingenuity in building the house. When Quinn wanted to go to college, his father refused to pay for anything unless Quinn attended a nearby community college. Instead, Quinn obtained a scholarship at a private liberal arts college in another state and worked to pay all his other expenses.

Quinn's mother was apparently a more giving person, but she seems to have stayed in the background for much of Quinn's childhood, unable to stem the tide of his father's many tirades. She dressed Quinn inappropriately in elaborate "Little Lord Fauntleroy" outfits she sewed herself; these were the cause of many schoolyard taunts until at age seven Quinn refused to wear them any more.

Quinn's memories of childhood molestation by his grandfather returned to him in a rush while he was watching a television show about sexual abuse. The memories had a horribly overwhelming clarity, but he told no one about them for years. Eventually, his sister, although unaware of his abuse history, became concerned about his anger, depression, and mood swings, and she convinced him to enter therapy.

Shortly after starting therapy, Quinn disclosed to his family that he had been sexually abused by his grandfather. No one expressed doubts about his revelation, but his mother was unnerved and claimed to have had no previous knowledge that her father was capable of such acts. His father minimized the impact of the abuse on Quinn, saying that the grandfather had also abused the father by never repaying a sum of money the father once lent him. Quinn's sisters were supportive, and recalled that the grandfather had often showed them the photos he had taken of Quinn as a young boy, exclaiming about Quinn's beauty and how much he loved his grandson.

For the first few years in my group for sexually abused men, Quinn's stance was nearly static. He had periods of massive depression, and when he talked it was about how angry he was at his father and grandfather, how images of his grandfather's molestation kept haunting him while he was asleep and awake, how infuriated he was when anyone said he should be forgiving and/or "move on." He often brought up media depictions of sexual abuse, which depressed him if they were supportive of abuse allegations and enraged him if they questioned the validity of any accusations. It was difficult to work with him on these issues except to listen and be supportive. Pointing out how he was stuck in his anger was perceived as undermining his victimhood, even though he counterphobically maintained that he no longer considered himself a victim. Yet eventually group members expressed open frustration at how fiercely he held on to his positions and did not address the current problems in his life.

During this same period, however, Quinn started a business related to his early interest in construction work. At first immensely insecure about his skills and ability to negotiate the business world, he had many fits and starts in this work before becoming moderately successful at it. The group supported him in his efforts, often giving him sound advice based on their own business experiences. Quinn also improved his ability to relate to his girlfriend during this time. While the relationship remained tempestuous, he became far better able to tell her about his needs and to attend to hers; eventually, the two parted ways in a relatively amicable manner. Finally, his relationship with his father slowly improved as Quinn noticed that his father had softened over the years. He was forced to differentiate between the harsh, dismissive, and challenging father he had grown up with and the sickly older man who now wanted Quinn's love and was marginally better able to be loving in return.

A crucial turning point in Quinn's treatment occurred three years after we first met. He had heretofore always talked about "my grandfather and what he did to me." One day, however, he referred to "Grandpa" in this context. I asked him about this term of affection, noting that he had never used it for his grandfather before. He began to reminisce about how Grandpa had adored him, in marked contrast to his father's aggression and hostility. The relative warmth his father was now showing him reminded him of those early feelings with Grandpa. In a very different tone than usual, he talked about how he had felt comforted and loved in Grandpa's embrace. As he spoke, he sounded shy and said he was scared that others would deride him for loving Grandpa, his abuser. He then said that, while he had never liked the sexuality with Grandpa, it had seemed a small price to pay to obtain the tenderness he craved.

Recognizing his affectional needs had a dramatic effect on Quinn. For the first time, he was willing to consider antidepressant medication, which was effective in lifting his mood and stabilizing his oscillating self-esteem. His continuing rage subsided somewhat, and he was able to promote his business more productively. He also noted that he was no longer as obsessed by external media depictions of sexual abuse. Instead, he finally reached inside for the hurt that had been covered by his fury. A few months after his father finally died, Quinn wept as he murmured, "Why didn't they help me? Why didn't they help me?"

Acknowledging his needs for tenderness and love, particularly from a father figure, helped free Quinn from his furious and constant demands that his molestation be the center of everyone's relationship with him. To his surprise, he was then finally able to start putting together a life in which his history of sexual abuse remained an important influence but was no longer the primary focus of his daily experience.

Isaac: Emotional Neediness, Hero Worship, and Loss

Unlike Quinn, Isaac had multiple victimizers over time, but he also felt ambivalent about an abuser. Emotionally needy when his parents divorced, he retained a naïveté that set him up for exploitation. Looking for older boys and men who could protect him and help him find his way in the world, he repeatedly encountered sexual predators instead. When he found a young man who seemed to like and nurture him, Isaac idolized him. But this relationship turned abusive as well, and, having had to cut himself off from what had been a source of support, Isaac unconsciously mourned this loss for years.

At age six, Isaac was sent to boarding school when his parents' marriage broke up. He stayed there till he was eight. At this school, Isaac was raped on two occasions by two different eighth grade boys at night in the dormitory. Both times he was on his way to the bathroom, which required passing the dormitory where the older boys slept. On the first occasion, he was grabbed and taken into a laundry room and anally raped on piles of dirty laundry. On the second occasion, he was forced to fellate an older boy in the dark hallway. Isaac disclosed these rapes with embarrassment but with little other affect. The experiences must have been terrifying, but his voice was flat and dissociated as he described them to me.

In the years after leaving boarding school, Isaac continued to be sexually victimized. A lonely and naïve child, he lacked male role models and sought them out. His father moved to a distant city. His mother remarried, but his stepfather was a distant figure in Isaac's childhood, although he became supportive in later years. Isaac could remember ten additional separate occasions between the ages of eight and seventeen when he was approached sexually by older boys or men in intimidating circumstances. These ranged from being groped on a train by a stranger to being lured to a lonely cabin in the woods by two military veterans who nearly raped him before they stopped because of his terrified pleading. It is difficult to ascertain whether as time went on Isaac related to men in an eroticized manner that could have been interpreted as a sexual invitation. This may well have become the case as he learned that some men were interested in him when he was sexual with them, but he did not present it this way.

When Isaac was seventeen, he grew close to Ned, a man who worked for Isaac's stepfather in a business that operated in their home. Ned, a man in his early thirties, was the stepfather's nephew by marriage. Isaac idealized Ned as a mentor and older brother figure. Ned took an interest in Isaac's sports activities and talked to him in a manner Isaac considered flatteringly adult. He felt like he had finally found the older brother or father he had been seeking.

One evening, they were alone in the house after Isaac came home from sports practice. Ned offered to give Isaac a haircut, an offer he had made many times but which Isaac had never accepted. At Ned's direction, Isaac stripped to the waist and Ned cut his hair. He then suggested they watch TV together on Isaac's parents' bed. He offered Isaac a back massage, which Isaac accepted. As Ned worked his way down to the top of Isaac's cutoffs, he asked Isaac in a joking tone if he were shy about him going further. Isaac said he wasn't shy but that Ned shouldn't go too far down. Then Ned motioned for them to sit with their backs against the headboard and began to stroke Isaac's belly. Isaac says he froze at that point, finally realizing that this was a sexual approach. Ned took Isaac's passivity for consent and began to stroke Isaac's genitals, first through the jeans, then opening Isaac's zipper and using lotion as a lubricant. Isaac experienced a dissociative episode, sensing an enormous physical distance between his brain, which was repulsed by what was happening, and his pelvic area, which was excited. "I seemed to be watching my genitals through the wrong end of a telescope. I felt aroused, but my excitement seemed far away." He started to shake uncontrollably, and Ned asked what was wrong. Suddenly, Isaac wrenched himself out of his passivity and yelled, "Hey man, I ain't no homo!" Ned stopped and, seemingly deflated, told Isaac he could go. Isaac somehow felt he had let Ned down. "I wonder why I spoke that way? Like a child might. I was old enough and smart enough to speak in a more grown-up way about homosexuality." I suggested to Isaac that it had been out of a kind of strength that he resorted to the language of the streets, because it was an effective way to get Ned to stop. He responded sadly, "I guess so, but it made me lose him too." And Isaac started to mourn the relationship with Ned.

Soon after this incident, Isaac visited his father in another state where he lived with his second wife and Isaac's half-sister and two half-brothers. Uncertain about what might happen with Ned if he returned home, Isaac precipitously decided to live with his father for his senior year of high school. By the time he next visited his mother, Ned had separated from his wife and no longer worked for Isaac's stepfather. Isaac never saw Ned again.

In the next section of this chapter, I will recount Isaac's abuse of his sister during the year he lived with his father. At the end of high school, Isaac went away to college in a distant state. There, he got heavily involved in pot smoking and flunked out. He moved to New York City, where he remained underemployed for many years in a low-level service industry job. Attending college sporadically over many years, he finally graduated at the age of forty-one, six years after first beginning psychotherapy.

ABUSIVE RELATIONSHIPS

Abusive relationships, whether overtly sexual or not, are another possible legacy of childhood sexual abuse. Dimock (n. d.) has commented that in his experience, which is different from mine, most sexually victimized men have also been physically or sexually abusive to someone else. When this is the case, even if there was only a single episode in childhood and adolescence, it often creates a barrier to recovery because of the man's subsequent guilt and shame.

As I have said, the men I have worked with have not included adult abusers. An extensive literature exists about working with this population (see, for example, Maletzky, 1991). I have, however, worked with a number of men who as children or adolescents enacted sexual abuse with other children. Other men I have treated were covertly abusive or exploitative in their adult relationships.

Abusiveness is a product of identification with an internalized image of the victimizer, a clear example of identification with the aggressor. In Chapter 2, I discussed Ed's abuse of his sister (see pp. 48–51), and in Chapters 6 and 7, I described Patrick's sexual relationship with his three-year-younger brother (see pp. 141–142 and 186). Now let's look at some other men's experiences:

In the previous section, we saw that Isaac lived with his father during his senior year of high school, following a sexual approach in his mother's home by a relative he had idolized. During this year, he initiated sexual activity with his ten-year-younger half-sister. Its aftermath left him guilt-ridden for decades, ashamed of himself and terrified of ever acting spontaneously on impulse. One day, his sister came into his bedroom while he was lying on his bed masturbating. He quickly covered himself but then asked her to come into the bathroom, where he locked the door. Lying on the floor, he told her to straddle his face, and he licked her vagina while he masturbated behind her. This sequence was repeated a second time a few weeks later. He does not remember either of them speaking during the abuse, except once when she told him not to press so hard with his tongue because it hurt her.

When Isaac was forty, he thought his sister alluded to her abuse in a conversation when she said she always used to get scared when she went into the room that had been his bedroom. He was reluctant to pursue the topic, telling himself that he did not really know if she was ready to talk about it. When I wondered whether her allusions indicated that she actually wanted to talk about the abuse, he acknowledged that it was he who was ashamed and unable to talk to her. As of this writing, three years later, Isaac, who remains blocked from fulfilling his potential in many areas of his life, has not spoken to his sister about the molestations.

Following earlier abuse by his mother's lovers and husbands, Willem also molested his sister during a crucial period of their lives. Shortly after his mother and her third husband divorced, when he was twelve, his mother died suddenly. He and his two-year-younger sister lived thereafter with their intimidating maternal grandparents. Willem became visibly depressed and was sent without warning to a large city for a psychological evaluation. On the night of his return, confused and unhappy, he turned to the family's minister for solace, at which point the minister tried unsuccessfully to seduce him.

Willem was relieved when he was sent away to boarding school after a year and a half. With guilty pain, however, he related that during these eighteen months at his grandparents' home he abused his sister by engaging in sexual intercourse with her. In explanation, he said this was his way of clinging to the only human relationship he treasured. Yet he also acknowledged that his sister was an unwilling participant in the sexual activity. He said, in fact, that the need to escape his memories of abusing her was a major factor in his decision to come to this country at age twenty. When we first met, he had never again spoken to his sister. Indeed, he said he had barely any memory for the period of his life prior to his mother's death. In our work together, he began to piece together his childhood. Eventually, he made contact with his sister, who was eager to reestablish a relationship with him. He needed to proceed very slowly on this path, knowing his own tendency to pull back suddenly when overwhelmed by previously dissociated material. He continued contact by letter and then by phone, hoping eventually to visit her and talk to her about the abuse.

Another man, Felix, became both abuser and nurturer to his young sister. His parents had married as teenagers. By age twenty-seven, they had had six children, of whom Felix was the eldest. They divorced when Felix was twelve. Felix's premature erotic experience consisted of walking in on his mother and her lover in bed when he unexpectedly came home from school for lunch at age eleven. He was seen by them both before he slammed the bedroom door shut. This incident was an overstimulating and confusing sexual betrayal, if not actually abusive as the term is usually interpreted. It was never alluded to by Felix, his mother, or her lover, for whom his mother left Felix's father a year later. Shortly thereafter, when Felix was twelve and a half, he once touched and caressed his sleeping five-year-old sister's vagina. He believed she slept through the molestation. When he shamefacedly related this incident to me twenty-six years later, it was the first time he had told anyone his guilty secret. In discussing his relationship with this sister and his other siblings, Felix described how he often acted as their parent after their parents' divorce. His mother was competent and well-meaning, but was distracted and seems not to have been a particularly nurturing parent anyway. In any case, she was overwhelmed by the task of working while raising six children. Felix made sure his brothers and sisters were dressed for school, and he was their caretaker in the afternoons and often in the evenings as well. Indeed, the sister whom he abused once said to him as an adult, "I always think I should send two cards on Mother's Day, one to Mom, and the big one to you." Telling me this, he cried as he described again how he had abused her, betraying the trust everyone had in him. His own loneliness and the crushing burden of being both caretaker to his siblings and carrier of the secret of his mother's infidelity had, it appears, made him feel starved for any close human contact. This may explain why he did what he did to his sister, but, as he repeated over and over to me, it does not excuse his behavior. With time, Felix gained some perspective on both his abusiveness and his nurturance, and he acknowledged how inappropriate the demands had been that he behave as an adult. While he did not forgive himself for his abusive act, he began to see it in the larger context of his behavior toward his sister and allowed the abuse to recede in importance so he could go on with his life.

In addition to the overt abuse that Ed, Patrick, Willem, Isaac, and Felix enacted, abusiveness can be reenacted subtly in everyday relationships. We will see in Chapter 11 that Victor was an overt victimizer as an adolescent, but he was also subtly exploitative as an adult while rationalizing to himself that as a victim he was blameless and had the right to do whatever he felt he needed to do:

"It's hard to think of myself as selfish. I like to think of myself as just a kid, and my mother and father as the ones doing the bad things. But then I see in here that I manipulate people and lie to them. I don't like that."

"You'd rather think of yourself as an innocent who just does what he needs to protect himself. So if you lie to your mother, somehow it's her fault."

"Yes. I hear how ridiculous that sounds, but, still, when you say it, I feel comforted. As though nothing I do is bad, she's the bad one. I'm just a kid. I really like thinking of the world that way. On the other hand, it's terrible to think of myself like that—I'm thirty-four-years old. I can't be this little kid forever. I'll never grow up if I keep on like that—I'll never become the person I want to be."

Keith gives a further illustration of subtle manipulativeness and exploitation (see also my discussion of Yale in Chapters 5 and 9). Seemingly well-related, he managed to maintain a personal remoteness from others.

Keith worked freelance in an industry in which people tend to be partially involved in a number of projects simultaneously, knowing that only some of them will materialize into paying work. Therefore, a certain amount of juggling of business ventures is necessary, and occasionally people have to back out after they have done a great deal of work on a project. After two situations occurred in which he withdrew from ventures because of more definite and substantial offers elsewhere, he talked with some surprise about the bitterness he encountered from the people who had expected to work with him. These people felt he had made a personal commitment to them and had then gone on to deceive and betray them. The sense of treachery went far beyond what might be expected in a business situation, and initially Keith was perplexed by it. As we explored how he cultivated business relationships, Keith conceded that he "seduced" potential work partners into wanting to work with him. "I feel they won't want me on the basis of my skills, so I pull out all stops. I show them how incredibly I understand their needs. I make sure they bond to me. Then if I pull out of a commitment or a semi-commitment for reasons that are totally understandable from a career point of view, they feel *personally* betrayed. I never understand why, and I never get it that I'm hurting them. And if I do get it, I don't care. *I'm* always the victim—I can't imagine anyone else being victimized, and certainly not that I'm doing the victimizing." Keith said this matter-of-factly, communicating little sense even then that he really cared about whether he hurt people.

Keith had considerable charm and sweetness, and in general was well liked by associates. Yet he felt he had no friends except for his wife, and indeed he often felt walled off from her too. He had strong interpersonal relationships with some colleagues, but did not consider them friends. As soon as they asked about anything personal or revealed anything personal about themselves, he withdrew. His work was such that he dealt intensively with groups of people for a concentrated period of time, then moved on to other, similar groups. While involved with these people, he had dinner with them every night and talked at great length about the work they were doing, creating what he called "a little family." But once he moved on, he might never see these people again. This pattern was very comfortable for him, especially because it had a side benefit of allowing him to keep his distance from his wife. He was often invited to industry parties, where, since he no longer drank, he had little to do. Once there, he networked as necessary, then withdrew into a corner, surveying the others and waiting till it was late enough to leave. Apparently popular and certainly successful, he remained a stranger while surrounded by illusory friends he could not allow into his private space.

SADISTIC AND MASOCHISTIC THEMES

A natural next step from repeatedly entering abusive relationships is actively to seek sadomasochistic sexual contacts (Wright, 1997a; see also Ehrenberg, 1992). My experience with this subculture is small but two different gay men have told me that every man they knew who (like themselves) was deeply involved in bondage and other sadomasochistic practices had been sexually or otherwise abused in childhood. While their claims may well have been exaggerations, they do suggest that clinicians should explore for a history of sexual abuse with patients involved in sadomasochistic behaviors.

Sadistic fantasies not acted upon are also common. Victor reluctantly told me after several years of treatment that he had recurring sadistic fantasies of tying men up and either tickling them till they screamed or bringing them nearly to orgasm but not allowing the orgasm to take place. He had never considered the possible connection between these fantasies and the fact that, in his own abuse, his grandparents had tickled him mercilessly as part of a sexual game, and that later, when his father abused him, Victor kept himself from reaching orgasm, in part to frustrate his father.

Jared had a seductive relationship with his father and a sexually abusive one with a teenager when he was five. As an adult, he was only interested in partners who were twenty to forty years older than he. This is a not-infrequent dynamic for sexually abused men. The reasons are complex, and not necessarily negative. Some of these reasons have nothing to do with abuse As we saw earlier in this chapter, however, there sometimes has been a positive relationship with the abuser in addition to the abusive one. This may lead to a complicated ambivalence about people who remind the victim of the abuser, whether because of age or other factors. Or, having been abused in the past by someone who had real or imagined control over his fate, he may need a sense of being able to handle himself better in a situation similar to the abusive one in order to restore a sense of mastery over himself and his fate. However, there is a danger of simply repeating the abusive pattern, perhaps in a disguised, seemingly benign way. In such situations it is imperative that he make absolutely sure it's what *he* wants rather than what he assumes the other wants before proceeding with a potentially exploitative relationship.

Many men who have been abused develop lifetime patterns of allowing themselves to be exploited in ways that are not explicitly eroticized. Abe and Owen demonstrate both erotic and nonerotic masochistic relatedness.

Abe: Searching for the Abuse That Feels Like Home

Abe was a forty-five-year-old semicloseted gay man who worked in the creative arts. At the beginning of treatment with me, he had been chronically depressed and anxious for many years; had been in some form of psychotherapy his entire adult life with limited results; complained of recurring abuse and exploitation by colleagues, friends, and family; and had been in recovery from alcohol and drug addiction for nine years. He continued to have problems with overeating for which he compensated with hours of competitive sports daily.

Engaging, humorous, and self-deprecating, Abe recounted a familial situation in which his self-effacing but vindictive father was frightened of his mother's rages and emotionality. The father explicitly told Abe that it was his job to be his mother's caretaker since the father could not deal with her. A typical horrifying example of this occurred when his father without explanation pushed four-year-old Abe into the mother's bedroom, where she was hysterically grieving, minutes after hearing about her own mother's unexpected death. His father told a petrified Abe to "take care" of his mother, and then the father himself left the house.

Abe's mother, both alcoholic and addicted to pills, was hospitalized twice for psychiatric reasons during Abe's childhood. A beautiful, sensuous, fascinating, and demanding woman, she openly had multiple affairs until she died in her early seventies. She wanted a girl when Abe was born, and she frequently and laughingly recounted that when Abe was first brought to her in the hospital as an infant she yelled, "Take him away! I don't want him!"

Narcissistic in the extreme, Abe's mother masturbated with candles that she then left around the house. Abe found these misshapened candles, was excited by the vaginal smell, eventually realized what they had been used for, and continued to feel excitement mixed with deep shame and revulsion. His mother encouraged Abe and his brother to vie for permission to sleep with her when the father was away on business trips. The boys were beaten severely for minor transgressions when the mother was drunk, and Abe recalls his brother being tied spread-eagled to a bed prior to at least one such beating. This brother had been severely scalded as a child through severe parental neglect, and had suffered extensive disfigurement. In addition, on several occasions Abe walked in on his father masturbating the family dog and encouraging the dog to lick the father's penis.

Abe's relationship with his mother had been stimulating, exciting, and arousing. He was never bored when he was with her; he felt he was her "best beau" and leaped at any chance to spend time with her. He never stopped trying to keep her happy, and it was only after he became sober that he began to think about the sacrifices he had made to remain her caretaker. He also recognized for the first time that his vivacious, vindictive, charming mother was vicious, deeply depressed, and incapable of thinking about him, his needs, and his identity as separate from hers.

He remembered, for example, that his parents tended to send their children to different summer camps every year, depending on what seemed popular in their often-changing network of friends. Abe was often unhappy at these camps, and one year he said he wanted to go to a particular camp that a friend of his attended. His mother agreed, but then told him that she and his father would never visit him at this camp, and would only visit his brother at the camp the mother chose. He did not believe her and attended camp with his friend; his mother kept to her word and did not visit. Abe was especially miserable that summer and never attempted that kind of openly independent stance with her again.

By age twelve, Abe was regularly looking to be picked up by older men. Many of these men were interpersonally cold and hurtful to Abe during sexual encounters. They thus were abusive emotionally in addition to being pedophiles. At the time, however, Abe felt good about being chosen by them. It did not occur to him until decades later that he had perpetuated with them a pattern of being exploited and abused, and that they had been criminal offenders who took advantage of his neediness. Indeed, they were the first in a long line of inaccessible people with whom he reenacted the dynamic he had lived with both parents, especially his mother. He craved the love of these parent substitutes even as he chose them because they were incapable of giving it.

In treatment with me, Abe began to think about his identification with his mother's underlying depression. He remembered telling her as a young teenager that he was depressed and unhappy, and that he wanted to see a psychiatrist. In response, she said, "Unhappy? You think you're unhappy? Just wait till you're older and then you'll know what unhappiness is!" Other than his being given this ironically prophetic pronouncement, his request was ignored. Thirty-five years after saying this, when she was near death, his mother suddenly turned to him and asked whether he had ever gotten rid of the depression he had complained about as a teenager. Abe could not remember her ever asking about his psychological state before. He was astounded that she remembered the original interchange, that she had any curiosity about him at all. After remembering this comment of hers, he had the following dream: "I'm lying in bed. I'm very sick, I'm dying. My mother is there. She looks at me with no expression and says she's going out. I say 'If you go out, I'll be dead by the time you get back.' She shrugs—like 'So what?'—and turns and goes. Yes, that's the way it really was."

Abe also recalled that when he seemed happy in the morning his mother repeated a home-grown aphorism, "If you laugh before breakfast, you'll cry by dark." She would then say she was telling him this for his own good. Abe began to realize that to feel anything but depressed and hopeless seemed like a betrayal of his mother, and we began to track his masochistic fantasies and behaviors in light of this recognition. He often felt especially masochistic after he was most capable or pleased with himself. On one such occasion, he had successfully confronted a difficult colleague, finished a long-term project, and capped his day by attending a concert he enjoyed, when he suddenly longed to be beaten physically. When we spoke about this scenario, he said, "Feeling good is a betrayal of my mother—so being humiliated and in pain is an act of loyalty to her. It's amazing—after all this time, I still feel that if I'm happy I'll lose her support and love—even though I know I never had it."

As an adult, Abe felt profound shame about his body and his sexuality. He was involved in a difficult but devoted relationship with another semicloseted man that had lasted for over ten years but had not included any sex after the first year. Sexuality was reserved mostly for anonymous, compulsive, unpleasurable encounters or short, intense affairs with extraordinarily inappropriate and uncaring men. Though not sexually interested in women, he seemed to avoid places where a positive sense of gay identity might be fostered.

In the past, Abe had engaged in sadomasochistic and dangerous sexual behaviors, including being tied up and anally fisted during anonymous encounters. He recounted these incidents with great shame, never having told anyone about them before. He described a brief affair he had once had with a man who broke it off by saying he was disturbed by how much Abe wanted to be hurt and how much he had grown to want to hurt Abe. Though startled by the man's words, Abe did not take in their meaning until an incident some years later, when he found himself in a sadomasochistic sexual encounter with a man whose hands were at Abe's throat. Abe suddenly understood that he liked being choked this way. The implications of this discovery had a powerful effect on him and were influential in getting him to stop his alcohol and drug abuse, as he realized these substances promoted his pursuing to their furthest extremes the dangerous sexual behaviors he craved.

On another occasion, a few years later, Abe took to the streets one night, desperately cruising for men to pick up in bitter cold weather after an agitated dispute with a colleague. Not having found anyone willing to come home with him, he discovered to his horror in the morning that a man he had spent a long time trying to solicit was in fact a homeless, filthy, and possibly psychotic derelict. That day, Abe, who had been in long-term psychotherapy several times, decided to seek treatment specifically for sexual abuse. "I realized that even though I no longer took drugs I was still acting as though I did. I preferred walking those frigid streets looking for degrading sex than going into the gay bars I was passing, where I might have felt some companionship in addition to any sex we were having. And I was so far into abuse that even a derelict's body was acceptable."

In our work, Abe was initially shy and guarded. Over time, he reported that whenever he left individual or group sessions he was overwhelmed with inchoate feeling. He said he liked this, since it meant he was feeling emotion and was no longer numb or depressed. He said feeling anything was better than enduring his usual living death. Abe later told me that in the initial six months of treatment he had felt wide swings in his feelings about me. Why was I interested in him? What did I want from him? How might I use him? What was I pushing him to do? Similar questions recurred cyclically throughout our work.

It was not until the third year of treatment that Abe trusted me enough to shout at me how much he truly distrusted me, even while sobbing that he trusted me more than nearly anyone else in his life. I found that any interpersonal move on my part might be interpreted by Abe as abusive. On many mornings I heard middle-of-the-night messages on my answering machine detailing my tone, my timing, my attitude, my questioning his decision to take a vacation, or whatever else Abe felt had wounded him. All of these qualities, Abe would maintain, reflected my coldness, my tendency toward abusiveness, and my inability to be empathic. No doubt in each case he was picking up on some real aspect of my behavior, but his cataclysmic reactions went far beyond the realities of what I had said or done. In his attacking mode, he often pressed my own psychological buttons, and at times I reacted defensively and argued with him about what he had perceived in me. Our relationship became thorny and recurrently tempestuous. He frequently threatened to leave treatment, and I sometimes thought he would do so. Occasionally I was even relieved to think that if he left we would finally end our painful interchanges. Yet somehow we got through each of these crises, and both of us grew from our encounters. With time, Abe noted how unusual it was in his life to have a relationship in which he could confront someone and not have to end the relationship.

Meanwhile, and not by coincidence, he began to have his greatest success professionally in a venture in which he felt he was more assertive than in the past. Yet he continued a people-pleasing mode of relating while agonizing over it and comparing it to his job in the family of placating his mother and keeping her rages in check. Unable to stop himself, he tracked with self-deprecating humor his inappropriately friendly responses to people's coldness or, at times, abuse. Abe noted mordantly that his father and brother showed absolutely no interest in his success, and did not read reviews of his work, ask about it, or see it. He commented that he could take no pleasure in the praise his work received: "I search for my parents among those who look at my work. I look for abuse and dismissal. There can be 198 people who like my work and two who don't. I'll listen to those two. For me, the abusive people are the only important ones there."

In talking about the way he related in "grown-up" situations with people he experienced as powerful, Abe plaintively said, "I wish I could stop disappearing." He felt that when a demand was made on him he had to acquiesce, and that when someone was angry at him he had to be the placater. Thus, in work situations he brought flowers or gifts to people whom he felt had abused him, and he accepted the blame when there was a problem not of his making. He felt responsible for keeping people content and pleased with him, occasionally compromising his work to appease an exploitative collaborator or colleague. At such times, he felt like he no longer existed, that he was an extension of another person's needs and self. The parallel to his early life with his mother was self-evident.

These themes recurred throughout his treatment, but began to recede in importance after many interpretations of how Abe repeated the placating patterns of his childhood and prodding about how he continued to do so with me. Eventually, he openly and angrily questioned my judgment and abilities, saying I was not gentle and supportive enough with him. My countertransferential frustration about this attack led me to feel I was relating to a burn victim, that no matter how delicately I "touched" him it would be excruciating for him because his skin was too damaged to protect him. When I shared this perception with Abe, he reminded me that his brother had been physically scalded as a child. He acknowledged that he felt psychologically scalded, and that he had a deep need to control interpersonal relationships, particularly those that seemed affectionate. This perception seemed to calm Abe considerably, and allowed him to relax some of his interpersonal wariness. (See Chapter 9 for further discussion of the vicissitudes of my relationship with Abe.)

He reported a flowering in his professional work and in the quality of his interpersonal life. His knees began to shake uncontrollably during therapy, which he said was a sign that he was in touch with feeling and expressing it. "I've always been closeted about my feelings and needs— not just my sexuality or my gayness, but my feelings. I have a problem exposing who I am to *myself*."

Two years after beginning treatment, Abe noted one day with surprise and suspicion that he had not engaged in anonymous sex for many months; this behavior has not recurred in the six years since then. Recalling his earlier statement that he wished he could "stop disappearing," he said after five years of treatment, "I've stopped disappearing now—and now I'm anxious all the time. I see why I had to keep disappearing—but it's better this way."

Abe's relationship with his father was nearly as problematic as that with his mother. I have recounted how his father explicitly told Abe that it was his job to be his mother's caretaker; he added that Abe did not need to take care of him. But Abe eventually saw that his father also wanted to be taken care of. No less narcissistic than Abe's mother, he was spiteful and mean if he felt slighted. The relationship between Abe and his father was painful, even into the father's old age, but we were able to address it partially before the father died. "I never thought change was possible—certainly not about my feelings toward my father. He was bitter, belittling, self-serving—and grandiose and insecure. When I first did my qualification at AA, I said, 'I hated my father from the moment I saw him.' I never even *wanted* to forgive him. My old therapist used to tell me I had to forgive him and I finally told him that if he ever again brought up the word 'forgive' in relation to my father I'd walk out and never return. Then, two years after I got sober I had an epiphany—I realized I wanted my father's love. So later I talked about it here, and I made a change. I never forgave him for what he did, but I grew to like him as an old man. I told him he *had* to put his arms around me and hug me when I saw him. I forced him—I actually took his arms and placed them around my waist—but he did it, and I liked it, and I saw that he liked it. When I called, he was glad to hear from me, and I liked that, too, even though it never made up for what he did while I was growing up. I didn't forgive him, but I was at peace with him when he died." Abe had always felt his father *wanted* him to fail in life, that he considered it an affront if Abe had any success. But, a year after his father's death, Abe suddenly saw that his father, like his mother, had not had the capacity to think about anyone beside himself. "Maybe it wasn't that he hated me. Maybe he just couldn't ever consider anyone's concerns but his own. He just didn't *notice* what he was doing to me."

In the year following this insight, Abe talked about how he continued to re-create his family in interpersonal situations. One day he said with great emotion that he realized he could not walk away from a particular professional group of people who over the years had ignored or derided his achievements. Poised to enter a new contractual arrangement with them, he was astounded and horrified to note that, while he saw very clearly how little he could ever get from these people, at the same time he was unable to give up on them. He cried out with passion, "I have to get them to recognize my worth! They become my mother and father, people who have no capacity to see beyond themselves, who care nothing for me, who don't even *think* about me when I'm not there. But I keep trying to change them, I keep hoping they'll turn around and say, 'Abe really has something there—we were wrong about him—look, he's terrific!' And, *even as I see that there is zero chance that they will do that, I also can't give up on the possibility!* I see it all, but it does no good—I can't stop myself from repeating it yet again!" I suggested that if he did let go of the possibility that these parent substitutes would express appreciation of him, he would then also have to grieve about feeling so unimportant to his parents. He wept as he clenched and unclenched his fists, repeating over and over that he knew he could expect nothing from these people but was just not capable of leaving them. Yet, in all this, we also saw that he had managed to encapsulate the abusive repetition to an important but isolated area of his life, and was simultaneously behaving very differently in other areas of his personal and professional worlds. And, indeed, he resigned from his work with this abusive group a few months later.

After six years of therapy, Abe finally began to address his masochism directly. Following a successful professional endeavor, he was overcome with sadomasochistic fantasies, and clipped an advertisement for a leather-oriented dominator from the back pages of a gay newspaper. He did not act on his wish, but brought it up in therapy instead. We explored the multiple meanings of the fantasy: He wanted to be in pain, first, because he felt he *should* feel pain rather than good feelings about his success, since that was his familiar role. Indeed, he said he felt it was a betrayal of his mother to feel positively about himself. Second, he wanted to feel a more defined pain than the foggy suffering he experienced after good feedback about his work. Third, he said that perhaps if it got bad enough, he would be moved to say "Enough!" and stop it. And, fourth, by choosing to be in pain and by making it explicit and defined, he felt in control of it, rather than lost in its maelstrom.

Referring to his masochism and hypervigilance about possible abuse from others, Abe said, "I carry my abuse around with me. Whether or not abuse is really taking place, I'm going to see it there, because that's what I bring to every relationship." After that, he continued to suffer anxiety, depression, and despair in interpersonal situations where confrontation was in the air, and could never altogether stop his people-pleasing mode of relating. He noted it when it happened, however, and was often able to disentangle himself from it more quickly. Periodically, though with diminishing frequency, he still blew up at me, threatening to leave treatment, feeling misunderstood, abused, and not accepted or cared about by me. And this helped him continue to go out into his world and stand up for himself in both professional and personal interactions.

Eventually, after seven years of treatment, Abe noted that he had not felt unbridled rage in relation to me for a long time. Moreover, he said, his attempts to stand up for himself in the world were no longer solely fueled by fury, but more often came from a less volatile capacity and wish to assert himself. Reflecting on his life and his treatment, Abe declared, "I'm still scared, inhibited, ashamed of my body. But I'm expressive, more than I ever, *ever*, EVER, *EVER* thought I could be. I don't consider myself unlucky at all."

Owen: Expecting and Finding Exploitation in Intimacy

In Chapters 2 and 4, I recounted Owen's history, which included a long-term "affair" beginning at age twelve with a man seventeen years his senior named Calvin, and a lengthy heterosexual marriage despite a clear homosexual orientation. Owen's therapy with me lasted for a number of years, and of course we focused on numerous themes having no obvious link with his sense of being exploited or his worries about intimacy and sexuality. These, however, are the themes on which I focus in this section.

Owen mourned his failure to establish a positive long-term relationship with another man, and felt that at age sixty-eight he was now too old ever to do so. About a year and a half after we started to work together, however, he came in one day agitated and ashen-faced. He said he was afraid he might be considered a child molester. He had met a teenager, Jimi, that week in an area frequented by gay men. Jimi initiated an encounter and followed Owen home.

A seventeen-year-old high school student, Jimi was born in a poor third world country and had come to the United States with his family five years earlier. He spoke broken English and claimed never to have had sex with a man before. Nevertheless, he aggressively pursued Owen, who was astounded, frightened, and intrigued. Owen wondered why Jimi would be as interested as he claimed to be in a man fifty-one years his senior. He considered whether he was being suckered by a young hustler. Alternatively, he asked how to find out whether it would be illegal to be sexually involved with someone Jimi's age.

After he found out that Jimi was over the age of consent in New York State, we began to talk about what it would mean psychologically for Owen to encourage the relationship. The parallel to the "affair" between Owen and Calvin was of course unmistakeable. We talked about the similarities as well as the differences in the two relationships as he began a liaison with Jimi. Jimi came from a culture that venerated older people, a fact that Owen could not comprehend. In addition, Jimi seemed instinctively to see Owen as a mentor who would introduce him to an Americanized culture that was totally foreign to Jimi's parents, who spoke no English and worked long hours at menial jobs. Owen, who considered himself ugly and undesirable, was both flattered and suspicious of Jimi's attentions, and constantly worried that he was being exploited for his money. Indeed, Owen did spend a great deal of money on Jimi, who had virtually none, and he alternated between feeling generous and foolish for doing so.

As Owen developed and deepened his relationship with Jimi, we had the opportunity to examine and analyze many of the themes of

Owen's life. Jimi was very demanding of Owen's time and attention. He often arrived at Owen's home early in the morning and expected to spend all day with Owen. Owen felt invaded by Jimi's presence, and wanted Jimi to be more aware of Owen's needs for privacy and interpersonal space. This forced Owen to look again at his historical difficulty in setting limits with people. Also, Owen felt uncomfortable walking down the street with Jimi, even in gay neighborhoods. He thought everyone who saw them realized both that he was gay, which he had mixed feelings about acknowledging publicly, and that they were lovers. He was afraid they considered him a foolish old man who was paying a young boy for his favors. Always hyperaware of public opinion about himself, particularly in relation to his sexual orientation, Owen had to come to terms with accepting a more public gay persona.

Another complication for Owen was the divergence of their interests and the inequality of their socioeconomic positions. Jimi, unsophisticated and uneducated, was interested in action movies and sports. Owen had sophisticated tastes in music, movies, theater, and food. He had to negotiate with Jimi how they would spend their time so that each was satisfied. In addition, Owen tried to educate Jimi, teach him English, and orient him to going to college after he finished high school. He paid for tutoring of various kinds, as well as for sports equipment. While he felt this was the right thing to do for someone he cared about, he continued to worry that he was being used.

It appeared that Jimi did genuinely care for Owen, and, while he profited from the relationship, he also gave a great deal to it. He forced a companionship on Owen for which Owen had always yearned but had never had with a man. He was an eager and insistent sexual partner; again, Owen had always wanted such a lover but had not had one since Calvin. Owen learned, somewhat to his surprise, that he did not always welcome either the companionship or the sexuality. This made him reconsider why he had never had a successful long-term relationship with a man, as well as his deep ambivalence about intimacy. Perhaps, he thought, he really preferred being alone.

Eventually, this led us back to the history of Owen's relationships with Calvin and with his parents. Owen continued to see Calvin as not having abused him, since he enjoyed the sex, but he did finally recognize the exploitative aspects of the relationship. Owen acknowledged that he would never have been interested in Calvin had Calvin not pursued him, and he knew his youth and vulnerability had attracted Calvin, who took advantage of them. Owen also looked differently at his parents' role in the relationship. In many ways, they had acquiesced in the "affair," despite the father's pro forma questioning about whether anything inappropriate was happening. Indeed, the parents profited from the relationship themselves by using Calvin's car, accepting Calvin's gifts, and going on vacations with him that they could never have afforded themselves. Owen also began to feel his parents had taken advantage of him by asking him to act as a parent to his younger siblings so that they could give their full efforts to caring for his sick sister.

A subtle lifelong pattern had thus begun in which Owen learned to expect exploitation and to acquiesce automatically to others' needs. We looked at how this had been true with his parents, his wife, his previous analyst, friends, various former lovers, and me. He continued to look out for the needs of his siblings and, to a lesser extent, their children, with the interesting exception of the once-invalided sister. In each case, and again with Jimi, Owen's fear was that love would be withdrawn if the other's needs were not satisfied. This was intolerable for Owen, and so he had allowed many subtly exploitative relationships to develop in his life.

Intimacy with Jimi became a testing ground for Owen's abilities to change these patterns. He had to limit Jimi's insatiable desire to take up his free time, to say no to requests for overly expensive gifts, to insist on going to cultural events that interested him whether or not Jimi came along. He continued to question the appropriateness of their relationship, especially given how different their interests were; but he recognized that the openness of Jimi's love and affection were a strong aphrodisiac for him. As had happened earlier in his life, it was unbearable for him to turn down someone who offered him such love. With this understanding on Owen's part, the relationship between Jimi and Owen continued for several years, including an extended period when Jimi attended an out-of-town college. At times, it seemed that Owen loved Jimi no more than he had loved Calvin, and that their relationship continued only because Jimi desired it. At other times, it appeared that only under such circumstances could Owen own his desire for intimacy.

In the next chapter, we will look at how the problems sexually abused men develop about interpersonal relating affect the therapeutic relationship.

CHAPTER 9

The Patient–Therapist Dyad

Childhood sexual abuse almost invariably involves a rupture in a critically important relationship with a parent or someone who is a parent substitute, either in fact or in the child's perception. The child then integrates abuse into his developing ability to relate, especially to authorities. We saw in Chapter 8 how this fissure informs a child's everyday relationships as he matures. In this chapter, we will examine how expectations of abuse affect the man's evolving attachment to a therapist. We will first focus on the vicissitudes of the patient–therapist dyad. Then we will consider how the therapeutic relationship becomes a vehicle for change in the man's capacity to enter and maintain other relationships. Simultaneously, we will look at the effect this arduous work may have on the therapist.

Many clinical discussions about treating sexually abused adults address the difficult transference/countertransference predicaments ubiquitous in the work (for example, Courtois, 1988; Briere, 1989; Lisman-Pieczanski, 1990; Davies and Frawley, 1992, 1994; Gabbard, 1992; Ehrenberg, 1992; Fields, 1994; Marcuse, 1994; Price, 1994, 1997; Hegeman, 1995a, 1995b; Diamond, 1997a; Daskovsky, 1998). Childhood sexual abuse obscures and distorts interpersonal relationships, and enactments of these distortions in the therapeutic relationship often lead to an intense, stormy atmosphere (Price, 1994). Frequently, and *necessarily*, a therapist gets caught up in these tempests and finds him- or herself furiously wishing to retaliate against the patient. Therapists are forced to encounter and accept these aspects of their own negative countertransference as part of the work with sexually abused adults.

Typical therapist reactions to this atmosphere noted by Courtois (1988) include fear, dread, and horror; denial and avoidance; shame, pity, or disgust; guilt; rage; grief and mourning; viewing the patient as *only* needy or *only* self-sufficient; generalizing victimhood to include everyone; using euphemisms to mute the affective impact of abuse experiences; secondary PTSD in the therapist; a sense of privileged voyeurism; and sexualization of the therapeutic relationship. Davies and Frawley (1994) have systematically identified a series of common problematic transference/countertransference paradigms encountered in the treatment of sexually abused patients, which I will discuss later in this chapter. Clearly, there are many pitfalls possible for therapists working with this population.

On the other hand, the relationship with the therapist is frequently seen as a potent agent of change for sexually abused patients, as is also clear in the cases described by Davies and Frawley and others. Hegeman (1995a) speaks forcefully of the need to begin work early on reviving the patient's capacity for relationship in order to allow the therapeutic dyad to be the vessel in which the abuse gets resolved. Briere (1995), however, highlights a conundrum inherent in these efforts. Noting that healing takes place in a damaged intimacy channel of relating, Briere emphasizes the sexually abused man's need to establish an ability to relate but also reminds us that paradoxically this is exactly what is most difficult for such a man to do.

CONTEMPORARY VIEWS OF THE THERAPEUTIC RELATIONSHIP

As a psychoanalyst, I think about the therapeutic relationship through the lens of a contemporary relational and interpersonal psychoanalytic model of treatment, particularly in regard to countertransference (Winnicott, 1949; Tauber, 1954; Wolstein, 1954, 1959; Greenberg and Mitchell, 1983; Stern, 1989; Maroda, 1991; Hirsch, 1993, 1995; Fiscalini, 1995). In this model, according to Hirsch (1995), "the analyst is seen as not only affectively influenced by the patient but as inevitably *enacting* this influence in the context of the transference–countertransference matrix, as well as acting as an agent of influence" (p. 656). The therapeutic relationship itself is considered above all to be dyadic and co-constructed by patient and therapist. In this co-construction process, patient and therapist also co-create the transference and countertransference of the treatment.

"Transference" in this model refers to all feelings and reactions to the therapist, conscious and unconscious, enacted or not, reality- or fantasy-based, that originate and are located in the patient. "Countertransference" refers to all feelings and reactions to the patient, conscious and unconscious, enacted or not, reality- or fantasy-based, that originate and are located in the therapist. Neither transference nor countertransference is necessarily neurotic. Both may be valuable sources of information about each participant, about their relationship, and about how to proceed in the treatment. Interpersonal and relational models of transference and countertransference emphasize that countertransferential reactions provide "a powerful ongoing source of data—a forced invitation into the patient's world" (Bromberg, 1995b, p. 148).

In considering countertransferential reactions, it is crucial that a therapist carefully reflect on his or her own usual relational patterns and how they may be affecting the relationship being co-constructed with a patient. With these serving as background, the therapist can see more easily when he or she begins to behave or react in uncharacteristic ways with a patient. This leads to awareness of interpersonal pulls from the patient that can help the therapist understand the patient's relational patterns. As Siegel (1996) puts it, "[T]he feelings induced in me by my patients' transferences represent a possible source of the reactivation of my past conflicts and a way to deal further with my own pathological defenses. More important, I view these feelings as indicators (not as proof!) of what might be going on in the patient at that time" (pp. 7–8).

I want to emphasize again that both transference and countertransference may be either reality- or fantasy-based. If, for example, a patient perceives, correctly, that I am sitting closer to him than usual, that is a reality-based part of his transference to me. This is true whatever conclusions he draws about my reasons for sitting closer to him. He may, for example, believe I am trying to seduce him, a fantasy-based part of his transference. But the reality-based part of his perception contributes to his transference whatever the reasons for my behavior actually are. For example, I may have placed my chair closer than usual to the patient chair because my previous patient was hard of hearing; nevertheless, the perception that I am closer than usual is part of the patient's transference to me. If I am sitting at my usual distance from him, the perception that I am unusually close to him is a fantasy-based part of his transference to me. In that case, his transference reaction may be based on some memory or incident in his history or current life, or on his current feelings about me and our relationship.

In nearly every case, a patient's transferential reaction is at least in part a response to some real aspect of my behavior, even if he distorts the importance of that behavior or if his conclusions about the reasons for it are erroneous from my point of view. For example, my chair may be in its usual spot, but I may be leaning slightly more forward than is typical for me. This countertransferential behavior on my part may derive from a variety of "real" reasons, whether reactive to him (for example, perhaps he is talking more softly than usual), ordinary (for example, perhaps my back feels stiff and I have shifted my position to stretch it), or peculiar to my own psychology (for example, perhaps I am feeling a need to feel closer to him).

If, on my side, I become aware that I am distracted in a session, that is part of my countertransference. I may then reflect on the sources for my distraction. Am I pulling back from the patient because he is talking about painful experiences? Has he brought up an issue that has personal meaning for me, and am I now involved in a personal thought process having to do with those reactions? Does that thought process lead me to associations that are relevant to the patient's situation, or are they idiosyncratic and unique to my own circumstance? Have I heard bad news just before the session? In that case, my distraction has little or no connection to the patient, but it may become relevant to our treatment.

This last situation occurred during my work with Uri. Minutes before a session with him, I heard that a friend in her late twenties had just died after a devastating illness. Uri began to speak in the session, then stopped and asked me if I was all right. I asked what was behind his question, and he said I looked gray and my eyes looked almost vacant. Instantly, I realized that the shock I had just received was showing on my face, and, uncharacteristically, I made a decision to validate his perception before going on to ask about his reactions to it. I felt that to do otherwise, to withhold the information for which he asked confirmation, would be both cruel and mystifying. His reality had often enough been denied by members of his family. I told him briefly that I had heard of a friend's death shortly before he came into my office, and that undoubtably my reactions to this sad news were showing on my face. He asked a question or two, and I expanded the information I gave him slightly, saying that my friend's death, while expected, had tragically occurred while she was a young adult. He asked if I wanted him to leave so I could collect myself. I said I had no wish for him to go, that I felt I could continue working with him. Then I asked if he wanted to leave, and about his reactions to my disclosing this information. He said he wanted to stay if I felt comfortable continuing, then voiced both his relief and his bitterness at hearing that his perceptions were accurate. "I almost can't believe you told it to me like it is. In my family, everyone always told me I was imagining things. Then maybe a year later I would realize that I had been right. My parents *were* fighting, there *was* a problem about money, my mother *did* invade my life and touch me inappropriately. But I never knew where I stood, I always wondered if I was crazy." This led us to a dialogue about how he perceives things in his current life, whether he tries to confirm or disconfirm his reality, and what happens if he does or does not make this attempt.

Would we have gotten to the same place had I not told him about the death of my friend? Perhaps. I certainly am aware that by telling him I took some risks and foreclosed some options.[1] But telling him freed me up emotionally to work actively with the issue then and there, which I do not believe I would otherwise have been capable of doing. Equally important, it gave us a joint relational interchange in which he experienced an alternative to the pattern of familial mystification he knew so well.

In this vignette, Uri's perception of my distraction was transferential, even though it had a basis in reality. My distraction was countertransferential, although I believe it had nothing to do with Uri. His expectation that I would withhold information or lie about it was transferential, stemming from childhood experiences as well as later ones. My decision to tell him the truth was countertransferential, arising from a variety of sources, some having to do with Uri, others having to do with me. These sources included my need to tell someone about my friend as well as my instinctive sense that I would be repeating a damaging interpersonal pattern in Uri's life if I did not confirm or disconfirm his perceptions. Our interaction about his perception was a co-construction that inaugurated a new interpersonal script in his life as well as in our work together, one we came back to again and again as we later considered his relationships with others and with me.

RELATIONAL RECONSTRUCTION
IN THE THERAPEUTIC DYAD

The primary need of a patient who has experienced incest or other childhood sexual trauma is to gain the capacity to relate to others in more functional ways. Cognitive restructuring, abreaction, rethinking gender roles, and other themes and techniques described in this book and elsewhere are meaningful and helpful in resolving sexual abuse, but they do not address this need. *Relational restructuring occurs above all through the interactive and current relationship between patient and therapist.*

The relational wound created by childhood sexual abuse means the

---

[1] See Mitchell's (1998) reflections on telling patients information confirming their perceptions about the therapist.

patient is likely to enter treatment "with fear, trepidation and ambivalence, as well as eagerness, desperation and immediate involvement and attachment" to the therapist (Price, 1994, p. 216). The decision to be in therapy itself may be experienced as a betrayal of oneself or of one's family, since the task of the patient in therapy is to tell the secret he has been forbidden to tell. Attention must be paid early in treatment to enhancing the patient's ability to relate (Davies and Frawley, 1992, 1994; Hegeman, 1995a), a critical factor because it is in the present, emotionally alive therapeutic relationship that the scenario for abuse gets rewritten. And this can occur only if patient and therapist are able to co-construct a meaningful intimate relationship. This conception of psychological treatment draws on the work of Sandor Ferenczi (1930), who wrote about using transference to help the patient effect an active mastery of a traumatic past through the immediacy of an emotional relationship with the therapist (see Balint, 1968; Bromberg, 1991; Hegeman, 1995a).[2]

A sexually abused man is thus less in need of "insight" about his history and its aftereffects than of a relationship that permits him to let himself be known intimately without fear of surrendering himself to the other person. This is one reason that the relationship between therapist and patient must be active and genuine. In it, the therapist encounters the patient directly, in all his multiple self-states (Bromberg, 1995a, 1995b), as described in the following section. The relationship with the therapist then becomes a catalyst that allows the patient to envision healing bridges over the spaces between his dissociated self-states.[3] In the experiential field of the therapeutic relationship, the patient connects dissociated aspects of self, including both internal and external realities. This is how he comes to "know" himself (Bromberg, 1991).

The therapeutic relationship also gives the man a laboratory in which to reenact his old abusive relational scripts, but with new outcomes. If, for example, he relates through distrust because of his abuse

---

[2] Franz Alexander (1948; Alexander and French, 1946) wrote about the "corrective emotional experience," a somewhat related theoretical concept. The difference is that Alexander believed that a patient learns emotionally about relationships through engagement with a therapist who behaves very differently than the patient's parents did. The therapist's behavior is thought to be more mature than the parents' was, and the patient has a corrective emotional experience through identification with the therapist's healthier attitudes. By contrast with Alexander's conceptualization, I am talking here about the therapist and patient mutually examining their co-constructed relationship. The patient actively discovers how the past affects this intimate bond and masters traumatic material through direct engagement with it in live interactions with the therapist.

[3] A similar point has been made specifically about the treatment of sexually abused men by Fitzgerald (Morris et al., 1997).

experiences, he has conceptualized relationships as invariably headed toward some kind of betrayal. If he cannot trust, it makes sense that he will feel that the therapist is malevolent. He has an internal narrative in which life leads inevitably to traumatic conclusions. Encountering the therapist within an intimate relationship where distrust is not warranted, at least not in the way it was when he was a child, he experiences a new perceptual truth that propels him to resymbolize his conception of relatedness. He is changed because of a relational encounter that is *experientially*, not only conceptually, different from what he knew before (Bromberg, 1993). As he retells his history, he is also able to reconstruct and reconcile formerly bewildering and contradictory events in a new relational context. Traditional efforts at "reconstruction" without this new relational reality fail because the patient's internal core personality remains untouched (Bromberg, 1995b).

Why is it that a new relational experience with a therapist, combined with an opportunity to recount his history in that new context, leads to relational restructuring and a reintegration of events in the patient's history? Interpersonal psychoanalytic theory posits that human experience is affected and changed by the relational context in which it happens. In Chapters 5 and 7, we saw the implications of Conte's and Gilgun's findings that sexually abused boys who had a confidant in childhood were less likely to become rapists or other violent criminals. These boys had the opportunity to process their ordeals cognitively at a time close to the events themselves, and had encoded their abuse in language. This encoding in a relational context seems to ameliorate the worst outcomes of abuse. The therapeutic relationship offers the patient in adulthood this possibility of symbolizing his experience. (For an example of this, see my discussion later in this chapter of the abuser/victim dynamic that existed between Abe and me.)

RELATING TO A PATIENT'S
MULTIPLE SELF-STATES

In Chapter 7, I described the contemporary psychoanalytic concept of a universal multiplicity of self-states rather than a single unified self. This model proceeds from the assumption that all people dissociate at times, and that dissociation is central to character formation. The abrupt changes in mood and behavior often seen in traumatized men (see, for examples, my descriptions of Patrick, pp. 141–144 and 184–186, and Abe, pp. 221–228, 245–247, and 254) can be conceptualized in this paradigm as attempts by one or more of the self-states to interrupt any positive relational flow. This need arises from that self-state's conviction that intimate relating is dangerously hazardous and that it is therefore imperative to destroy any hope that a good relationship is possible. Thus, at one point Abe told me that when he was relatively optimistic about his interpersonal world there was a constant voice in his head saying, "Get out of here! What are you doing here? Don't say that! Stop being a fool!"

According to this view, a therapist is always encountering the patient's multiple self-states, whether he or she is aware of them or not. Change is only possible when the therapist has the capacity to relate directly to all the multiple self-states the patient presents to him (Bromberg, 1995a, 1995b). When this happens, the patient's ability to bridge the gaps between his multiple realities is created or enhanced.

To accomplish relational restructuring, Davies and Frawley (1992, 1994), like Bromberg (1991), advocate speaking directly to each of the dissociated self-states, which are akin to separate personalities. This establishes immediate alliances between the therapist and, for example, the dissociated child-self that experienced trauma. These writers are not talking about a child-self being brought into the therapy metaphorically. Rather, they say a child-self must be contacted *directly*, not talked *about* to the more evolved, rational adult self that initially came for treatment. If such direct contact is not made, the therapy becomes an ineffectual attempt to achieve pseudoadulthood (Bromberg, 1991). There is thus a need for the therapist to forge a relationship with each of the multiple self-states in order for change to occur. When this happens, the patient can internalize a new therapeutic object relationship based on the experience *each* of the self-states has with the therapist. Bromberg (1991) notes that this direct contact between therapist and a patient's dissociated self-states "is important for most patients but *vital* for some" (p. 417, footnote).

But if a patient overlooks for even a moment his deeply held belief that being intimately related to his therapist inevitably leads to betrayal and a fractured sense of self, he abandons his "hard-won coterie of protective inner voices" (Bromberg, 1995a, p. 515). These voices remind him forcibly of his jeopardy. A rapid switch from one self-state to another, often happening at exactly the moment when things seem to be going well in the therapeutic relationship, represents a predictable and self-protective reminder from another self-state that intimate relatedness is perilous. As Bromberg (1995c) observes, progress in the therapeutic relationship is both " 'good news and bad news.' The 'bad news,' in one form or another, will be experienced and communicated as such by parts of self that do not feel gratitude for having been relationally 'enlivened' but feel threatened at having been 'invaded and betrayed.' Those parts of self would like to be able to comfortably and routinely return to the familiar dissociated structure—that is, to the ability to see life as a disaster waiting to happen—and to mechanically deal with the potential failure of the environment to protect the patient from trauma" (p. 189).

To illustrate: After two years of treatment, Victor told me he was afraid to allow his tremendous anger into our sessions, afraid it would overwhelm both me and him. As we explored this declaration, he suddenly said, "It's as if there's another voice inside me, telling me to be careful of you, telling me you're dangerous." I asked whether he could speak to me in that voice. After a long hesitation, he said, "I've protected Victor all this time. He would have died without me. Now you want to destroy me and leave Victor helpless and friendless. You have no idea what I've shielded him from going through!" I replied, "You *have* protected him, and I honor the good job you've done. But you've been overworked. He's older now and I think his world may be different. I do *not* want to destroy you. What I'm asking is that you see whether Victor can handle some of the things you've protected him from. You'll still be there when he needs you—but I don't think he needs you as often as he used to." Victor closed his eyes for a moment and then said, "It's as though that voice is really another person inside me, fighting to be heard. It helps to know what he thinks. It helps to know what the stakes are, what I'm really afraid of."

In this vignette, we see in rapid succession the existence of multiple self-states in a patient without dissociative identity disorder; the attempt by the patient to create a relationship with the therapist; the swift appearance of another voice to stop this alliance; and the work by the therapist to encounter directly this dissociated self-state in order to forge a relationship with it and encourage it to be a collaborator rather than an enemy in the therapeutic work.

The key in this aspect of the treatment is to remember the parts are there and to honor them for the work they have done and continue to do. This was beautifully brought home to me by Abe, who made an analogy between therapy and the *Oresteia*. In the Greek tragedy, Orestes kills his mother, then is haunted by the Furies and goes mad. In order to regain his sanity, he must give the Furies an honored place in his life. These Furies are similar to the parts of self that must be honored in order for the individual to feel whole.

Two weeks after the interchange reported above, Victor told me he had always had mixed reactions to hearing my voice, which he characterized as soothing, soft-spoken, and lulling. He said he had begun to realize that it reminded him of his father's voice during his abuse as his father told him how big and strong he was, how the father did this because he loved Victor and knew Victor wanted this to happen as much as he did. "So I've always been suspicious of you underneath it all, wondering if you had ulterior motives, if you cared about me or what I had to say." Victor said he had begun to think differently after I talked to the part of him that felt I was dangerous. "You didn't say that I don't need that suspicious part of me. You just asked me to see if I needed it as much. Those words have been reverberating in my head ever since. I've begun to hear you differently, to notice that even though you are soft-spoken you don't tell me what I feel. Instead, you really ask me to tell you what's going on inside of me. It's completely different from my father—I could never let myself see that before."

TRANSFERENCE, COUNTERTRANSFERENCE, AND REENACTMENT

Recurrent themes affecting the transference and countertransference with sexually abused patients start with the patient's wariness of the therapist and the dangers involved in intimacy. In addition, dependency, reliance, and counterdependent and counterphobic defenses tend to emerge, often cloaked in overt idealization of the therapist. In this idealization, patients may expect the therapist to be the all-attentive, nurturing, nonseductive, and nonabusing parent who will heal and undo the trauma. All these themes tend to appear in concerns about boundaries, secrecy, control, and power, and in discussions of fees, confidentiality, and other issues related to the frame of the treatment (Price, 1994).

Behavioral reenactments in treatment allow a patient to communicate previously dissociated, and therefore unsymbolized, material to the therapist. By analyzing verbally what has been communicated through behavior, the therapist and patient initiate a process by which the dissociated material becomes encoded in language, and therefore available for conscious consideration.

Behaviors associated with a reenactment in therapy are unconscious messages from the patient to the therapist and to himself about a traumatic past (Bromberg, 1991, 1993; Hegeman, 1995a). They represent an attempt to bypass the need for symbolized experience. Reenactments are most likely to occur when the patient has a reduced capacity for self-reflection, another result of being unable to verbalize traumatic experiences that were never encoded when they first occurred. Memories became "trapped, encased within a wordless world" (Davies and Frawley, 1994, p. 210). Incapable of articulating what he has never symbolized verbally, the patient repeats *behaviorally,* or reenacts, an aspect of his dissociated trauma. Thus, when Isaac went into my refrigerator and used my milk for his coffee, he brought the issue of boundary violations directly into our relationship. When Patrick took his pants off during a session, he forced us to address openly his sexual relationship with his father.

Such reenactments are crucial disclosures about unintegrated, unsymbolized, unformulated experience. Understanding the unconscious communication within a reenactment is often a pivotal point in therapy with a sexually abused adult. Bromberg (1993) argues that symbolization can be produced via reenactment within a psychotherapeutic relationship. Working through reenactments of trauma makes the previously dissociated experience "thinkable" (Bromberg, 1995b).

Seen in this light, enactment is a way for the patient to allow himself to be known by co-constructing, with the therapist, a means of living out a new, less disabling version of the original trauma. In this co-construction, cognitive symbolization of trauma occurs when the trauma is reenacted within a therapeutic relationship, reproducing the original interpersonal context but not leading to the original outcome (Davies and Frawley, 1992; Bromberg, 1994). Once this happens, dissociated experience is transformed to internal conflict and human relatedness, which are more available for verbal consideration in psychotherapy. By working through reenactments, the therapist thus gradually obtains access to the patient's various multiple dissociated self-states.

The analysis of a reenactment is embedded in the therapeutic relationship. Davies (1994) describes how the therapist is both the magnet that draws out the reenactment and the architect of a transitional arena in which the patient's experiences of self and other can be reconfigured in more harmonious ways. "We assume—indeed, we rely upon—the hope that analyst and patient together will become enmeshed in complicated reenactments of early unformulated experiences with significant others that can shed light upon the patient's current interpersonal and intrapsychic difficulties by reopening in the analytic relationship prematurely foreclosed areas of experience" (p. 156). If the reenactment is to be integrated as other than the original trauma, however, "something essentially different must happen to render this reenactment only a partial one" (p. 157).

Davies and Frawley (1994) identify four paradigms recurringly found in therapeutic relationships with sexually abused women. The four paradigms Davies and Frawley describe are:

- The sadistic victimizer relating to a furious but helpless victim,
- The collaborator in a seductive relationship where one participant is the seducer and the other is seduced,
- The powerful but idealized rescuer of an entitled child who demands rescue, and
- The nonabusing but uninvolved parent relating to an unseen and neglected child.

In addition, Frawley (now Frawley-O'Dea, personal communication), suggests a fifth paradigm in which one participant is a certain believer and the other is a chronic doubter. In this dynamic, both patient and therapist oscillate between absolute certainty and absolute tortured doubt about the abuse, finding it nearly impossible to attain comfort with the normal degree of ambiguity we all must tolerate about past and present events.

These four paradigms all involve two complementary relational models, each of which may be alternately enacted by both patient and therapist as they relate to one another. Thus, over the course of time the patient may enact the victimizer while the therapist enacts the victim; then the patient may enact the victim while the therapist enacts the victimizer; then the patient is the seducer while the therapist is seduced; then the therapist is the seducer while the patient is seduced; and so on. Through these models, patient and therapist fluctuate between the two roles in each paradigm, and in a single treatment every one of the models may occur at some point.

The relational models of transference and countertransference posited by Davies and Frawley are reenactments of different aspects of the dissociated relationships involved in victimization by a parent or caretaker. Indeed, as previously noted, Davies and Frawley assert that abusive countertransferential reenactments are an inevitable part of the treatment of sexually abused patients (see also Diamond, 1997a).

Transference–countertransference reenactments are vehicles for communication to the therapist about the internal relational experience of the child as he was being abused. As such, they are powerful tools, but they are also forceful and often coercive catalysts in the therapeutic relationship. Reenactment compels the therapist to experience the patient's original reactions to abuse, reactions that are his dissociated aftermath to a deeply traumatic childhood experience. To heal the patient of the trauma, the therapist must experience that trauma is some way. The reenactment may be symbolic of the abuse, but the feelings engendered in the therapist are very real. These may include helplessness, impotence, rage, inadequacy, shame, guilt, idealization, omnipotence, overstimulation, humiliation, torture, and fear (Price, 1994)—all internal states with which the patient is very familiar.

Thus, treating patients whose relationships and personalities are organized by dissociation involves a challenging psychological encounter with the trauma that caused the dissociation in the first place. Therapists can easily feel traumatized themselves under such circumstances, as I will discuss below. Yet it is important to remember that neither reenactments nor countertransference reactions to them are necessarily "mistakes."

Rather, they are unavoidable phases in the treatment of traumatized, dissociated patients.

In the next sections of this chapter I will discuss and illustrate each of Davies and Frawley's four transference–countertransference paradigms. In the descriptions of treatments throughout this book, however, we can see the ubiquity in the work of their four paradigms as well as the fifth one suggested by Frawley-O'Dea.

THE ABUSER AND THE ABUSED VICTIM

It has commonly been noted that abused patients tend to identify with their abusers and then to be transferentially abusive to their therapists. In doing this, they are repeating with the therapist what happened to them as children. The abuser–victim relational configuration is particularly upsetting to work with for both patient and therapist because of its ubiquitous intense transference and countertransference enactments.

When the patient takes the position of the abuser, he retains a bond to the victimizer through unconscious identification. This stance also allows the patient to keep at bay his feelings of helplessness. He projects this helplessness onto the therapist, whom he may then devalue. In this context, the patient may demand special treatment from the clinician. Boundary violations of the therapist, such as making contact with people or institutions in the therapist's personal life, are also likely at such times. When this happens, the clinician feels intruded upon and penetrated, often coming to dread therapy sessions. Yet it is crucial for this enactment to occur. In dealing with it, the therapist must walk a tightrope between ignoring the man's abusive behavior, and thus becoming the unseeing parent, and expressing a feeling of victimization that may evoke excessive guilt in the patient.

Alternating and concurrent with abusive behavior toward the therapist is a dynamic in which the patient repeats a victimized relationship with the therapist, and the therapist reenacts the abuser's role, usually (but not always) in some symbolic way. Gabbard and Twemlow (1994), for example, describe a man with a history of maternal incest who tended to experience his therapist's comments as "biting and injurious" (p. 185). While they imply that this was the patient's distortion, we must remember that patients' transferential perceptions almost always have a basis in some reality of the relationship, and therapists are commonly drawn into playing an abusive role that is often, but not always, symbolic.

When the therapist enacts the abuser and the patient becomes a victim, the patient may react to the inequality of their relationship, feel victimized by the fee, or otherwise feel exploited by the therapist. In turn, the therapist may become intrusive or controlling. Often, a therapist who has usually been the victim in the transference–countertransference enactment may explode after months of abuse, instantly reversing the abuser–abused dynamic in the relationship.

The transferential reenactment of abuse can be subtle and symbolic. It may come through as a tendency to manipulate and exploit the therapist in covert ways. Recall, for example, that Yale told me after being in treatment for a few months that he had originally consulted me with the idea that I would have to testify in a court case if he decided to sue the Catholic Church because of his childhood sexual abuse by a nun. It had not occurred to him to say this directly to me when we first met, even though (or, perhaps, *because*) he believed I might not want to testify in such circumstances. This manipulative enactment in the transference revealed a great deal about how Yale related to others, as I discussed in Chapter 5.

The abuser–victim dynamic can be direct and overt as well. Witness my relationship with Abe in the fifth year of his treatment. This was at a midpoint in his shift away from being a perennial victim. A man who had perceived, found, or created abuse in nearly every interpersonal situation, Abe had evolved to a point where he was no longer blaming all his troubles on others. Instead, he had just begun to see how he participated in setting up abusive relationships. During this period, we repeatedly delved into his expectations of abuse from me. Each of us experienced the other as abusive on occasion, and it was the live interactions between us about these feelings that got through to him.

For example, one day Abe exploded in rage when he felt I had not comprehended the extent of his vulnerability when I commented on his abrasiveness. I assume he was correct that there was at least a partial failure of empathy in my remark, though his reaction to it seemed nearly out of control. Abe snarled about my inability to empathize, and then castigated me about my defensiveness in the face of his attack. I felt assaulted, and no doubt I was defensive and counterattacking at least to some degree in my reaction. Yet, in general I remained attuned to him, continuing to talk to him, giving my point of view without invalidating his perceptions of me. Our interchange got very heated on both sides. I pointed out in several ways how he had escalated and compounded any abuse that might have existed in my original comment.

At the end of what had nearly become a screaming match, we both felt spent, but we had also somehow arrived at a point of mutual respect. I had been at least symbolically abusive in my original remark, helping to create Davies and Frawley's abuser–victim dynamic, which they note is inevitable in working with an abused patient. I had nevertheless reacted to his subsequent transferential victimization of me in a way that served as a model for how one can remain in a significant relationship but not permit mistreatment. On his side, he felt that I heard him. When we talked about our clash during the next session, I said at one point that I hated our arguments, that I found them difficult and draining, but that I simultaneously welcomed them, because they gave us an opportunity for a live encounter in which we affected one another, with each of us surviving and growing from it.

Abe brought up this comment a number of times in subsequent years as a revelation to him, a sign that I cared about him enough to endure a taxing and painful emotional state. He recalled the screaming marathons in his house as he grew up, which typically ended in violence, brutal punishment, or threatened suicide. He found it impossible to believe I cared enough about him to endure what had passed for human interaction in his family.

This led him to think differently about our relationship, and about relating in general. He saw that his negativity about interpersonal situations developed even when things were going relatively well. He became able to assert himself at times, to move away from rather than toward abusive situations, and to avoid most exploitative relationships. Yet he still feared being around people, and was often sure he had been or would be manipulated and misused.

In reflective moments, Abe was able to see that these reactions had not changed since treatment began—indeed, not since childhood—even though the stimuli were different. In the midst of his continuing despair, he said he was glad it was so clear that real abuse was no longer occurring. It made him realize that he carried around his abuse history and assumed it was recurring even when he "knew" it was not. As he said, this was an important differentiation.

What in our relationship helped him get to this point? It is true that I sat and listened to him for years, pointing out over and over how he was "arranging" continuing abuse, and noting things he might have done or said in a given situation to stop what he considered to be exploitation. At times, I rehearsed with him how to deal with tense interpersonal situations. I believe, however, that Abe's most important shifts came from his over-arching direct experience of our relationship as basically nonabusive. Especially compelling for him was my willingness, when things heated up between us, to stay related to him and even to acknowledge some personal shortcomings and errors. With time, Abe developed an enhanced capacity for tolerating the ambiguity of a relationship in which both highly positive and highly negative qualities coexisted. In addition, our relationship offered him the opportunity to encode linguistically his interpersonal experiences with me and with others.

Two years after the incident when I told him I simultaneously hated and welcomed our arguments, Abe brought up an idealized therapeutic relationship portrayed in a popular movie, and said, "That has nothing to do with therapy! I didn't need some wonderful person who could withstand whatever I dished out—I needed someone with an edge, someone who engaged me at my level, who'd fight it out with me if necessary, who'd tell me if he thought I abused him—it didn't matter whether you were right or I was right—it mattered that I knew you would stick it out with me anyway." At a still later point in the treatment, Abe pointed out that his shifts had not come from talking about relationships outside my office. "I talked *about* things in therapy before. But it was living them out with you, having to face the abuse I felt in our relationship, here, alive, with you, that forced me to change."

THE SEDUCED AND THE SEDUCER

Particularly noteworthy in any discussion of transference and countertransference in work with sexually abused men is the sexualized transference and its sequelae. Like many sexually abused women, men with a history of sexual abuse tend to expect every relationship to involve seduction by one party or the other (see Siegel, 1996). Children who are molested by parents or other caretakers are oedipal "winners" in a distorted, pathological sense, and, as my first child analytic supervisor told me, there is no one as seductive as an oedipal child. Such a child often grows up to be a seductive and seduceable adult.

How does being a childhood oedipal winner of this magnitude translate into how an adult relates in psychotherapy? In Chapter 8, I noted that sexually abused children learn that sexuality is their interpersonal currency, a means of bonding to authority figures whose love they long for, need, and fear. As adults in psychodynamic treatment they reenact this dynamic again and again, and the concentration of seductive energy in the therapy can overwhelm both patient and therapist. They bring their intensely seductive manner of relating to their treatment, sometimes to the point of outright attempts at seduction of the therapist. It is therefore not surprising that adults sexually abused in childhood have been found to be more often subject to sexual abuse by their therapists than other patients (Smith, 1984; Gabbard, 1989; Kluft, 1990; Lymberis, 1994). These, obviously, are "real" abusive countertransferential reenactments.

As Price (1994) puts it, "[T]he sessions and the office may be cloaked in an erotic atmosphere and tension that may be difficult for the analyst to contain and tolerate" (p. 225). This may happen in the total absence of overt sexual content in the session. Explorative and probing questions by the therapist may be experienced as sexual or abusive by the patient, or may become so as the therapist is inducted into a seducer–abuser role in the relationship.

Thus, the ambiance of the treatment is filled with a sense of seduction, and therapist and patient each recurrently feels seduced by the other. The patient may be afraid of being flirtatious or seductive, fearing that this will bring on abuse. Concurrently, however, he may feel that this is the only way to get what he needs, having been trained to seduce in order to maintain a primary relationship. The therapist may feel both attacked and aroused by this behavior. Should the clinician feel sexual arousal from the eroticism of the material being presented, he or she may feel guilty and exploitative, and may want to withdraw emotionally from the overstimulating emotional field of the therapeutic relationship. Nonetheless, it is imperative that the therapist remain emotionally available. This must happen concurrent with the therapist conveying to the patient the idea that sexual feelings are acceptable and not instilling guilt and shame about the erotic energy in the relationship. Simultaneously, it must be communicated that one can set boundaries, not act on sexual feelings, but also not deny them.

In such instances the therapist must be careful to monitor countertransferential feelings about sexuality, love, nurturance, affection, and abuse, the same feelings the patient has trouble differentiating. It is important to articulate the differences among these feelings over and over, and to demonstrate, for example, that it is possible to be nurturant without having sexual designs. To do this with a sexually abused man, though, the therapist may have to sort through the same kinds of intense, inchoate feelings about the patient that the patient experiences in virtually every relationship of his life.

For example, my treatment of Patrick required me to find new capacities to work with his enactments in many interpersonal spheres, but particularly in our sexualized transference–countertransference relationship. Patrick was the victim of profound sexual abuse by his father for several years starting at age two or three, as described in Chapter 6. His dissociated defensive style was discussed in Chapter 7. I will here focus on the dynamic of seducer and seduced victim enacted in our transference and countertransference.

Patrick was openly seductive with me, frequently referring to me as his lover and jauntily offering to have sex with me. At such times, his manner was brittle and mocking, as though he were daring me to take his offers seriously. He laughingly recounted how he told his friends details of his sexual fantasies about me. On the occasions we were able to explore these fantasies in a more sober vein, what emerged was an image of me as an eroticized but loving father figure. He imagined he would feel safe in my arms, and was eager to perform all kinds of sexual acts on me to secure my permission for him to stay close to me. He imagined I would protect and support him, both emotionally and financially. At this point, at least, there was no hint of the other side of this transference, namely, that I would be the abusing and hurtful father as well.

In our work together, Patrick brought in all the eroticized themes of his life, often reenacting them with me so that I felt traumatized, disturbed, and exhausted. A subtle example occurred one day when he heard me cough and offered with a faraway smile to listen to my chest with a stethoscope for signs of bronchitis. On the face of it, this was a caring, if inappropriate, offer. But his dissociated smile, followed by a wolfish grin, made it clear that he was seductively interested in molesting me by invading my boundaries in the guise of taking care of me.

A far more glaring example occurred one day when he suddenly removed his trousers in a session, supposedly to show me exactly what happened when he tried to seduce his father. When I told him to put his pants back on, he became angry, ridiculed me for being sexually constricted, and finally accused me of shaming him about his abuse experience. Outwardly, I worked with him in a reasonable manner about this, asking what he was trying to accomplish by taking his pants off, what he imagined my response would be, and what the meaning could be of his engaging in what he knew was unacceptable behavior with me.

But my interior life was chaotic as we struggled about the meaning of what he had done. I felt tantalized and seduced, stimulated to have exciting but bewildering feelings while feeling dimly that I might be humiliated because of the inappropriateness of those feelings to the situation. I felt Patrick had suddenly reversed the power relationships in the room by standing up while I remained seated and by being sexually aggressive, even though he remained affectively disconnected from his predatory sexuality. At the same time, however, he experienced me as abusing him by shaming him about early sexual experiences. I wondered how true it was that I was too constricted to deal with the complexities of sexual experience Patrick described and enacted. I wondered what would happen if my colleagues found out that my patient had partially disrobed during a session. I wondered whether in some way I had been unconsciously seductive with Patrick, and whether his getting undressed was a response to inappropriate behavior on my part. I wondered who Patrick would tell about what he had done, and what they would think. I imagined him ridiculing me to them, blandly and amusedly telling them how nonplused I had been when he had acted so flamboyantly and seductively with me. In short, I countertransferentially felt the anger, ridicule, abuse, excitement, coercion, arousal, and shame that Patrick had felt first as a child, and then again with me. This is what Herman (1992) would call my "traumatic countertransference" to Patrick (see my discussion of this phenomenon later in this chapter).

What was the transferential meaning of Patrick's behavior? As I see it, his disrobing was an attempt to seduce me as a reenactment of his relationship with his father. I believe Patrick was deeply ambivalent about the response he wanted from me. He was testing me to see if I would molest him, but he did not know what kind of outcome he hoped for. Remember that Patrick as a young man had actually tried to seduce his father, who apparently was no longer interested in him as a sexual partner, possibly because of Patrick's age or the greater likelihood that the relationship would be publicly revealed. Patrick's attempt to reestablish a sexual bond with his father seems to have come from a longing for the closeness that had accompanied the abuse, at least on a symbolic level.

Through his seductive behavior, therefore, Patrick wanted me to enact a seduction, on the one hand, in order to reexperience the painful intimacy he had once had with his father. Yet he was also hoping I would stop the reenactment. This would help him create a new narrative about the abuse. It would help him experience the possibility of a different outcome, an outcome in which his father substitute set limits on the sexuality in their relationship but not on the intimacy.

Reenacting the relationship with his father in the therapy was also a way for Patrick finally to symbolize his abuse experiences. Committing these actions as an adult permitted him to put into words what had never been verbally encoded in childhood. This was ultimately a means of further giving up the dissociation about his abuse by connecting to it through linguistically encoded expression rather than solely through reenactment.

A final point about Patrick's dissociation from his sexualized reenactment is that in the absence of his experiencing the erotic elements of our relationship, I experienced them with greater intensity. This frequently happens in any relationship when one of the participants disowns feelings: the other person experiences an augmented but distorted aspect of those disowned feelings. Therefore, when Patrick could not acknowledge his erotic feelings, I came closest to feeling overwhelmed by them. As those experiences got encoded in language, he became more disturbed about them, while I became more relaxed.

THE RESCUER AND THE NEEDY CHILD

It is easy for therapists to be drawn into the role of omnipotent savior, as Davies and Frawley note, since "we have chosen, after all, to live our lives as professional helpers" (1994, p. 178). The therapist's wish to heal deprivation and emotional starvation is magnified many times over when a man's circumstances include a history of having been abused, neglected, violated, or otherwise victimized as a child. After all, in boyhood the man did need rescue but did not get it. The urge to make psychological reparations can be strong, and is further intensified by the man's corresponding wish to find a caretaker who will, finally, protect and deliver him from his trauma.

Thus, the therapist becomes the rescuer in a therapeutic relationship when the horrors of the abuse elicit internal caretaking responses. Rescue fantasies recur throughout treatment, but they are especially likely when the patient is beginning to integrate experiences and mourn. At such a time, the therapist may get caught up in the poignancy of the patient's situation. The patient may become like a wounded child who demands that he get recompense for his suffering. He may want to replace his childhood with a wonderful new one given to him by the therapist. If this happens, clinicians must try to balance their reactions, allowing the man's long-buried yearnings for relatedness to emerge while also permitting him to rail against his original losses.

The flip side of this equation occurs when the therapist is needy in some way, and the patient tries to make things better. The therapist may feel, for example, that he or she has given and given to the patient, but is unappreciated. At such a moment, the clinician may have the impulse to retaliate through emotional withdrawal. On the other hand, when the patient becomes the rescuer, he is often acutely attuned to the moods and needs of the therapist. He may act to help the therapist partly out of a fear that if he does not do so the therapist will be unable to give to him. But he may also be acting out of loving wishes to nourish the therapist. Accomplishing this may have the added benefit of making him feel capable of being a nurturer.

Some of these dynamics occurred with Uri in the example described earlier in this chapter when he discerned that I was in shock and I acknowledged that I had just heard about the death of a friend. We decided to continue the session, and, along with the other work we accomplished, there was the thread of his helping me through an emotionally difficult period. By the end of the session, I was over the initial blow of the news I heard, and was glad I had spent the time in his company. On his side, in addition to being relieved that I had been straightforward with him, he felt competent and capable because he was able to give to me emotionally, reversing the usual flow in our relationship.

To illustrate some of the ramifications of the patient's wish for an idealized rescuer, consider Harris, whom I will discuss further in Chapters 10 and 11. A highly intelligent, self-contained professional man in his forties, Harris had been abused by an alcoholic father for a period of years during latency. His father, who normally spent no time with his children, would take Harris to the park and engage in mutual masturbation with him there. Otherwise, the father spent much of his time drinking, and never held a steady job. Harris grew up in a psychological fog, overresponsible for his mother and brothers but with no real goals in his own life. After serving in the army, Harris returned to his parents' poverty-stricken home. For the next seven years, especially after his father's death, he led a life grimly similar to his father's. He never worked steadily, took occasional courses at schools, and led what he called an "indolent" life, spending his evenings in bars picking up women for one-night stands.

By the time he was thirty, Harris was profoundly frightened. He started treatment with a woman analyst and began to work for a living, initially at a humiliatingly low-level job as a stockboy in a store. He put himself through college and professional school, marrying when he was about forty. Despite these obviously positive changes in his life, Harris maintained much of his psychological fog, with occasional flashes of inchoate rage, usually suppressed quickly or directed inward in some self-destructive manner.

He was referred to my group for sexually abused men by his female analyst. Having had a history of difficult relationships with male authorities, he was initially wary of me. But he quickly saw me as an expert who would save him from the aftermath of sexual abuse he was just beginning to face. In his first months in the group, he looked to me to be his nurturer, and protected me from attacks by other group members. He swiftly developed an idealized view of me as a fathering figure who was giving him what he had sorely lacked all his life from his own father. He defended me from criticism by other group members, often using methods so subtle I only detected them in retrospect.

This became apparent when Abe, another group member, attacked me in the last moments of a group session because he did not like my practice of making summarizing comments at the end of a group. Because time did not permit us to deal with the issue, I elected not to make any such remarks that night. Harris came to the next group session in a fury, declaring that Abe had deprived him of what he needed from me.

At first, Harris raged chiefly at Abe, who saw me in individual treatment and who Harris therefore experienced as being more favored by me. In his fury, Harris reenacted his father's bullying role in his own family. Indeed, he much later acknowledged that as an adolescent and young man he had taken a similar ogrelike bullying stance in relation to his younger brothers as well. But it was clear that Harris's anger was as much with me, his transferential father, as with Abe, his transferential sibling. He felt I had capitulated to unreasonable demands and was therefore favoring Abe while cutting Harris off from a primary source of nurturing from me. His struggle with these feelings helped us both to recognize the enormity of Harris's neediness, but it also signaled the end of his view of me as his rescuer. (In Chapter 11, I will further discuss the mutual sibling transference between these two men.)

With time, Harris dropped his idealization of me and instead voiced directly the transferential rage that had always lurked beneath it. Our relationship became a reenactment of the abusive one Harris had had with his father, and in a flash either of us could become the abuser or the victim. During this period, Harris was painfully sensitized to any change in my tone, particularly one that conveyed to him a wavering of empathy, a condescension, or a patronizing attitude. Sometimes he startled me with the immediate fury of his response. At other times he kept his anger hidden, then spit it out at me later when I least expected it. During the individual sessions I periodically schedule with group members he told me about my many shortcomings as a therapist. He particularly focused on what he called my callousness and inability to see how hurtful I was, as demonstrated by my ignoring his directives about how to listen to him and my repeated failures to meet his needs. He said he now saw me as impeding his progress in the group, as a necessary evil he had to endure because the group experience was so important to him. In order to maximize the group's effectiveness, he said, he now had to screen out my existence as much as possible. I will return to these themes in Chapters 10 and 11.

THE INEFFECTIVE PARENT
AND THE NEGLECTED CHILD

As Davies and Frawley (1994) note, "Whenever a child is sexually abused, someone's eyes are closed" (p. 168). If a boy grows up with a parent unable, unwilling, or not caring enough to see what is happening and save him from harm, he has to find a way to resolve this relational injury. A relationship between a nonabusing but nonseeing, ineffective, and uninvolved parent and a neglected, unseen, and unprotected child may result in profound attachment trauma that precedes any sexual abuse.

Because the parent is loved and needed by the child, this relational constellation is split off from consciousness, with the child preserving the image of a loving, available parent. But, while he preserves the parent consciously as devoted and capable, unconsciously he may set up relationships in which people who seem accessible and loving are actually uncaring, unavailable, or unfeeling. If this kind of dynamic is replicated in the therapeutic relationship, the man creates a situation in which he seems to be establishing a positive relationship, but experiences the therapist as cold, callous, or rejecting. Out of this pain, the man may become alienated, hurt, and despondent. Eventually, these feelings may turn to anger, and he may retaliate.

When a patient enacts the neglected child, he denies his own wishes and protects and caters to the therapist, feeling this is the only way to get his needs met. Therapists may not easily see the falseness of this presentation because it is initially experienced as positive relatedness from the patient. Over time, however, the patient becomes deeply disappointed in the therapist, and this disappointment can turn to covert rage. Eventually, he may develop an openly hostile transference, experiencing the therapist as not seeing him, not remembering important things about him, and not caring sufficiently about him.

All the aspects of this pattern came into play in my work with Abe, whose narcissistic parents were unable to see or care about his needs. He had always seen them as malevolent and hateful, but with time he acknowledged that perhaps they hardly knew he existed in the world. In a way, this was a graver injury to his self-esteem than thinking they wished him harm. In our work, Abe often seemed able to relate warmly to me, but he was quick to notice any failings on my part, and was then alternately hurt, depressed, and attacking. He saw me as he saw his parents, and he fluctuated between thinking I did not want him to succeed in life and believing I was not capable of feeling empathy for him. On my side, I frequently found myself burdened by the complicated interpersonal field we lived in, and periodically pulled back emotionally for relief from it.

On the other hand, a man may identify with the unavailable parent and turn on others who had expected emotional resonance from him. In the therapeutic relationship, he may seem indifferent, compassionless, or cruel. The clinician then becomes the neglected child countertransferentially, experiencing him- or herself as unwanted, unimportant, and unconnected to the patient. It is crucial that the therapist not abandon the patient emotionally during these periods. However, feeling wounded, unappreciated, or depressed, he or she may eventually be pulled to behave callously toward the patient, becoming, for example, sleepy or forgetful during sessions.

Both sides of the ineffective parent–neglected child paradigm were played out in my work with Patrick, whose overburdened mother managed to provide physical caretaking for her nine children but otherwise lived in a depressed, alcoholic haze. She continued to deny that the family had severe problems into her old age. Witness the oscillations in my relationship with Patrick as we approached the premature termination of his psychoanalysis:

After four and a half years, Patrick's therapy benefits were cut off by his insurance company. He and I went through several appeal processes, but we were eventually given a cutoff date for his treatment. He had made some remarkable changes. He had nearly completed a demanding graduate program while maintaining his full-time job. He had had one six-month-long relationship with a man which, while it ended unhappily, represented the closest he had ever come to an intimate love relationship. He had dropped a number of superficial friendships while developing a few that appeared to have some depth. He had confided in most of his siblings about his abuse history, and had been surprised by the support shown by several of them, including a brother who made himself emotionally available to Patrick in unexpected new ways and a sister who revealed that she also had been sexual abused by their father.

Yet, Patrick was often moody, depressed, and isolated. He was highly changeable in his feelings about me and the treatment, and continued at times to question the veracity of his memories. He had developed a highly structured work and school life in part so he did not have to deal with emotional relationships.

As it became clear that the treatment would end, Patrick's strong dissociative defenses reemerged and predominated in our work. He had, of course, never lost his ability to dissociate altogether. Indeed, everyone needs some ability to dissociate in order to cope with unexpected trauma. The predominating dissociation now seemed more potent than ever, and in retrospect I see that he was preparing himself for what was indeed a major trauma. The difference, however, was that now I was able to break through the dissociation at times, and he sometimes expressed relief when I did.

Patrick had always voiced some ambivalence about the therapeutic process. It was demanding and painful, often leaving him depressed, frightened, and wondering if his memories were themselves simply a reflection of his craziness. He passively allowed the insurance company to resolve his ambivalence about treatment by dictating that he would stop. He never investigated whether he would be able to pay for his therapy privately after his graduation, when he would be working two jobs, nor did he ever ask me whether I would consider lowering my fees. When I brought up these two possibilities, he dismissed them. He seemed to feel it was natural that he not be cared for, and this combined with his usual resistance to treatment, making him proceed implacably toward the conclusion of our work.

As we approached our final session, I tried to talk to Patrick about his feelings about the termination. He responded formally in general terms. When I pressed him toward the end of a session about how he felt about our relationship ending, he said coolly, "Ours has been a professional relationship. You have always behaved as I would expect a competent professional to act."

I felt stung, and, internally, I recoiled. I recognized that on one level he was telling me that he was grateful I had acted appropriately and kept our boundaries clear by maintaining the professional frame of our work despite his efforts to break it. Yet I also felt his interpersonal distance repudiated the intensity of our therapeutic relationship. After the session, I felt enraged at what seemed to be a calm dismissal of all the work we had done together. As I thought through my reactions, however, it occurred to me that Patrick was resorting to his usual dissociated way of reacting to anxiety and pain. In addition, he was reestablishing the rigid boundaries between us (indeed, between himself and everyone) that he felt were necessary in order for him to function in the world. I realized that I had to ask more about his reactions. We had been alternating in the roles of unavailable, ineffective, and cold caregiver and needy, depressed, and wounded child. When he was feeling needy, as when he wanted my help in order for his medical benefits to continue, I was ineffective, and probably at that time he experienced me as unavailable and cold. When he was cold, I felt abused, wounded, and enraged. Each of us activated such responses in the other.

In the next session, I asked Patrick further about his feelings, reminding him of the many emotional ups and downs we had experienced, and doubting that his statement reflected everything that was going on inside him. He closed his eyes and was silent for a moment, then said quietly, but passionately, "I have been abused by my father and my brother. My other brother died of AIDS in my arms, and I had to go choose clothes for him to wear for his cremation, then scatter his ashes alone. My mother continues to act as though everything has always been fine in the family. If I can get through all that, I can certainly handle not seeing you!" Then he burst into tears and sobbed about all his losses as I sat with him, my own eyes filled with tears.

This declaration had many meanings. It was a needed rebuilding of boundaries between us. It was an affirmation for Patrick that he could indeed survive. But it was also a demonstration of a new ability to symbolize his trauma verbally rather than to dissociatively sleepwalk through it. He broke out of his seemingly cold stance and grieved in this session and those that remained to us. His capacity to do this personified all the work we had done to allow him to mourn openly the childhood innocence he lost through abuse.

COUNTERTRANSFERENTIAL DENIAL

How do therapists react to the chronic intensity of treatment with sexually abused adults? According to Price (1994), they "often find themselves in situations that test deeply held beliefs regarding themselves, the world, and psychoanalytic treatment" (p. 211). As Kluft (1990a) recognizes, "[M]y ignorance did not become awareness, understanding, and knowledge without going through prolonged and recurrent phases of skepticism, disbelief, and denial" (p. 11). Therapists frequently experience the impulse to reel back from the shock and deny the horror of the material being described. This is a natural reaction in any therapist who is empathically attuned to the patient:

> [The] thrill of the explorer . . . was largely overwhelmed by the fear and horror of it all. I did not want to know this information. It scared me. . . . How could this be true? How could there be so much child abuse? . . . Worst of all, it made us sick—sick at heart, sick in our souls, and sick to our stomachs. . . . When people "remember" previous trauma, . . . they relive it, or, more often, . . . live it for the first time. It is terrible for them, extremely painful, embarrassing, and disgusting. . . . The participant-observer is completely unprepared for what is coming and inevitably experiences some kind of secondary or "vicarious" traumatization at witnessing the horror and trauma of a past time intruding into the present. (Bloom, 1997, p. 7)

Like the patient, the therapist may try to keep the experience unformulated and unsynthesized. After all, trauma by definition is an event that seemed impossible in the patient's worldview, and may seem equally impossible to the therapist. The dilemma, as Daskovsky (1998) conveys, is that it is in experiencing the therapist's struggle to listen to the impossible that the patient gets freed from it:

> Working with abused patients requires that therapists learn to sit with unbearable tension between intolerable choices. . . . The paradox here is that by stopping trying to escape the helplessness, we might actually be able to offer something that is truly helpful. What is required is a tall order for those of us whose stock in trade is to hope and help: We need to tolerate the reality of our patients' and our own hopelessness and helplessness without acting to defend against their intolerable feelings. If we can succeed in doing this, we can help our patients to mourn for the choices they never had as children and to see more clearly the ones they do have in the present. (p. 13)

Stories of transgressions, atrocities, and abuse may cause therapists to react by feeling disbelief, pain, sadness, anxiety, and rage (Price, 1994). They may become disillusioned and hopeless about the world, about humanity, and about the family (see the discussion of therapists' vicarious traumatization in the next section). While these may be projective identifications, a taking in of the patient's own disillusionment, they are also human, caring responses to hearing true stories about rape, violence, and the exploitation of children. Price notes that therapists' difficulty tolerating these internal states may make them move away from the affects, blame the patient, or shield both patient and therapist from experiencing the feelings.

Accompanying this is the wish to hurry the patient toward awareness and insight. Such a wish represents the therapist's countertransferential need to make a shortcut through the material so that neither patient nor therapist has to endure the pain of what is being re-experienced. In this instance, the therapist has partially formulated the trauma, but, like many patients, he or she is compartmentalizing terror, dissociatively putting it into a mental box in order to keep its affect out of experience. At such times, the therapist must make great efforts to maintain psychological boundaries while staying attuned to the patient, neither merging with the material nor denying it. Otherwise, the work on the trauma will have no real emotional resonance for either patient or therapist.

For example, one day as I worked with Patrick, I noticed that as he reached for the words to recall early abuse he kept making a constricted "Khh-khh-khh" sound. It sounded like coughing, and I wondered if he were ill. He continued making this guttural vocalization, and then I had a sudden insight about this sound. Dry and strangled, it sounded as though he were gagging, and I abruptly wondered whether it was a reenactment of his choking attempts to accommodate his father's penis during fellatio at age three. I immediately felt enraged at Patrick's father, but also experienced disgust and nausea. I began to dissociate from my own thoughts and feelings, and I berated myself for having such ideas. I could not breathe easily. At the same time, I began to think Patrick was being histrionic, that this could not have happened. Aghast and appalled, I was experiencing both the symptoms and the doubts that Patrick himself felt. Only with pain and difficulty could I allow myself not to interrupt, neither to deflect Patrick from this topic nor to railroad him into a too-quick acceptance of my insight. I forced myself to remain silent, and a few sessions later he began to voice a similar nearly unbearable recognition of what his choking sound must have meant.

VICARIOUS TRAUMATIZATION
OF THE THERAPIST

How can any therapist listen to "impossible," overwhelming experiences without feeling his own boundaries have been invaded, without feeling infected by the horror of what he is hearing (Caruth, 1995)? Therapists may feel traumatized both by the manifest content of the material they are hearing and by the interpersonal process between therapist and patient. Simon (1992) has described this "severe countertransferential distress" as the "traumatization of the analyst by the traumatized patient" (p. 964). Others have called it "traumatic countertransference" (Herman, 1992), "contact victimization" (Courtois, 1988), and "vicarious traumatization" (McCann and Pearlman, 1990).

In their illuminating book, *Trauma and the Therapist,* Pearlman and Saakvitne (1995) define vicarious traumatization as "a process through which the therapist's inner experience is negatively transformed through empathic engagement with clients' trauma material" (p. 279). Empathy in these situations may be *cognitive,* involving an understanding of what the patient describes and understands about his abuse history, and *affective,* involving a connection to the full range of emotions evoked by the abuse experience. Empathy, a quality that is essential to foster a working relationship between patient and therapist, can paradoxically also be a liability that creates traumatic responses in the therapist. Through empathic engagement with the patient's experience, the therapist's "fundamental frame of reference and schemas are repeatedly challenged [as stories of intentional cruelty take their toll]. . . . How can one hold the illusion of safety, which allows him to walk down the street alone, sleep in a house with his windows open, and drive at night with the doors unlocked, after daily confrontations with the dangers faced by women and children in this society?" (Pearlman and Saakvitne, 1995, p. 298).

It is important to recognize and accept the reality that vicarious traumatization exists and that it is a natural occupational hazard of working with trauma (Pearlman and Saakvitne, 1995). When this understanding is permitted, therapists feel more comfortable acknowledging to themselves that they do feel traumatized at times. This is particularly likely for therapists who themselves suffered childhood sexual betrayal. They may have a heightened capacity for empathy with the patient's situation. On the other hand, they are at greatest risk for strong and disturbing reactions, whether conscious or unconscious, to what they are hearing.

At such times, therapists must be aware of the need to care for themselves. Self-care should occur in both the professional and the personal arenas. In terms of the work itself, therapists can avoid isolation and burnout through professional growth and education. Because of the likelihood of being pulled into reenactments of abuse dynamics and the grueling effect of listening to stories of betrayal, it is essential to have colleagues to whom one can turn for supervision and consultation about working with this population. In terms of personal self-care, involvement in one's own therapy, knowing one's limits, defining one's boundaries, creating balance in one's work life, seeking spiritual renewal, advocating for social change, and making sure one's own life has satisfactions with time for rest and play can all help the therapist feel grounded and renewed (Pearlman and Saakvitne, 1995; see also Crowder, 1995).

On the other hand, experiences with traumatized patients offer the therapist an opportunity to expand the boundaries of his or her "creativity, flexibility, self-discipline, humility, and maturity" (Bromberg, 1995b, pp. 143–144), and to be moved to a more authentic level of self-awareness and personal understanding of the human mind, his or her own as well as the patient's. The therapist may be transformed both as a professional and as a human being.

My work with Zak, like the work with Patrick described elsewhere in this book, evoked for me both these aspects of countertransference. It required me to find inside myself enormous patience and an ability to empathize with experiences that were almost unimaginably abusive. To work with him, it was essential that I expand my capacity for self-reflection in many areas. I repeatedly felt traumatized by the material I was hearing, and yet my relationship with him impelled me to enlarge the limits of my understanding of human nature in both its most repellent and its most inspiring manifestations. I felt profound fury, depression, disillusionment, and helplessness, on the one hand, and humility, admiration, and respect for the resilience of the human spirit on the other. I was torn between overidentification with his victimhood and incredulity about his story.

Zak's sexual abuse by his adoptive father took place in the context of a life so full of trauma that the sexual molestation, horrifying though it was, hardly stood out among the many blows he received. He warily but compellingly told me his history over a period of many months, having come reluctantly to see me after his wife had urged him to do so for over two years. In the following narrative, rather than detail the process of our therapeutic work, I will focus on his story and my reactions to hearing it.

An appealing and whimsical man of about forty, Zak's evocative and complex use of language belied the fact that he had never attended college. He opened our initial consultation by telling me that as a baby he had been sold by his biological parents to his adoptive parents for $1,000. A year later, the biological parents tried to get him back in order to extort an additional $250 from the adoptive parents, who moved to another state, where they were able to obtain legal adoption papers without the consent of the biological parents. The couple had already adopted another baby boy after the death of a biological son. His adoptive father was physically abusive to Zak in grotesque and shocking ways, and as an adult Zak bore numerous scars and physical afflictions related to the abuse. For example, he told me he still had pieces of bone floating behind his eye from a childhood beating with a belt buckle that splintered his eye socket bone. He almost never received medical attention for his wounds. His abuse was noticed by school personnel, but Zak always backed up his parents' stories about how he got his recurring bruises and broken bones from accidents. He felt at the time that to do otherwise was to court certain death from his father. Some of Zak's teachers knew Zak was being abused, and they told him explicitly that if he confirmed their suspicions he would be removed from his family. One school administrator even offered Zak a home with his own family if Zak wished, but Zak did not fully believe him and was unable to bring himself to leave his adoptive parents. As an adult he blamed himself for not escaping his family, but at the time he was suspicious that had he left he would eventually have been returned to his home and brutalized in even worse ways.

Zak described his father as a monstrously sadistic man who had himself been sodomized by both parents as a child. As we progressed through the initial weeks and months of our work together, Zak slowly allowed me to see the extent of the nightmare that had been his childhood. Although it is possible that some of the incidents he related were exaggerated or partially distorted by his memory, I do not doubt the core depiction of his barbarous childhood. One extreme example of his abuse occurred when he was about eight and involved a punishment for having used Magic Marker on a painting by his adoptive father. The father, a dentist, took Zak to his office and without anesthesia drilled random holes in his teeth. The holes remained unfilled for a week before he put fillings in them. Zak did not go to a dentist for years as an adult, and when he did go he went into shock, passed out, and had to be taken to an emergency room. When finally a dentist did see his teeth, he asked Zak sharply about the work that had been done. Zak was too ashamed to tell his story.

It was a very long time before Zak told me about his father's sexual violations. The father regularly raped Zak anally on Saturday afternoon visits to his office. On one such occasion, the father inserted a pistol that he said was loaded into Zak's rectum. Later, he made Zak hold this gun in his mouth while he was being raped. The father seems to have been in a seizurelike rage while the rapes took place. He screamed ferociously during his frenzied violations of Zak, then seemed limp afterward when the furious paroxysm was over. He would then tell Zak to get out of his sight, but otherwise appeared to be in a fugue state, not speaking or relating to anything for an extended period of time.

Zak described his adoptive mother as anxious to appear like a good parent publicly but unable to relate to her children on any but the most superficial level. He could not explain why she allowed the father's abuse to go on; it may be that she was not aware of its most horrific details. He believed she was afraid she would be the object of the father's fury if she intervened, and that she allowed Zak to substitute for her. When Zak was about eleven, the father did physically abuse the mother. Only at that point did they separate. Zak bitterly noted that his mother protected herself but not him. Zak was not altogether sure of the circumstances of their divorce, but he never saw his father again. Afraid of the fury he would feel toward his father if he found him, Zak made no effort as an adult to locate him.

His mother then began to live with another man who was involved in drugs and who took Zak and his brother to places where they clearly were in physical peril as well as subject to further sexual abuse. At this point, when he was fourteen, Zak ran away from home and took to the streets.

Zak lived on the streets for two years, hustling for money in a variety of ways while trying to attend high school. Eventually he dropped out of school, not obtaining a general equivalency diploma until adulthood. Zak did not believe his adoptive mother made any real effort to find him during the two years he was a runaway. After his teenage girlfriend, also a runaway, died in his arms, he returned to his adoptive mother's home. There, he found she had rented out his old room, so that initially he had nowhere to stay. In addition, his mother had given away nearly all his possessions, including nearly every photograph of him as a child. He showed me one of the few photos that survived, a Christmas snapshot of him and his brother in which his brother's blackened eye was clearly visible.

Zak married his wife when he was seventeen. Several years older than he, she seems to have been a stabilizing and nurturing force in his life. He was immensely grateful to her, although in later years he felt she had pushed him into a more conventional middle-class existence than he could manage. Over his protests, they had a child when Zak was about thirty. Zak then gave up, at least for the time being, artistic aspirations in a creative career that had begun to bear fruit. He instead became a talented craftsman and supported his family, albeit in a financially precarious manner. His ability to relate to his wife and child was limited, however, and at times he behaved in eccentric and even bizarre ways. For example, he could not eat in other people's presence. He would sit with his family as they ate, facing partially away from them, and then would eat by himself later, alone. On the other hand, he worked hard at developing a good, loving bond with his child, and seemed to have succeeded.

Zak's wife had been given my name by her therapist over two years before he first called me. Although he was in a severe crisis at the time, he could not bring himself to phone. The crisis was precipitated by a friend locating Zak's biological mother and bringing her from another state to meet him as "a surprise birthday present." The meeting was a disaster. She told Zak that when she got pregnant with him at age sixteen she tried many times to abort him, but he had held on tenaciously to life, and she had not been able to kill him. Although she said she was proud of him, she expressed surprise that he did not seem to have been damaged by her attempts to rid herself of the pregnancy. Zak heard hostility in these words, and felt she still hated him. This was partly confirmed when she then told him about his having been sold to his adoptive parents, and asked him, "What does it feel like to be bought and sold like a nigger?" Within a short time, his biological mother began behaving in an inappropriate, sexualized manner with Zak, and described endemic sexual abuse and bizarre behavior throughout her extended family of origin. Zak became highly anxious, and asked his wife never to leave them alone together in the remaining days that his mother stayed with them.

Later, during our work together, Zak began to see that as a child he had created a fantasy biological mother who loved, nurtured, and supported him. He held on to this idealized image throughout his years of vicious abuse, and the fantasy was a comfort to him. In essence, he had created a mother to nurture him during a time when he had no other nurturers at all, and in this sense he became his own mother. When faced with the reality of his inadequate and out-of-control real biological mother, Zak broke down and had what seems to have been a manic episode. He met someone on the Internet, a woman who was a substitute for the fantasy mother he had lost. Abandoning the responsible and dependable persona he had projected for years, he precipitously flew half-way around the world to meet her. His family and business were left in a shambles while he spent time with this other woman. Once he discovered that she was not the soul mate he'd imagined her to be, he returned home, massively depressed and almost totally alienated from his wife.

At this point, Zak was in communication with both his biological parents and the several half-siblings about whose existence he had never known. His biological parents had not stayed together long, and each had had other relationships that produced offspring. His biological mother lived a hermitlike existence in a rural area. She seems to have had severe dissociative difficulties, and was also diagnosed manic–depressive. She had not been on medication at the time she first met Zak and behaved so inappropriately. When she restabilized on medication, she remained fragile, but became increasingly more attuned psychologi-

cally to Zak. Their relationship eventually developed into one in which
there was some mutual nurturance. His biological father was a paranoid
schizophrenic with a fixed and full-blown delusional system. He frightened Zak the one time they met face to face, and phoned him repeatedly
with demands for money that Zak was able to fend off. Several of his
half-siblings were more responsive to Zak, who had desperately wanted
to find a family to whom he could relate.

Zak was very aware of the genetic implications of his biological
parents' mental illnesses. At my suggestion, he started on medication
shortly after we began to work together. At that time, he had a sleep disturbance in addition to mood swings. He was initially put on a mood
stabilizer; later an antidepressant was added. But he was highly conflicted about taking medication. He felt taking it was giving up his ability to control his own fate, and he began to tinker with the dosages,
stopping one medication without telling the psychopharmacologist. This
had nearly fatal consequences, as he began to have wildly oscillating
mood swings and briefly became overtly delusional. In this state, he took
a massive overdose of medication, was hospitalized, and nearly died.
The overdose did not seem to be a conscious suicide attempt, but instead
appeared to be part of a psychotic reaction related to his mood swings
and abrupt self-administered changes of medication. When he recovered,
he had no memory of the period before taking the overdose or his mental state at the time.

This crisis paradoxically had the effect of making Zak more agree-
able to following the medication regime prescribed by his psychopharmacologist. Having decided that he did indeed suffer from a bipolar
disorder and that he needed to take care of himself in ways neither biological parent had ever taken care of their own mental illnesses, Zak
became meticulous about taking his medication exactly as prescribed.
This was, of course, a far more adaptive way to express his need to exert
control over his life than the self-medicating that preceded his overdose.
Eventually, his mood became more and more stable, and Zak was in a
far better position to make the life decisions he faced.

Emerging from sessions with Zak, I felt paralyzed and dissociated,
as a soldier might feel after witnessing a brutal massacre. With time, I
began to schedule breaks after his sessions, feeling I could not see
another patient without personal recovery time. I learned to treat myself
well in a variety of ways as I dealt with my own oscillating feelings about
working with Zak. His personally appealing qualities made me warm to
him, and I admired the strength that enabled him to endure the horrors
life had brought him. At times, though, I doubted parts of his story, or
pulled back emotionally from their impact. I understood his stubborn-
ness and determination to stay in control, but they could be frustrating

and agitating to me. A prime example of this was his decision to stop his medication without consulting either me or his psychopharmacologist, which led to his drug overdose.

Luckily, I have a network of gifted colleagues experienced in working with abuse, and I was able to consult with them to help myself process the material I was hearing. Like Zak, I needed witnesses for the trauma I was experiencing. I needed other clinicians to listen, to hear me, to corroborate what I was feeling.

I also needed to consider how I was listening and behaving. When did I find myself backing off and disbelieving Zak? When did I listen without asking the questions that would encourage him to talk more? When did I overidentify with him or think of him as a victim rather than a person? When did I overidealize him for his capacity to overcome extreme adversity? When did I ignore or underestimate the negative impact of his actions on the people around him, today or in the past? When did I sentimentalize a history that sounded at times like a Dickensian tale of unremitting horror and woe? When did I tune out, or want to? Addressing these questions kept me from succumbing to the vicarious traumatization of reliving Zak's story with him.

In the next chapter, we will consider how the treatment of sexually abused men is affected by his seeing either a male or a female therapist.

CHAPTER 10

Gender and the
Therapeutic Relationship

with Sue A. Shapiro

The sex of the therapist significantly informs the treatment of any
patient, but it is especially influential in work with sexually abused
adults. When a sexually abused man chooses a therapist and decides that
it is important to him whether the therapist is a man or a woman, many
factors are involved in his decision, some having nothing to do with his
abuse history. But, whatever the sex of the therapist, gender issues are
likely to figure prominently and problematically in the treatment of a
sexually abused man (or woman), especially in relation to transference
and countertransference. This is true whether he chooses a therapist
whom he feels is different from or like his abuser or himself. It is true no
matter how rational or distorted his reasons for choosing a male or
female therapist. The therapist must inquire into these reasons and perceptions, and deal with the material as it emerges from the patient.

In this chapter, I have invited my friend and colleague Dr. Sue A.

Sue A. Shapiro, PhD, is a supervising analyst at the Postdoctoral Program in Psychotherapy and Psychoanalysis at New York University. She was also the founder of the Incest and
Abuse Treatment Center at the Manhattan Institute for Psychoanalysis. She is a psychologist and psychoanalyst practicing in New York City.

Shapiro to join me in discussing the impact of the therapist's sex and gender on work with sexually abused men. In the first part of the chapter, I will discuss the experience of being a male therapist who treats sexually abused men. In the second part of the chapter Dr. Shapiro will comment on being a female therapist working with this population.

CHOOSING A MALE OR A FEMALE THERAPIST

For any individual choosing a therapist, the choice may hinge on the therapist's biological sex. While many people in therapy do not seem to care about the sex of their therapist, most sexually abused individuals do state preferences. As I describe some of the themes that influence these choices for sexually abused men, it will become clear that the same decision about the sex of the therapist may be made for diametrically opposite reasons by different men. Thus, there are contradictory possibilities about the perspective from which a man may approach both the biological sex and the presumed gender characteristics and attitudes of his therapist (see Chapter 3 for a discussion of the difference between sex and gender). Therapists must therefore explore the reasons for a man's preference, and not assume it has an unambiguous, predictable meaning. Explorations of how the man arrived at his decision regarding therapist sex will yield the specific implications of this choice for the treatment and the therapeutic relationship.

Some writers have expressed doubts about whether male therapists can ever work well with abused patients. Courtois (1988), for example, who writes chiefly about sexually abused women, feels that women therapists are more likely "to understand the victimization of the abuse without excusing or rationalizing it" (p. 239). She acknowledges, however, that "some male therapists, with adequate attention to abuse issues and countertransference, can productively treat incest survivors" (p. 239). Courtois further concedes that for the sexually abused woman "past learning and mistrust can be countered by an experience with a man who draws clear distinctions between caring about her and exploiting her" (p. 241).

Evans (1990, p. 71), on the other hand, in writing about work with both sexually abused men and male Vietnam veterans, addresses this question from a different perspective, concluding that "gender attitudes" and "gender stereotyping" by therapist and client are more important in establishing therapist/client fit than the biological sex of the therapist. He notes, for example, that the therapist must be flexible about gender role, and in particular must not perceive men as less able than women to be emotionally expressive and to address personal concerns. Relevant here is Briere's (1989) comments about common power dynamics when male therapists work with sexually abused male patients. Briere argues that these men tend to take either "one-down" positions in which they are relatively passive with the male therapist, or "one-up" positions, in which they are aggressive, hostile, and hypermasculine.

One opinion often expressed about therapist choice for sexually abused patients is that the therapist should be of the same sex as the patient. This view is overly simplistic, as Hunter (1990a) points out. He does, however, convincingly make the related argument that "men learn about being men best from other men" (p. 137). On the other hand, male therapists must be careful not to perpetuate gender stereotypes while engaged in teaching and learning about being men. This would continue the kind of gender role stereotypy that has undermined a sexually abused man's capacity to deal with his victimization in the first place.

Crowder (1995) also disagrees with the position that sexually abused men should always work with male therapists, describing it as based on social learning theory and gender politics. Yet those who argue for it say that the working through is deeper with a man; that only a male therapist can help restore a healthy sense of masculinity; and that men injured by men need to heal from their hurt by interacting with a man who is skilled and nurturant. In addition, according to this position, the sexually abused man may have difficulty talking about sexual matters to a woman. Or he may feel less embarrassed about being in a feminized victim position when talking to a man. Other men, however, may choose a woman therapist for exactly the same reasons.

Struve (Morris et al., 1997) acknowledges that sexually abused men can benefit greatly from being in treatment with female therapists. He also contends, however, that therapy with a male therapist can provide an opportunity to face same-gender intimacy in a more direct and experiential way than is possible with a woman. Feeling shamed about acknowledging his "feminization" to a man, the man may believe he can only talk to a woman about being victimized. In such a case, working with a male therapist gives him the added experience of having a male model for allowing himself to experience the "feminine" emotions. Of course, many men are simply unable to do this during the early stages of dealing with their victimization.

The argument that the therapist should be of the opposite biological sex from the abuser is another naïve point of view. This does not take into account that the abuser may have been a chief source of nurturance for the child as well as the cause of deep anxiety and terror. For example, a father who abused a child may also have been the more nurturing parent, while the mother may have been unavailable emotionally and may have passively or even actively allowed the abuse to take place. In such a case, a therapist of the same sex as the abuser, while likely to be the object of conflicting, complicated transferences, may be the best choice (see Bolton et al., 1989; Hunter, 1990a).

Some sexually abused adults may deliberately choose a therapist of the same sex as their abuser in order to deal directly in treatment with the transferences they know inhibit many of their interpersonal relationships. I have found these patients likely to be more evolved in their thinking about the abuse experience than the patient who is only first acknowledging his history of abuse. This evolution has often happened in the course of treatment with a therapist of the opposite sex from the abuser. Thus, some men abused by a man in boyhood may choose to work with a male therapist after an initial period of treatment with a woman. This has been true of many of the patients who have been referred to my groups for sexually abused men. Of the twenty men not initially in my own practice who entered my groups in the first seven years I conducted them, fourteen were seeing female individual therapists. All fourteen had been abused in childhood by men, and were referred to me for inclusion in my group only when they reached the point of feeling prepared to work with a man about the abuse.

It seems intuitively obvious that a boy abused by a man would later be wary of a male therapist. What about men abused by women? Do they become phobic about female authorities and choose male therapists? Some do seem to prefer male therapists (for example, Yale, Abe, and Keith). But men who were abused by women may be as reluctant to see a male therapist for treatment as those abused by men. I once supervised a group for sexually abused men led by a male/female cotherapy team. Seven out of the eight group members were seeing female therapists in individual therapy. Of these seven, three were abused in childhood by women.

Such patients may choose female therapists because the female abuser was also a source of comfort and excitement. Their choice may also be influenced, however, by stereotypes that affect the transference to both the therapist and the abuser (Lisak, 1993, 1995). For example, in our culture, men are more typically seen as predators than women. Even a man who was abused by a woman may experience her as a masculine figure, or, as some might call her, a "phallic woman." In order to preserve his sense of women as nurturers, he may unconsciously transform his female abuser into a male figure.

There are no hard-and-fast rules about the meaning of the therapist's sex in these situations, nor should there be (Courtois, 1988; Hunter, 1990a). As Crowder (1995) sensibly notes, "Eventually, survivors need to embrace both genders; at some time in the recovery process, they will probably find it helpful to work with their less preferred gender. The only rule that must be followed is that clients never be forced to work with a clinician they don't feel safe with, be this gender-based or otherwise, because this replicates the original abuse dynamic" (pp. 122–123; in this passage, Crowder is using the word "gender" to connote what I mean by "biological sex").

WHEN THE THERAPIST IS A MAN

The patient's conception of masculinity, and especially his conception of and attitude toward male authority figures, permeates how he relates to his male therapist. Questions about the meaning of maleness, as we saw in Chapters 2 and 3, point the way to some of the treatment issues for men who have been sexually abused. If men are conceived to be untrustworthy aggressors, what does that say about the therapist as well as about the patient himself? If the patient unconsciously accepts social stereotypes about women being victims and men being predators, how can he relate to a man as neither a victim nor a predator? Can he somehow develop a healthy perception of himself and his therapist as men?

We have seen that a victimized patient may see himself as "not male" because he subscribes to cultural views of victims as passive and female. Thus, a boy who was abused by either a man or a woman may identify with women victims and feel "unmanned" by his own victimization. He may be ashamed to reveal to another man, especially one experienced as powerful and authoritative, that he is a "feminized" man who has succumbed or acquiesced to sexual abuse. When he is in treatment with a male therapist, he may identify the therapist with aggressive and predatory men. Or he may envy the therapist's assumed freedom to be a "real man," since he believes the therapist has not had to cope with the traumas the patient himself has faced. On the other hand, he may contemptuously think of the therapist's interest in emotion and interpersonal process as indicative of the therapist's own feminization. It is therefore essential for the male therapist to monitor his patients' messages to him about both patient and therapist as men.

Willem articulated the conflictual feelings a man may feel about therapist gender. I had originally referred him to a female therapist when he said he could only work with a woman because of his feelings about men. Some time later, she referred him back to my group for sexually abused men. Six months after entering the group, he described his continuing ambivalence about me, and contrasted his feelings with those he had about his female individual therapist: "I feel different when I speak to you than when I talk to her. She's a woman. You are male—to me that means you are powerful, in charge. You can do whatever you want, and that scares me. Plus, there's your professional neutrality—that adds somehow to my sense that I'm not in charge, that I can't read you well enough. I like you—it's not that. But each time we meet, or especially when we talk on the phone, I find I become defensive and nervy until I somehow remind myself—if I can—that it's been OK here with you."

Terror, Desire, and Shame

I listened to the message on my answering machine and heard a man gasping. He did not speak, and then he hung up after about thirty seconds. The next day, I got another message. There was more gasping, and then an intense, strangled-sounding man's voice asked me to call. When I telephoned, the man said he'd heard I work with men who have been sexually abused. He sounded terribly frightened, but he did finally make an appointment to see me. When I asked his name, he replied, "Frank." I asked for a surname, and he hesitated, then quickly said "Smith" in a low voice. I assumed this was a false name. I was not surprised when Frank did not show up for the consultation, but I decided to call him because he had been in such distress when we spoke. When I reached him, he sounded less panicky, but also depressed. He apologized for not calling, and said he realized he was in no way ready to talk to a man about his history of sexual abuse.

I never met Frank, and I know nothing about his abuse history, but the terror in his voice has stayed with me for years. Why was Frank unable to speak about sexual abuse to a man? I do not know the answer, of course, but for me he embodies the terror of male authority that I have heard over and over from my sexually abused male patients. This terror suffuses the treatment and informs the nature of our therapeutic relationship. In addition, the male patient's frequent and persistent feelings of shame about being sexually abused may create specific transferential problems. Shame makes it difficult for people to disclose abuse to anyone, but particularly to an authority figure. This occurs regularly with male therapists, but, often less obviously, also with female therapists.

Seth's molestation left him excruciatingly anxious, fearful, and shamed if he felt singled out in any way, particularly by a man. He explained, "Being noticed means I'm a prime target." I once commented at the end of a group session that he was an "interesting man," referring at the time to his need for attention in the group coupled with his anxiety about being the center of attention for too long. In the next session, he told me he had been anxious all week, wondering what such a comment meant. "I was especially worried because you're a man. I kept thinking that your office is in a hotel and that your couch could be a bed—it reminds me too much of how I was abused in that hotel room."

Greg provides a further clinical example of the reactions a sexually abused man may have when he feels exposed and vulnerable with a male therapist. He was referred by his female therapist to my group for sexually abused men. When he came to see me for what was to have been the first of three consultations I usually have before accepting a patient into the group, he said he was "terrified" of me. A gay, forty-year-old, divorced father of three, he had vague memories of sexual abuse by his father as well as a clear memory of his grandfather exposing himself to Greg. He assumed, as I do, that these early experiences led him to accede to later abuse by the pastor of a communal fundamentalist religious cult he had joined. This pastor heard about Greg's sexual conflicts during confession. Greg had come to him in a tearful panic after having had his first homosexual experience since getting married. The pastor told Greg he could act on his impulses to have sex with men, but only with him. He indicated that this was something he was doing on Greg's behalf: he was willing to descend to Greg's level and to sin in order to save Greg's soul. Though neither attracted to the pastor nor understanding this reasoning, Greg felt vulnerable, clung to the pastor, and complied with his offer for several years. During this period, the pastor did Greg special favors and gave him an honored position within the cult. When Greg tried to stop their liaison, however, the pastor humiliated him publicly and viciously in a men's group that met as part of the cult's activities. He proclaimed Greg's "faggotry" to the group, without acknowledging his own role in the sexual activity. Greg was shunned by the cult and had to leave.

Greg openly saw me in the pastor's image. We were approximately the same age, and my office reminded Greg of the room in which the cult's men's group had met. He trusted his therapist's recommendation that he should work with me, however; that trust in her was all he could hold on to in order to keep himself from fleeing my office. I was struck by the courage he exhibited in staying and telling me about his two-sided dread of me. He was nearly convinced I would indeed try to molest him, and was sure that if I did he would comply. This was one side of the dread. The other was that I might *not* want him sexually. He believed that if I was not interested in abusing him, I would have no interest in him or use for him at all, and therefore he would not get the help he needed from me.

This was Greg's dilemma: his sexuality had been his passport to special treatment from the powerful men who had molested him. He needed me, and felt that he could only get my help if I abused my power and sexually abused him. If I molested him, he would be a victim again. If I did not, he would not get what he needed. Either way, he would lose.

Greg was so disturbed by our first meeting that we decided to have an extra consultation a few days later. In that session, he told me that, while he did not trust me at all, he had noted that I seemed to treat him well and he was going to force himself to work with me and face the feelings I brought up in him. Because of Greg's extreme initial reactions to me, I decided to have several consultations with him over a period of a few months before he joined the men's group. In these meetings, we talked about Greg's concern that he would sexualize relationships with other group members as well as with me. We examined further the very shadowy memories he had of abuse by his father and grandfather. We also discussed his worries that straight men in the group would condemn him for being gay and for having "allowed" his father, grandfather, and pastor to sexually abuse him.

When he did join the group, Greg again said he was "terrified." He had given himself a short, uneven, and ugly haircut just before starting the group, with the conscious intention of making himself less attractive to the other men. For several weeks he was an eerie, silent, odd-looking presence. I later learned that he left each session filled with inchoate emotion and went to his individual therapy nearly incoherent as he attempted to articulate his panicky reactions to the experience of being in a room filled with men. As the weeks went on, however, he made timid connections to the other group members, and began to voice his rage about his abuse experiences.

When we met individually for our first follow-up session after he had been in the group for three months, Greg said he was only able to function in group by making believe I didn't exist. He dissociated his feelings about my presence in order to make use of the group. When I asked him to try to voice those feelings about me, he said he continued to distrust me as much as ever. Though he saw I made supportive and useful comments, he continued to wait for me to show my true colors and become abusive. I felt that at this point he had additional, more positive feelings about me, which he could not yet articulate to himself or to me. I therefore decided to make a statement that he could add to the cauldron of information and fantasy he had about me. In a manner suggested by Lew (1993), I said, "I know you can't believe this right now, and maybe you never will, but I will never, ever sexually abuse you. I may hurt you unintentionally—that happens in human interactions—but I will never abuse you." He looked at me, eyes filled with tears, said he heard me and thanked me, but then said that for the moment he needed to "scramble away" and not think about what I had said.

I was talking here about frank sexual abuse, not the inevitable abusive countertransference reenactments described by Davies and Frawley

(1994) that I discussed in Chapter 9. Nevertheless, I took a risk in making this declaration to Greg: I might be stopping his expressions of fear rather than dealing with the fears themselves. On the contrary, however, while Greg continued to maintain his distance from me, he became more likely to voice and describe his terror of me. Meanwhile, his connections to the other men in the group, as well as, I believe, his surveillance of my behavior with them and him, helped him behave and feel differently outside of therapy. He began to stand up to authorities and set limits with colleagues. After six months in the group, he said his terror of me was gone, at least for the time being. Reflecting on his initial feelings about me and the men in the group, he was disturbed and shaken as he saw how his severe transferential distortions had ruled his relationships for decades.

Fear and Longing

While Greg represents in a nearly pure form the terror sexually abused men can feel with a male therapist, other such patients bring an even more complicated mixture of fear and longing to the treatment relationship. For example, Jared and Lewis, both in individual treatment with me, were both also wary of my possibly being interested in them sexually. However, each felt indignant and bereft when I did *not* sexualize our relationships.

A forty-year-old gay man who had never had a long-term relationship, Jared was abused by a seventeen-year-old neighbor, Kris, for two years starting at age five. From the beginning, Jared, who said he already had a strong sense of being sexually oriented toward men, found the time with Kris exciting; he claimed to have been a willing participant in the sex, which mostly consisted of Jared fellating Kris. Yet as an adult he considered himself to have been sexually abused because of the drastic effects the overall experience had had on his emotional and sexual relationships.

One day, Jared and Kris were nearly discovered having sex in Kris's bedroom. Kris panicked and pushed Jared into a closet. He told Jared to put his clothes on there, then lowered him out the first-floor window and told him to go home. Jared, age seven, wandered around alone for hours, crying. He claimed that for the first time he felt that what they had been doing was wrong. He was ashamed of himself, and was cut off from his relationship with Kris, which stopped abruptly at that point. This shame about sexuality and fear of imminent desertion by a loved one continued into adulthood, when he was involved with a series of much older men to whom he was initially attracted but could not commit.

Another, more insidious result of Jared's experience with Kris had to do with how it informed Jared's relationship with his own father. When he was a child, Jared's father often walked around the house nude. Jared remembered his father coming in semidressed to kiss him good night. Afterward, Jared would cry himself to sleep because his father never attempted to have sex with him. He would sob to himself, "Why won't Daddy love me the way Kris does?" Having learned that sex was an appropriate way to express love, he concluded that he was unloveable to his father because his father did not engage in overt sexual acts with him. As an adult, he has, of course, had to deal with his memories of his father's seductiveness, including the likelihood that the overstimulating relationship with his father made him more receptive to Kris's advances than he might otherwise have been. His difficulty in dealing with these feelings about his father, however, was exacerbated by his experiences with Kris so that he continuously felt unloveable when men did not respond sexually to him. This was true even when he was neither attracted to them himself nor prepared to engage in sex. All of these feelings entered into our individual therapeutic work, where he both longed for and feared sexual interest from me.

This transferential dilemma was articulated by Lewis, a man who was physically and sexually abused for three years by various members of a family that baby-sat for him from ages three to six. Lewis was an attractive gay man, a recovering alcoholic who had shaved his head in order to look fierce and unapproachable. He was almost totally unable to be physically vulnerable, even with men he knew well and cared about, and had at times thrown lovers across the room during sex if he momentarily felt overpowered by them. When he stopped drinking, he could no longer have sexual relationships at all. At one point, I said to Lewis, as I had to Greg, that I wanted him to hear from me, even though he might not ever believe it or fully take it in, that I would never sexually abuse him. He was silent at first, but then said, "I know I should be relieved to hear that, and I suppose that in some ways I am. But I have to confess to you that my first reaction was to think, 'Why not? Aren't you attracted to me?' "

These vignettes point up that many men who were sexually abused as boys have learned to use sexuality as interpersonal currency. For them, sexualized relating is a way to appease, gratify, and cling to authority figures whose love they both desire and distrust (see Chapter 8). It is frightening at a (usually) unconscious level for such a man to be told that the relationship with the therapist will not be sexualized, for he has learned that only in sexualized relationships will he get what he needs in life. Much as he may dread this abuse, he believes he must exist in it in order to survive.

Aggression and the Need for Connection

Transference to a male therapist, or to fellow members of a men's group, may, on the other hand, be a vehicle for discovering an alive and dynamic male identity. Thus, the man who has been sexually abused may discover that men can be nurturers as well as victims or perpetrators, humanistic and ethical as well as abusive. Consider Harris, a man who had been abused by his alcoholic father for several years:

After two failed attempts to work with male therapists for various adjunctive therapies, Harris was referred by his female therapist to my group. I was struck by his articulate, energetic, no-nonsense approach to meeting me, though his latent sadness and rage were also apparent. He had no intimate relationships with other men, but yearned for that possibility, and so was eager to join the group. He was wary of me, but we were able to establish enough of an alliance for me to feel we could work together in the group. I describe in Chapters 9 and 11 how his history was reenacted in the group and specifically in relation to me. His work with me and the group about these reenactments led to remarkable changes in how he experienced all men. In particular, he shifted dramatically in his feelings about himself and about men in authority.

The issue came to a head in an interchange between us following a group session. Harris was still in the waiting room as I came out of my office carrying a vase of flowers to take into my office kitchenette. He smiled in what I felt was a sardonic and mocking manner and, exaggeratedly imitating my gestures, said, "Ah, look at him holding his roses so tenderly!" I was caught off guard and, feeling stung and ridiculed, blurted out that there was nothing wrong with a man caring about flowers.

Harris came to our next group session in a rage. He maintained that his comment had been made in a spirit of wishing he could express his tender side as I was doing, that I had totally misinterpreted his tone, and that this was yet another example of my failure of empathy with him. I was confused, unsure whether my perceptions were accurate, and worried that I was indeed insensitive and not in control of my own reactions to possible humiliation as a man. We went over and over the incident, with neither of us willing to relinquish entirely his own view of what had happened. The parallels between this incident and the mutual mockery and ridicule in the relationship between Harris and his father were unmistakable to us both, yet it was impossible to sort out whose "fault" any piece of our struggle was. We had achieved the inevitable transference–countertransference reenactment of abuse that Davies and Frawley (1994) eloquently elaborate.

Our working through of this aspect of our relationship took a very long time. It had been partly completed when Harris decided to leave the group (though not his ongoing individual treatment with his female therapist), supposedly because of time and money pressures in his family related to the therapies needed by his wife and son. By that time, we had learned to talk about this dynamic between us without a blowup, and had come to a kind of understanding about the very sensitive nature of our feelings relating to ridicule and contempt. Harris said he was sorry to leave the group, and I realized that I was sorry to see him go.

(Three years later, Harris acknowledged that a strong unconscious motivation for his departure from the group was despair about feeling he could never establish a truly satisfying relationship with me. A few months after that, he began to muse about the incident with the flowers and suddenly said, "I was just looking for a way to ridicule and humiliate you. The flowers seemed like a natural way to do it. I didn't altogether realize it at the time—I was too defensive to acknowledge how much I related to you as if you were my father. But that's what was going on.")

During the next year, Harris called me several times. First, he let me know he was having problems doing the creative writing he was trying to substitute for the group experience in his growth process. Later, he told me of his failure to make the friendships with other men for which he yearned. Finally, he asked for a referral to a mixed-sex group that was not abuse-oriented. He was unable, however, to find a group in which he felt satisfied with both the therapist and the group focus. Depressed, chastened, and lonely, fifteen months after leaving he asked to return to my group. In our exploratory sessions prior to his reentry to the group— about three years after the incident with the flowers—we talked at length about our relationship. Harris conceded that had he not "basically" trusted me he would never have called me or wanted to rejoin the group. We nevertheless agreed that there was a stilted quality to our relating, as we were being careful not to get into the warfare that at one time had occasionally shattered our interactions. I noted to him that I did not always comment freely when I had an association to something he said or did, but instead tended to weigh its possible effects on him and us more than I wished. He became sad, said he did not want to lose the possibility of spontaneity in our relationship, and indicated that he wanted to stretch his ability to hear me since he did "basically" trust me.

We both began to understand that it was no accident that Harris had returned to my group rather than joining a different one, and that we still had important unfinished work to do. We therefore agreed that we needed to monitor our relationship far more closely than we had in the past, and decided to schedule individual contact on a more frequent basis than we had in the past. As of this writing, more than two years after Harris's reen-

try to the group, this structure has helped us track the continuing vicissitudes of our relationship. We have acknowledged the mutual regard that
had coexisted with the occasionally abrasive quality of our relatedness,
and the abrasiveness itself has disappeared. Harris has contrasted our relationship shifts with the unremitting fury and contempt that continued in
adulthood between him and his father till the father's death and beyond.
This has led him to reconceptualize whether relationships have to remain
static, and whether they can be repaired when breaches occur. In turn, this
has helped him at long last to think about what his father had to go
through in his own life, and to show some compassion for his father's
severe unhappiness and early alcoholism.

When the Therapist and the Patient Are Both Men

I have indicated in my discussion and case examples how my male
patients with histories of abuse brought into their therapy conflicting
feelings of terror, longing, desire, fear, rage, and a need for refathering.
These themes reverberated throughout our work. Some of the feelings
were buttressed by cultural stereotypes about men. Others were linked
directly to the patient's earlier traumatic life experiences. Often there
was an oscillation of strong positive and negative feeling both about
being a man himself and being in treatment with a man. This fluctuation
affected the transference process beyond what I have found with patients
with no history of sexual abuse.

The male therapist working with a sexually abused man must sen-
sitize himself to these personal, social, and cultural issues. He must
expect and allow his patient to relate to him as a monster, a hero, a
lover, a father, a rapist, a weakling, a savior, and even a son. He may
be feared as macho and unfeeling, and he may be despised as impotent
and effeminate. The patient, in coming to a male therapist, declares his
willingness to deal with these ambiguities. The therapist must be
equally courageous. Together, patient and therapist can then discover
how to develop a relationship where both feel like men and neither
feels abused.

The remainder of this chapter is written by Dr. Sue A. Shapiro. Her
discussion reflects her thoughts about gender issues as she has seen them
unfold in her own work with both sexually abused men and sexually
abused women. Dr. Shapiro at times introduces themes I have discussed
elsewhere in this book. At these points, I indicate where I discuss these
issues. Her perspective on them gives added depth to the points I have
developed. She will also comment on my case material in the first part of
this chapter.

WHEN THE THERAPIST IS A WOMAN
AND THE PATIENT IS A MAN

The gender and sexual orientation of both patient and analyst impact in numerous ways on the developing transference–countertransference in all treatments, but especially in treatments of abuse survivors. I would like to describe some of my experiences as a female therapist working with men who were sexually abused. My sample is small even when supplemented by my supervisory work, but nonetheless it is a start. In this discussion I use the terms "heterosexual" and "homosexual" in their contemporary ordinary meaning: a preference for sexual activity with members of the opposite or the same biological sex. Similarly, I use "male" and "female" in their conventional, ordinary usage. In an earlier discussion of Dr. Gartner's work and in other writings, I have critiqued these dichotomies. We have yet to fully explore and theorize the impact of varying sexualities and genders on the therapeutic encounter (see Gornick, 1986; Hirsch, 1993; Shapiro, 1993, 1994; Blechner, 1998). For example, many of Dr. Gartner's clinical vignettes described in this and previous chapters sound familiar to me and could have occurred in much the same manner even if the therapist were a woman. For the purposes of this chapter I will, for the most part, leave these concerns aside, focusing instead on those clinical moments when it seemed to make a difference that I was a woman in the consulting room with a man.

Transference and Countertransference to Sex and Gender

It is critical that we be aware of how our physicality and our gender are experienced by our patients. What are they aware of and how much do they let us know of this awareness? How congruent with our own sense of our physical and sexual selves is their perception of us?

In a parallel fashion, it is important to be aware of our perceptions and responses to our patients' physicality and sexuality. Rarely do we acknowledge in writing or even in colleagial discussion the visceral response we have to a patient's size, shape, smell, and body language. If we can't acknowledge and explore these reactions in ourselves, it will be hard to explore them in our patients. Bodies and gender role behavior permeate the consulting room.

As a female therapist, I have numerous choices regarding my style of physical presentation: pants, skirt or dress, hair style, makeup, neckline, perfume. All of these choices, in addition to my "vital statistics"— height, weight, age, and body shape—affect how I am perceived, and consequently the transferences I am likely to elicit. In clinical work it is important to be aware of the usual responses that my body and physical appearance as well as my body language elicit and to note any changes in my presentation. For example, I found myself paying more attention to my outfits on the days I was seeing a male patient whom I liked and found attractive. Not infrequently, my greater attention to my clothing is matched by my patient's increased awareness of how I look even when that hasn't been directly expressed in words. Several years after treatment ended, a male survivor of sexual abuse contacted me. While discussing our work together, he remarked on several of the outfits I had worn while he was seeing me.

Men who have been overstimulated or abused by women are exceedingly tuned in to my physical and psychological state. One such patient went into a serious depression and resumed using drugs when, in my life outside the office, I began a romantic relationship. His condition deteriorated dramatically, and when I tried to explore its origins, he said, "I think you started to love someone else." This man was acutely attuned to nuances in my quality of attention and always seemed to know when I was sad or preoccupied.

I have not had the experience of being pregnant during the treatment of a male survivor of sexual abuse by a woman. Judging from colleagues' experiences, however, I think that this level of physical and sexual intrusion is especially disturbing to such patients. Some of my female supervisees have reported sexually abused men terminating treatment during their pregnancies.

Gender-generated discomfort occurs frequently in our work. It is important to ask ourselves how we treat our male and female, straight and gay patients differently. Survivors of childhood sexual abuse often require modifications of the traditional analytic frame: They might need phone contact, extra sessions, longer sessions, hospitalization, or contact during vacations. To whom do we suggest a phone call between sessions in an emergency? To whom do we give out a home phone number? To whom do we extend a handshake? How do we respond to a request for a hug? Do we attempt to deny or delay the emergence of erotic material by interpreting "preoedipal" material? Or, alternatively, do we unconsciously bolster a patient's narcissism, and perhaps our own as well, by denying early maternal longings—misrepresenting them as sexual? How do the gender and sexual orientation of the patient determine how we respond? Significantly, for all our discomfort about erotic transference and countertransference toward opposite-sex patients, there is even less written about same-sex patient and analyst pairs. Dr. Gartner's work in this book is a significant exception to this generalization. All of these issues and questions are heightened when working with survivors of sexual abuse, especially when the therapist is the same gender as the perpetrator.

Rigidity and Playfulness about Gender

As Dimen (1991) and Harris (1991) have noted, we and our theory may be postmodern, but our clinical practice is usually much more conservative. The clinical situation seems to force us into a more traditional position—as though, being representatives of "health," we must obey the gender rules of polite society, or at least the quirky variations on these rules imposed by the therapeutic structure and culture. Especially in the case of sexual abuse survivors, sexual orientation and gender role are not areas easily amenable to playfulness—this may be a luxury that most survivors of abuse cannot afford, as seen in Dr. Gartner's patients' desire to learn how to be men. Certainly, the literature on male survivors that Dr. Gartner cites (for example, Briere, 1989; Hunter, 1990a) is suffused with commonsense notions of gender. Perhaps this is because the sexual abuse of children occurs when gender identity and sexual orientation are in the process of consolidation and the rules of gender-appropriate behavior are quite strict. It might also reflect a general constriction in these patients in the area of play and the desire to always be certain about what is real and what is fantasy.

Gender Role Stereotypy

Dr. Gartner describes the wish for a model of maleness. Men who were sexually abused as boys may not want to be "new men"—at least not until they can comfortably and confidently feel like "real" men in the old sense (see Blechner, 1998). At the start of treatment, they may be quite troubled by and feel inadequate in assuming a traditional male role. They might be tempted by Robert Bly (1992) and others who promise to enhance their sense of male power, but at the same time they may feel threatened by the emotional and physical closeness of other men.

Perhaps one of our functions as therapists is to lessen the tyranny of gender role stereotypes—just as we might try to weaken a harsh, primitive superego. This may be connected to Evans's (1990) description of the importance of the therapist's "gender attitudes." I realize that some men who have been victimized may feel feminized, but they may also fear that ordinary assertion and initiation of activity is an act of violation and thus struggle with the conflict between their own ideals and cultural ideals of masculinity. Are they "real" men if they fear hurting the other? Are they perpetrators if they enjoy being sexually assertive?[1]

Similarly, women who have been sexually abused may be conflicted about expressing or experiencing any sexual desire or excitement—Does

---

[1] See Chapter 3 (R. B. G.).

this mean they asked for it, does this mean they are whores? They may also be ambivalent about being desired. But are they "real" women if they don't like being flirted with by strangers? If these women become assertive in the work world, they may feel overly identified with traditional masculine attributes and fear that they are betraying their mothers.

On the other hand, both men and women who were sexually abused at times feel magically desirable, experiencing this sense of sexual desirability as well as their sense of sexual prowess as their trump card.[2] People who were sexually abused as children often fear that no one will like them, or be interested in them, unless they have sex with them (see, for example, the case of Jared). If they are exclusively heterosexual or homosexual in their orientation, this may mean that half the human race is unavailable for friendship.

I realize another element enters here as well: active or passive? top or bottom? desired or desiring? These qualities don't cohere with gender or with sexual orientation. Yet we assume that in cases of childhood sexual abuse the child is by definition the more passive participant. Whether or not he or she is on top or on the bottom, is desired or desiring at any moment, the overall experience for the abused is one of being on the bottom—not in control of the time, place, duration, or form of contact. In our culture, these aspects of experience tend to conform to stereotypic female gender roles. Girls who are "desired" by older women are in the same relationship to that desire as if they are "desired" by men, and in a similar relationship to desire that many women find themselves in as adults. Boys who are "desired" by women or men are in a different relationship than they think they should be as grown men.

In this sense, childhood sexual abuse does more damage to boys' sense of themselves as "men" than to girls' sense of themselves as "women."[3] Perhaps this is because being a victim is unfortunately congruent with traditional views of femininity. Female victims of abuse suffer more disturbances of sexual desire, and at times suffer a more general loss of desire and agency. But since historically in our culture a woman's lack of sexual desire was not uncommon, nor for that matter until recently was a more passive, masochistic stance in life, these consequences of sexual abuse are not as problematic to their sense of themselves as women. They may, however, feel that they are damaged goods, forever spoiled by their experience. Women collectively experience themselves as objects, not subjects, of desire (Benjamin, 1988; Dimen, 1991), and feeling helpless and victimized is unfortunately still consistent with cultural conceptions of femininity.

---

[2] See Chapter 8 (R. B. G.).

[3] See Chapter 3 (R. B. G.).

Gender Identity Anxiety

Anxiety about gender identity seems more likely to arise when the abuse occurs at a very young age, at a time when the child's conception of his body and his gender, as well as his understanding of the basic differences between the sexes, is not fully and complexly formed. Thus, for example, a young boy who is anally penetrated may fear becoming pregnant. This concern in turn may lead to questioning his identity as a male.

Anxiety over gender role behavior also extends to men who were sexually abused as older boys. Since so much of our cultural definition of masculinity is at risk for boys who are sexually abused by men, even established gender identity may be insufficient protection from gender role anxiety. After all, to be a victim, to be a sexual object, to feel helpless—all are experiences that are associated in our culture with being female. Butler's work on gender performativity (1990) and Goldner's description of gender identity as a culturally pervasive false self system (1991) can help to explain the compensatory use of hypermasculine stereotyped behavior by these boys when they grow up.[4]

A man who has doubts about his gender role behavior may experience talking about this abuse to a man in a position of authority as a replication and continuation of the original trauma. He may feel less a man than his male therapist and thus he may feel safer with a female therapist. Boys who were sexually abused by men may have difficulty as grown men being assertive, both in social relations and in sexual activity. To be assertive may feel like an identification with the aggressor and make them feel like perpetrators. On the other hand, an inability to be assertive and dominant may make them feel like less of a "man"—either insufficiently masculine or insufficiently heterosexual. Often these men fear being too "aggressive" or too "passive" in their relations with both men and women, wondering whether they are really man enough or, conversely, whether they have been overly masculine. They may simultaneously long to be and fear to be the aggressor—either the sexual perpetrator with women or the dominant "alpha" man among men. With men, they may fear being assertive lest they trigger a man's rage and get revictimized. On the other hand, if they are not sufficiently assertive, they reinforce their sense of being less manly and an easy victim. For these men, it might feel safer to work with a female therapist—they assume less assertiveness may be necessary to keep them on top and successfully in gender role.

My patient Bill presented with a complex "solution" to these issues. As a child, Bill had been sexually and physically abused by both his mother and male relatives. He became sexually active with both girls

---

[4] See Chapter 3 (R. B. G.).

and boys at an early age. By the time he came to treatment with me, he was HIV-positive; he had seroconverted during a long-term, live-in relationship with an older man whom he cared for during the terminal phase of his illness. He was a divorced, involved father of three girls and at the time of treatment was actively pursued by another woman from his hometown. Yet at the same time he was frequenting bathhouses where he was pursued by many men. Interestingly, he was mistaken by some of my patients who saw him in my waiting room as my boyfriend. He had two names for himself: Bill and Ron. Bill was a mild-mannered, health-conscious poet who liked both men and women as long as they were very clean. But Bill tended to be henpecked when he was with women. Ron was an aggressive angry guy whom you would be scared to meet on the street. Bill had enormous difficulty integrating these two aspects of himself and tended to impulsively switch between the two. While space doesn't permit me to fully explore the ways in which gender role behavior and sexual orientation carried multiple paradoxical meanings for Bill, I'll state just a few. His primary personality was gentle and poetic—a presentation he got teased about as a child by other children who called him a "faggot." As an adult, it was this personality that surfaced when he was with female friends and lovers and with male friends. This was the personality who presented himself for treatment. Later, I was introduced to the rough aggressive Ron, a personality who went to homosexual bathhouses and got even with men for their prior abuse of him by being only partially available to them. This tough raging style also expressed some of his deep-seated internalized homophobia.

Sexual Orientation Anxiety

Heterosexual men who were older boys when they were sexually abused by men may maintain an intact sense of gender identity but have fears regarding their sexual orientation, inspired by their questioning why they were picked for same-sex abuse.[5] This may manifest as homophobia or avoidance of any intimate contact with men—including emotional closeness. It may also lead to compulsive womanizing, or at least to constant sexualized awareness of women and a need for sexual recognition by women as a reassurance for their anxieties. This leads to specific countertransference anxieties and technical questions that I will discuss below.

Sexual abuse of both gay and straight boys by men is further complicated when the abuser is an intimate known to the boy as someone

---

[5] See Chapter 4 (R. B. G.).

who is publicly living a heterosexual existence.[6] The sexual activity with the boy is then doubly denied and ineffable since it violates several taboos—both generational and, for lack of a better word, "orientational." The object of this abuse may experience the unconscious shame and humiliation of the adult who is an important figure for male identification and is also denying his sexual interest in same-sex partners. In what other ways has this person been two-faced? What makes same-sex activity unspeakable? Did it happen with other people too? If I grow up to be a man like my father (or teacher or uncle), might I also be interested in both men and women?

Dr. Gartner notes that homosexual men who were abused by men when they were boys may have a difficult time acknowledging that they were abused since the abusive sexual activity may also have been their first experience of same-sex desire by another. There may have been some relief in knowing that they were not alone in experiencing same-sex desire, but at the same time the abusing adult is hardly an ideal role model.

The homosexual man who was abused by a man when he was young may be struggling not to see himself as a victim and in that sense as feminized. Here the choice of a female therapist may be the patient's effort at identifying and acknowledging that he was in fact a victim, while simultaneously hoping to reduce the chance that homosexuality will be devalued and pathologized by an unconsciously homophobic male therapist. Some research suggests that women are less homophobic than men (Herek, 1998; Kite and Whitley, 1998) in relation to both male and female homosexuality. Friday (1981, 1998; Friday and Rubenstein, 1993), in a series of books on men and women's sexual fantasies, finds that one of heterosexual women's most common sexual fantasies involves sex with other women. But same-sex fantasies are not commonly reported by heterosexual men.

Homosexual men who were abused as boys by men may be especially prone to revictimization by both male and female therapists who want to "straighten" them. Male therapists may do this aggressively through penetrating interpretations, or more subtly by selectively reinforcing any tentative interest in women (see Blechner, 1993, and D. Schwartz, 1993). Some female therapists may, in addition to the above, also become highly seductive in an unconscious effort to get the erotic attention they expect and demand from a man. This provocative seductiveness may mirror the frequently noted behavior of the mother of a young gay boy who is disappointed by the lack of romantic attention that she had anticipated from her son. Homosexual men who as children

---

[6] See the discussions of Lorenzo (pp. 166, 189, and 201) and Beau (pp. 100 and 107) (R. B. G.).

were abused by men may also fear an overly sexualized transference or countertransference with an openly homosexual male therapist.

Attitudes toward Women

As with all people who have been sexually abused as children, it can be very difficult to address the ways in which these men have identified with their aggressors and may belittle and abuse the people with whom they are intimately involved, including their therapists. This identification with the aggressor can be more difficult to unravel when the therapist is female and the patient male since in our culture the socially sanctioned role for men includes a degree of aggressiveness with which some women may be uncomfortable. The female therapist may often find it easier to identify and align herself with the patient as victim. And yet, if a man is feeling conflicted about being an assertive heterosexual guy, there may be times when his behaving in ways the female therapist finds mildly abusive or degrading is actually a movement toward a "healthier," normative masculine identity.

This feature of the heterosexual man who was sexually abused by a man causes an interesting clinical dilemma. The female therapist, wishing to be treated as a person, not as a sexual object, may understandably cringe and consider interpreting a male patient's sexist comments. But if she sees part of her goal as reinstating, or helping him resume, his "normal" development as a man, should she let some of this behavior go by uninterpreted—or at least differently interpreted and understood?

Often these men, while fearing being sexually aggressive, and indeed at times having sexual difficulties because of fears of their own power, nonetheless find other ways of expressing aggression and sadism toward women. Of course, we must keep in mind that frequently the boy who is sexually abused by a man has also been neglected and/or abused by his mother. Thus, his behavior as an adult man with female partners is also complexly determined.

Nonsexual Intimacy

Another issue that needs further discussion is that of nonsexual intimacy. We talk about the desire for fathering or mothering, but what of nonhierarchical relatedness? What of nonsexual same- and opposite-sex closeness? Dr. Gartner describes how difficult and compelling this quest for nonsexual intimacy can be in abuse survivors. Sullivan (1953) recognized the critical importance of "chumship" as a stage in development. I think we need to extend this idea in order to better describe the kind of vital, intimate, friendships that are so transformative in people's lives

(Shapiro, 1993). At times, patients may need to experience their therapists in an intimate but nonsexual, nonhierarchical manner. Too often,
therapists may think that the lack of an obvious oedipal or erotic transference means that the therapy is superficial. Patients frequently first find
this kind of safe, nonsexual, intimacy in twelve-step programs, intensive
group experiences, hospitalizations, or retreats.

Men Who Had Female Abusers

Men who as boys were sexually abused by women, especially by their
mothers, are often deeply disturbed by the experience, shifting from
intense rage to suicidal despair. The contradictions between what society
says they must have experienced during these encounters and what they
in fact experienced are deeply confusing. On the one hand, the professional literature has acted as though sexual abuse by mothers is exceedingly rare and an indication of extreme pathology on the mother's part.
On the other hand, contemporary cinema has picked up the story of sex
between a boy and his mother in ways that have alternately glorified it
(*Murmur of the Heart*) or altered the power relationship (*Spanking the
Monkey*). In this latter movie we get some sense of the deep psychological confusion that consummated mother–son incest can cause. In both
movies, sex with the mother is portrayed as an initiation rite in which
the adolescent boy goes on to be sexual with a same-age partner after the
initiation with the mother.[7]

These movies make it seem as though the boy's masculinity is
increased and he is empowered through this experience of "oedipal victory." In my experience, this has not at all been the case. It is true, however, that such men may have an uncanny appeal to women and know it.
An obese patient whom I would never have guessed was a ladies' man
said, "I must have the right scent"; he always had many female admirers.
This quality may lead to compulsive womanizing, an activity that serves
to both express hostility toward women and at the same time reassure a
man of his attractiveness and adequacy. But the womanizer is only as
powerful and sexually adequate as his last conquest, and as with any
addictive behavior, the need is never sated.[8]

The womanizer poses serious problems for the female therapist.
These men are often exceedingly charming and disarming, know how to
make a woman feel very important and understood, and at the same
time may exude an underlying vulnerability, thus appealing to both sex-

---

[7] See Chapter 2 (R. B. G.).

[8] See Chapter 8 (R. B. G.).

ual and nurturant desires of female therapists. Heterosexual men who were sexually abused by their mothers thus present an intense countertransference challenge to their female therapists. Many female therapists have described an overwhelming, intense blending of erotic maternal preoedipal countertransference with the oedipal countertransference. Often, in the course of these treatments, the female therapist is intensely engaged in a struggle to help save the life of a man who is both deeply despairing and simultaneously charming.

During these treatments, the female therapist may find herself privy to a degree of openness from a man that she rarely encounters outside the consulting room. Women in our culture generally have less experience handling the heady combination of idealization, need, and sexual adoration that is directed more frequently to men in power. It seems likely that, just as with female patients who were sexually abused by male therapists, these men who were previously abused by women are more vulnerable to abuse by female therapists. Ideally, judicious use of supervision will reduce the likelihood of such enactments. However, it is precisely in these treatments that a therapist may find it most difficult to seek consultation. Alfred Stanton (1973) used to say that when you start to feel like you have a very special relationship with a patient whom no one else would be able to understand, it's time to run to supervision. It's best to always have in place a colleague whom you deeply trust for just such emergencies.

Often men who were abused by their mothers, that is, treated more like lovers and confidants than like sons, seem exquisitely attuned to women's moods—a quality that makes them very desirable to women. However, once the initial attraction has done its job, the trouble begins. Fears of abandonment, infidelity, and inadequacy frequently plague the sexually abused man, and his unconscious and conscious rage at women's power and anticipated insatiable demands begin to be expressed. Men who as boys were not only sexually overstimulated by their mothers but were also forced to engage in overt adult sexual acts often feel intense humiliation, shame, and rage. The intensity of this rage frequently surprises and frightens the female therapist who had been more tuned in to the vulnerable, abused boy. I have been consulted by men with this history who feel they are at an impasse with their female therapists. I have been struck by the viciousness of their rage with their therapists, and by their therapists' denial and minimization of this rage. I think therapists do this at their own peril.

I worked with a man named Michael who had suffered covert maternal incest as well as chronic maternal physical abuse, and who felt deeply inadequate. This sense of inadequacy found literal expression when, upon being sober for several months, he went shopping for clothing. He repeatedly underestimated the size clothing he wore. His self-experience remained that of a little boy, one who was too small to satisfy his mother. During our treatment, Michael frequently made reference to friends of his who had developed sexual relationships with their female therapists. He often expressed his concern, both in dreams and in his waking statements, that he wasn't classy enough for me to find him interesting. In fact, I thought he was extremely bright, engaging, emotionally open, and vulnerable.

Whenever our work seemed to be going well, Michael would react by missing appointments, abusing drugs, or neglecting the practical demands of daily life. We came to understand this as his way of deliberately disappointing me, before he could be found lacking by me. I found these actions to be striking reminders that he was, despite his competent, engaging persona, in a lot of trouble. In his romantic relationships, he managed his fears of being inadequate by always having two long-term relationships going on simultaneously, with frequent additional one-night flirtations or short-lived sexual encounters. Michael would become depressed if he noticed he was not attracting the gazes of women on the street, and he found any withdrawal by a primary girlfriend completely intolerable. But his infidelities invariably led to retaliatory moves by his girlfriends. He was recurrently caught in a vicious cycle.

During the course of this treatment, Michael became involved with a very accomplished but emotionally unavailable woman. He was able to remain monogamous for the first time in his life, but we both felt his monogamy was only possible because of the intensity of our treatment. His girlfriend sensed this and expressed considerable jealousy of me. If I seemed to be taking him for granted—for example, by being a few minutes late to a session—he would arrive late to the next session and announce that he was sorry but he and his girlfriend had been having sex.

Our best work in therapy came during a period when Michael and his girlfriend accepted a referral for couple therapy and he agreed to take antidepressants. The medication not only curbed his suicidality and his rejection sensitivity, but also reduced the intensity of his sexual craving. This reduction in sexual desire came as a great relief. Unfortunately, I responded to this increased stability, and perhaps unconsciously to his decreased need for me, by becoming, in his view, less emotionally available. For example, I had normally been hypervigilant to any sign that he felt slighted and in the past had been quick to reassure him in the face of whatever narcissistic injury he experienced. He quickly sensed this change in me and increased his abuse of over-the-counter drugs and alcohol. As he put it, drugs were a perfect mistress.

The consequences of my reduction in emotional availability were quite dire. Michael required several hospitalizations to regain sobriety, and recurrently tested the consistency of my concern for him and whether I still found him worthwhile and adequate. Fortunately, years later I can say there was a good outcome, at least by conventional standards. Michael is married, has children, is a devoted father, and is highly respected in his field. But he still struggles with his need to retreat.

Choosing a Female Therapist

I have seen several heterosexual men who were molested as boys and/or adolescents by adult men. Some had been abused by relatives, others by strangers. These men specifically wanted to work with a female therapist who had had experience working with sexually abused adults. Often they had not disclosed their sexual abuse histories to previous male therapists. These patients knew that they had been abused but did not feel comfortable describing their experiences to their male therapists. In part, this discomfort seemed to arise from their own questioning of their sexual orientation and/or gender as a consequence of the abuse.[9] At other times, their silence was more reflective of what they experienced as their previous therapists' doubts about whether boys can really be sexually abused. For these heterosexual men, discomfort arising from questions regarding sexual orientation, gender identity confusion, and gender role anxiety seemed to be relieved by the presence of a female therapist in the consulting room.

Similarly, many men who have been molested as children feel that women can understand them better because women know what it is like to be abused, scared, and sexually victimized. The female therapist in this situation, pleased that the male patient is expressing a preference for working with a female, may fail to recognize the "dark" side of this preference. Perhaps she will miss the contempt with which she and all victims may be viewed by her male patient. It is vital that the female therapist resist any simplistic sense of being the "good guy" and explore the role of the women in these men's lives at the time of their sexual abuse as well as the dynamics between them and their lovers, wives, and other women in subsequent periods of their lives. Men's reactions to these women will be replayed in the transference/countertransference over the course of any successful treatment.

Experiencing the Woman Therapist as an Abuser

A challenge for female therapists working with sexually abused men is accepting and owning the relatively rare experience of being perceived and experienced as the abuser or rapist of a man. I have had patients

---

[9] See Chapters 3 and 4 (R. B. G.).

experience my words and interpretations as a penis being shoved in their mouth, and have had to repeatedly pass tests about my trustworthiness. We may think we are behaving in our standard way and yet suddenly the patient feels deeply violated, terrified, raped. As we struggle to work through these rough moments, reestablishing a therapeutic alliance, uncovering whatever past event has been triggered by our actions, we may self-consciously monitor our behavior, both verbal and nonverbal, wondering if our questions are prurient or intrusive, our statements defensive or illuminating. The clinical dilemma is how to explore these behavioral enactments without further traumatizing the patient. But if we do not do this detailed exploration then I think we cheat the patient.

When working with men who have been sexually abused by their mothers, I have at times experienced what for lack of a better term I would describe as a "two-way rape." I have felt raped by the intrusion through projective identification of intense sadomasochistic fantasies that were totally unfamiliar. Under these conditions, I have had highly disturbing fantasies. For example, I once had the fantasy of masturbating by using a baby's body as a penis, or teaching a child to sexually penetrate me. In these fantasies, I was insatiable. Upon reflection, I felt certain that the baby/child was a particular male patient who had experienced severe beatings and sexual stimulation by his mother. As a teenager, he was molested on several occasions by priests. His behavior with women suggested that he had also been the object of more direct sexual abuse by his mother than he had previously recalled. Although we were never able to know this with certainty, it seemed likely to both of us that these disturbing fantasies of mine represented something of his early experience with his mother.

Seductive Undercurrents

One of the dangers when working with abuse survivors is that we and they may distrust all sexual looks and all requests for attention. And yet it is part of "normal" development to be admired and adored, to know that you are Daddy's favorite little girl or Mommy's best little man. Is the absence of that sense of mutual attraction, either in the family of origin or within the therapeutic dyad, also pathogenic? The sexually abusive parent makes ordinary attraction and attractiveness unsafe. Perhaps part of the treatment of abuse survivors is to help them reclaim a sexuality that is their own, one that they can safely experience, explore, and share when they choose.

I have certainly had intense sexual feelings toward both men and women patients in my practice, but I think their experience and mine is different as a function of both sexual orientation and gender. The sense of danger and excitement is far greater when I am working with someone, either male or female, who was abused by another woman and is currently sexually interested in women. The mutual seductions seem closer to the edge, the tension is far greater.

The "ordinary" seductiveness that permeates a long, intimate relationship between two people can take on more intense and desperate dimensions in therapy with abuse survivors. For example, I saw a male patient who wore Bermuda shorts, despite the cool temperature, when I visited him in the psychiatric hospital. True, it was overheated in the hospital—but I'd never seen his legs before. I kept trying not to look. Months later, he spoke of wanting to cause me some discomfort, wanting to watch me try not to respond. In fairness, of course, I must add that I was always aware of what I wore to see him. Had I unconsciously been doing the same to him?

The paradox Dr. Gartner describes of the longing for and dread of sexual contact is very familiar and in my experience occurs in both same-sex and opposite-sex therapeutic dyads, and with heterosexual, bisexual, and homosexual patients. As one patient put it, "I will try everything in my power to seduce you, I don't trust any woman who doesn't want to sleep with me, but I will hate you if you succumb." I agree with Dr. Gartner that at times it is important to make a position statement about not abusing the patient even though, of course, he can't simply believe and trust you. I also think it is critical to find a nonjudgmental and nonhumiliating way to address his wish to be sexually wanted and his simultaneous dread of being desired. It can be very tricky to do this in a way that is neither coldly clinical and rejecting nor overstimulating; I refer the interested reader to Jody Davies's (1994) courageous discussion of these issues.

Dr. Gartner's Case Examples

Much of what Dr. Gartner describes in his work is familiar to me and doesn't seem specific to male patients or to male therapists. I've had female patients call for a consultation, too scared to give their real names, interviewing me on the phone, sending me letters to test my reactions, and then never coming in person. I don't know that they are more scared of me, a woman, than if I were a man. I never got close enough to find out. However, I am sure that the cultural identification of male with aggressor, sexual initiator, top person in the hierarchy, significantly alters the experience men have coming to see a man in authority.

In considering Dr. Gartner's clinical examples, I'm struck by how many of the issues the men deal with are equally characteristic of women. For example, Frank, the man who can barely speak of his need on the phone and fails to show for his first appointment, states that he is not yet ready to talk to a man about his abuse, but perhaps he is not yet ready to speak to a women either. At least he picked up the phone and called Dr. Gartner. Greg's conflicting fears of being molested and of not being sexually desired by Dr. Gartner are fears expressed by many of my heterosexual male patients who were abused by women, and my heterosexual female patients describe or enact similar conflicts with men in their lives or people in authority positions. Many female abuse survivors are so under the sway of these fears that for long periods of time they avoid all contact with men. I have not found this dynamic to be as central among my female patients, both straight and lesbian, who were abused by women when they were children.

Jared presents with a picture rarely seen among women: he claims that the sexual contact between him at age five and his seventeen-year-old neighbor was pleasurable and that only later did he consider it abusive. Dr. Gartner seems to understand the pleasure to stem in part from Jared's early sense of his homosexual orientation. I wonder how much retrospective coloring has been applied to these memories. If we substitute a heterosexually oriented five-year-old girl with a seventeen-year-old male neighbor in the vignettes of oral sex in which the child fellates the older boy, most of us would be surprised if the female patient focused on the pleasure and excitement of the event, although we know these feelings are often part of the experience. Dr. Gartner seems to imply that the sense of abuse stemmed mainly from the way the relationship ended: the near discovery, the older boy's fear, Jared's sense of rejection and abandonment. But I would wonder about Jared's conscious focus on the pleasurable aspects of his experience, given differences in size, initiation of activity, and expressions of desire. I wonder whether a male therapist is more likely to accept his male patient's descriptions of sexual activities as pleasurable? Is it ego dystonic for both male therapist and patient to experience themselves as helpless or as sexual victims? Conversely, might it be easier for male patients and therapists to acknowledge sexual arousal during abuse than for female patients and therapists to do so?

This vignette also raises questions about the impact of an early sense of sexual orientation that is different than one's parents' orientations. Dr. Gartner reports that after being pushed into a closet Jared began to realize "for the first time" that what he had been doing with Kris for two years was "wrong." But why did Jared keep his relationship with Kris secret from his parents (I'm assuming it was secret), because it was homosexual or because it was sexual?

Dr. Gartner's example of his work with Harris beautifully illustrates the value of group therapy with survivors of abuse.[10] Often patients can tolerate experiences in a group that they cannot yet manage in individual

---

[10] Dr. Shapiro is referring here to the material about Harris in Chapters 9 and 11 as well as in this chapter (R. B. G.).

treatment. Also, abuse survivors frequently were incapable of establishing same-sex friendships during childhood and adolescence, depriving themselves of the healing power of chumship that Sullivan (1953) has described. Often they have felt so unlike their peers, so much more grown up in some respects, and yet so scared and needy in others, that they were unable to make friends. If they did have friends, there were profound secrets standing between them and true intimacy. In addition, many survivors of childhood sexual abuse are so anxious and depressed as children, so desperately trying to get people to see the trouble they are in, that they behave in ways that set them apart from their peers. For example, they may have poor personal hygiene, idiosyncratic gestures, or preoccupation with a fantasy world. Same-sex group therapy affords an opportunity for reworking a critical stage of development.

SEX AND GENDER PARADOXES IN TREATMENT

In concluding this chapter, I want to emphasize what odd work we do. In our consulting rooms, men and women strive to be intimate and vital, but not overtly sexual. They are not defined by their gender, yet they are able to explore the impact of their respective genders. In many ways, the participants in a psychotherapeutic treatment become fully intimate, yet remain undisclosed. And therapists are inevitably voyeuristically gratified but should not actively seek to be turned on.

We struggle with these paradoxes continuously, most pointedly when we work with adults who were sexually abused as children. We struggle to know when we can ask questions and when these are intrusive. We expect to know if patients have sex, but can we ask how they do it? How they feel? What's important to them? Is it the same with all lovers? How is it different if they make love with men or with women? Do we need to know the answers to these questions, or do we just want to know? To be safe we could, like some therapists, refrain from asking any questions. But does that suggest to the patient that we don't want to know or can't imagine the answers? Do we ask about some areas of life but not others? Can I ask about sex without engaging in sex? I certainly can't ask without revealing my own standards, experiences, and expectations (see E. Singer, 1968). But then we're all supposed to act like it is not happening. Dialogues like this one help us become increasingly attuned to these constant paradoxes.

CHAPTER 11

— ·•·—

Group Therapy

Since sexual betrayal in early intimate relationships disrupts the sexually abused man's ability to form and maintain relationships, therapy must engender a capacity for interpersonal connections. This process must be ongoing throughout his treatment. The primary relationship with the individual therapist is the principal vehicle by which he experiences new possibilities in his ability to relate. A complementary and equally powerful means of effecting change in relatedness can be group therapy, especially when the group focuses on abuse and its aftereffects. Parker (1990) comments that, for this population, group therapy's "power to reduce isolation, enhance self esteem, and provide a boundary laboratory where stereotypes and dysfunctional patterns of intimacy can be met with a more appropriate systemic response seems to operate at an order of magnitude above individual therapy alone. What individual work provides in depth and particulars, group work provides in breadth and enhanced power" (p. 187). Some of these men have never revealed their history to a single person besides a therapist. Many experience great shame about it. In fact, questions raised by a history of sexual abuse regarding basic issues like masculinity, gender, and sexual identity can make them phobic about being in the company of other men at all. This phobia is heightened if their abuser was a man. For many men, these themes may be addressed more effectively in a group situation than in individual treatment.

The literature on group therapy with sexually abused men is scant, although some writers have addressed the issue at least in part (Bruckner and Johnson, 1987; Dimock, 1988, n. d.; Lew, 1988; Bolton et al., 1989; Pescosolido, 1989; K. Singer, 1989; Brown, 1990; Ganzarain and Buchele, 1990; Hunter, 1990a; Parker, 1990; Isely, 1992; Knight, 1993; Crowder, 1995; R. M. Friedman, 1995; Harrison and Morris, 1995; Gartner, 1997b; Horsley, 1997). The near-consensus has been that this population is best served in same-sex groups.[1] In general, these writers have drawn on the complex literatures about group therapy (for example, Yalom, 1975), gender (for example, Fast, 1984; Pollack, 1990, 1995), feminism and rape (for example, Brownmiller, 1975), homosexuality (for example, Sedgwick, 1990), masculine identity complexities (for example, Lisak, 1993, 1995; Levant, 1995), group work with abused women (for example, Mennon and Meadow, 1993), all-male group work (for example, Andronico, 1995), and individual treatment of sexually abused women and men (for example, Bolton et al., 1989; Davies and Frawley, 1994) in order to synthesize ways to think about working with sexually abused men in groups. Much of this literature is discussed earlier in this book.

In this chapter I will examine how group therapy parallels, supplements, and accelerates the work accomplished in individual dynamic therapy. In addition, I will focus on ways it can help a man attain goals that individual treatment can not always accomplish.

GROUP STRUCTURE AND GOALS

Yalom (1975), discussing group therapy as a modality, identifies its major benefits as "installation of hope, universality, imparting information, altruism, the corrective recapitulation of the primary family group, development of socializing techniques, and imitative behavior" (p. 3). Among these, universality—the confirmation that they are not unique—and symbolic recapitulation of the abuse with new outcomes are especially relevant for sexually abused adults (K. Singer, 1989; Horsley, 1997).

Many of the groups described in the literature on sexually abused men are time-limited in nature (Brown, 1990; Isely, 1992), though some writers suggest renewable short commitments to the group so that the experience can ultimately be long term (Harrison and Morris, 1995).

---

[1] See Brown (1990) and Knight (1993) for discussions of mixed-sex groups for sexually abused adults. An important advantage of mixed-sex groups is that group members can confront gender stereotypes *in vivo*, particularly stereotypy about gendered victim–victimizer perceptions. Advantages of same-sex groups are delineated throughout this chapter.

Some writers describe psychoeducationally oriented tasks used both to structure the group and to contain group members' anxiety (Isely, 1992). Other writers are more process-oriented (Parker, 1990; Harrison and Morris, 1995), and one recommends a two-stage group experience, with a time-limited group followed by an open-ended process-oriented group (Crowder, 1995). K. Singer (1989), R. M. Friedman (1995) and Gartner (1997b) have previously described psychodynamically oriented, open-ended group therapy models for sexually abused men. In groups like this, unconscious processes related to such issues as power, control, intimacy, shame, isolation, and guilt can be addressed over an extended period of time.

Writing about sexually abused women, Herman (1992) suggests a succession of three goals in their treatment that she feels are best addressed in group therapies with different structures: The initial goal is to establish safety in the present. Herman argues that this is most likely to happen in didactic groups and groups that focus on self-care. In such groups, the emphasis is cognitive and educational rather than psychologically exploratory. A second goal is to remember and mourn the abuse, focusing on the actual trauma. Herman advocates doing this work in trauma-focused groups that are highly structured and time-limited, with fixed goals and little emphasis on interaction among group members. The third goal is establishing a reconnection with oneself and others, including interpersonal relationships in the present and future. According to Herman, these goals are best accomplished in open-ended, psychodynamic groups where there is a here-and-now focus on long-entrenched interpersonal relationship patterns.

Herman's goals apply as much to group therapy with sexually abused men as to the group treatment of sexually abused women she discusses. I concur that structured, psychoeducational, or time-limited groups can all be very useful for men, particularly those in the early stages of dealing with their abuse. I believe, however, that all of Herman's goals may also be addressed at one time or another in open-ended, psychodynamic groups such as those I have run. Such groups primarily form the basis for my discussion in this chapter. In them, there may be psychoeducational components, especially at the beginning. Most of the men I have worked with, however, have reached a sufficient sense of safety elsewhere and are ready to address their abuse in a more emotionally oriented and less cognitively focused group setting. The main work of my groups has combined, first, work on trying to remember the abuse and mourn it, which is accomplished by concentrating on past experiences; and, second, addressing relational patterns, achieved by emphasizing the interpersonal events in the group itself. In my experience, combining these goals has not presented a problem.

Men who are just beginning to confront their abuse or their psychological issues in general may need the safety of a time-limited group. In time-limited groups for sexually abused men I have supervised, my experience is that by the end of the allotted time group members usually feel that time was too short (Herman reports a similar experience in time-limited groups with sexually abused women). However, these same group members acknowledge that they would have been too frightened to enter a group without a structured ending. Nevertheless, as K. Singer (1989) notes, "Short-term treatment is not adequate in helping them to identify the emotional and behavioral symptoms, recognize the negative messages from the past, and develop ways to alter the feelings and behavior that work against them" (p. 470).

For a man who has been addressing his abuse for some time, open-endedness in itself may create a sense of safety. He is willing to take risks if he trusts that the group will be there for him should he get in trouble. As Julian said in the second session of a newly formed group, "We have the luxury of time. Time to get to know each other—not having to try anything until we are truly ready. Time stretches out in front of us, and we can take the time to do this right."

Group treatment for sexually abused men, like their individual treatment, must particularly take into account how men's gender socialization affects their view of an abuse experience (see Chapter 3). Men's groups in general are thought to be places where men can learn to accept traits typically considered feminine, such as emotionality, empathy, and dependence, and to challenge assumptions about masculinity (Kupers, 1993).

Dimock (n. d.) writes about group therapy in a paper that appeared on the Internet web page maintained by the National Organization on Male Sexual Victimization. Although intended for men with sexual abuse histories, his thoughtful comments are equally useful to clinicians. Dimock argues that in groups sexually abused men redefine masculine stereotypes more easily; give themselves permission to be vulnerable; cultivate ways to release anger and use power appropriately; identify healthier role models; develop intimacy with other men; discover how to focus on process rather than end-product; learn to be interdependent rather than to fear dependence; and find out how they can compete appropriately, value the things men do, and gain a feeling of pride in being men.

In the all-male group situation, each member is forced to be in the company of other men. If he confronts his transferences to them and starts to change, his initially terrifying experience can be ultimately exhilarating as he finally finds a way to feel good about being a man. This happens when the core underlying issues associated with gender shame are brought up and thus made available for therapeutic intervention. At the heart of gender shame for many sexually abused men is a history of having no fathering because of a physically or emotionally absent or abusive father (Dimock, n. d.). A boy without a functioning father to guide him into the world of men may feel lost, isolated, inadequate, with no place in the world. Despite women's importance in the development of a boy's masculine identity, it may be that only other men can give the validation and acceptance a boy needs to feel like a man (Dimock, n. d.). A men's group can provide a forum for this to occur.

Other issues discussed throughout this book also take on added resonance in a group situation. It is particularly important to address in a group patients' preconceived notions about what constitutes sexual abuse, as well as the likelihood that they have equated victimization with femininity. Similarly, the confusion for many men who have been sexually abused by men about whether having been chosen for abuse means they are homosexual is an important consideration in forming a group, especially when deciding whether the group should mix heterosexual and homosexual men, an issue I discuss below. Most important, the group experience can be useful in combating sexually abused men's isolation, self-blame, interpersonal wariness, and reluctance to be self-disclosing, particularly with other men (Hunter, 1990a; Harrison and Morris, 1995; Mendel, 1995; Gartner, 1997a). For this population, these factors heighten the "customary dread" that Yalom (1975, p. 302) describes in all people entering a group therapy situation.

Horsley (1997) surveyed group therapists working with sexually abused men to interview them about their experiences. She focused on their beliefs about how groups with this population work and the essential elements for success with them. Because of her difficulty finding a sample of appropriate therapists, she used a nonrandom, convenience sampling technique in which respondents were located via a snowball method, using word-of-mouth referrals from other clinicians. She included only group therapists who had worked in all-male or mixed-sex groups designed to address sexual abuse issues. In all, she contacted 355 potential respondents, chiefly on the U.S. East and West Coasts, asking whether they ran a group for sexually abused men or knew someone who did. In a remarkable demonstration of the paucity of groups available to sexually abused men, she was able to include *only nine* therapists in her final sample. Her findings, while impressionistic, lend further credence to suggestions made by other clinicians who have written about these groups, particularly Dimock (1988, n. d.), Lew (1988), Bolton et al. (1989), Hunter (1990a), Crowder (1995), R. M. Friedman (1995), Harrison and Morris (1995), and Gartner (1997b). I will summarize Horsley's work here and refer to it elsewhere in this chapter.

Reviewing the literature about group therapy for sexually abused adults, Horsley notes that, like all group therapies, these groups are laboratories for learning new ways of relating to others. They are important for sexually abused men because they can teach them ways of interacting that are different from adaptations to familial abuse that are maladaptive outside the family. Horsley's respondents articulated five major themes that brought men into their groups: gender role confusion, expressing and managing emotions, sexuality, fears of becoming abusive, and relationship problems. This list naturally has a large overlap with the issues Horsley's respondents said were actually addressed in their groups: interpersonal relationships (especially with men), sexualization of friendships, problems with power and control, vulnerability related to intimacy and trust, shame and guilt, expression of anger, and fear of becoming perpetrators of abuse themselves.

Horsley also notes five factors thought to be curative by the therapists in her sample: rebuilding identity, reducing isolation, reworking family dysfunction, regaining power and control, and recognizing defenses. In particular, her respondents noted how in groups men could learn to distinguish their unhelpful defenses, such as isolation and numbness, as well as break down maladaptive defenses, reconceptualize behavior that was once adaptive, and confront shame, self-blame, and self-hate. Other curative factors identified by these clinicians included discovering the universality of the abuse experience, gaining new hope, testing self-degrading beliefs, learning how to express a wider range of emotions, understanding the limitations of gender socialization, allowing men to tell their stories for the first time, and providing a place for men to confront their fear and expectation that other men will judge them. In addition, Horsley's respondents noted that through group work men can appropriately incorporate victimization into their self-perception, much as sexual orientation, race, and ethnicity comprise part of their identity. The abuse thus becomes more "ordinary" in the men's experience, and therefore has less uncontrolled, unpredictable, and unconscious influence on how they live.

LEADERSHIP

In Chapters 9 and 10, we considered some of the themes underlying how a sexually abused man develops a relationship with a therapist, and also the common transference/countertransference paradigms in the work. All these issues also emerge in a group therapy situation. They may be magnified if a man has intense feelings about re-creating his family through the group and therefore relates to the therapist as to a parent.

Alternatively, they may be diminished if he relates more intensely to other group members than to the therapist.

When deciding on leadership parameters for a group, the number of therapists and their sex are the most obvious variables to consider. Groups are generally run either by a single therapist or a cotherapy team. Cotherapy teams are most often found in groups run in agency settings, because it is difficult logistically to have them in private practice situations. Much has been written about the advantage of male–female cotherapy teams in group therapy (Yalom, 1975), but I have also heard of successful groups for sexually abused men run by two male therapists, by a woman clinician working alone, and, more frequently, by a male therapist working alone, which is how mine are run.

Cotherapists are able to support one another and give one another perspective on what is happening in a group. On the other hand, it can be complicated to manage the dynamics between cotherapists, which may begin to resemble those in the families of the abused men. Male–female cotherapy teams may re-create a sense of family more easily than single-sex cotherapy teams or single therapists, but it is my sense that family transferences are inevitably set up in all therapy situations, particularly group therapies. What is most important is the therapists' ability to monitor these transferences and work with them in a relatively free and nondefensive manner. This has been an area of special concern to me in my groups because I include men I work with in individual treatment along with men seeing other therapists. This setup is not ideal, and I would prefer the luxury of working with a group made up entirely of men from my private practice or entirely of men in treatment with other therapists. The pragmatic realities of working in private practice have made this impossible (among Horsley's respondents, the only clinicians who were able to set up groups in the preferable manner worked in institutional settings). Mixing men from my own individual therapy practice with men seeing other therapists could potentially set up a complicated transference paradigm in which, for instance, some men may feel they are special to me while others may feel as though they are my step-children (see my discussion in Chapter 9 of the dispute between Harris and Abe). My vigilance and openness to hearing subtle transference messages has been crucial in dealing with these issues as they arise.

I feel it is generally better to have a male therapist working alone than a solo female therapist in these groups. Men can more easily address male gender shame with a male therapist, who offers a direct experience with a man that it is acceptable for men to be vulnerable, hurt, or victimized. Female therapists, however, have pointed out that they are often perceived as safer than men (Horsley, 1997), and even men abused by women may experience men as more dangerous than women. Some men are unable to work with a male therapist, as I have noted elsewhere in this book, but may benefit from a group experience with a woman therapist. Again, the therapist's flexibility and skill at monitoring dynamics elicited by gender issues are the most important variables here.

As with individual therapy, a group therapy situation may draw the therapist into reenactments of abuse dynamics, sometimes with several patients simultaneously. Because of both this likelihood and the painfully distressing effect that listening to multiple abuse stories can have on any empathic person, it is important that group therapists, like individual therapists working with this population, find professional support systems and attend to their own self-care (see Chapter 9). On the other hand, the group experience can be positive and personally rewarding and growth-inducing for the therapist. I reprint two responses given Horsley (1997) when she asked group therapists how leading a group for sexually abused men affected them:

> "[It has affected me] deeply. I've been moved, very depressed at times. It just stretched my own conception of what people can do to one another. There's obviously something about this situation that has personal meaning to me . . . , although I myself have not been abused in any overt way. I feel boundary violations are meaningful to me personally which is probably why I do this work. And I find it oddly very enlivening because it's really demonstrated to me in a most electric way . . . how people can overcome things. They haven't been crushed like you'd expect from these types of experiences." (p. 57)

> "[I]t was a very liberating experience. These guys had such resiliency and strength underneath these difficulties that . . . it was very inspiring. . . . [T]hey had the ability to go through all this stuff and negotiate this emotional turmoil for years and years all by themselves." (p. 57)

SCREENING GROUP MEMBERS

Establishing an early connection between therapist and group member enhances the likelihood that group members will commit to and stay in the group (Yalom, 1975). This attachment begins during the essential process of screening potential group members. During this process, the therapist meets with them to see if they are appropriate for the group and to prepare them for what they may encounter in the group's dynamics.

Sprei (1987) suggests guidelines for such screening of potential members of women's groups for incest survivors, and these guidelines are useful for men's groups as well. They include the need to evaluate for motivation, and to assess the individual's current life situation, needs from the group, and interpersonal skills. Sprei considers being in a current life crisis to be a contraindication for group membership. Other contraindications suggested by her include being actively psychotic, intensely paranoid, drug- or alcohol-addicted, acutely suicidal, and severely self-mutilating. She also discourages accepting group members who are unable to discuss incest without substantial dissociation, or who have poor impulse control, a life-threatening eating disorder, or a multiple personality disorder.

Writing specifically about incest recovery groups for men, Lew (1988) notes the importance of potential group members having established an appropriate, nonabusive relationship with an individual therapist that has lasted at least six months. In addition, Lew screens for substance abuse problems, requiring that group members have remained substance-free for at least six months to one year prior to beginning in a group. They must also have had no psychiatric hospitalizations for at least a year, and must currently not be in the middle of a major crisis, be living in an abusive environment, or be abusive of another person.

In screening for therapy groups with sexually abused adults, it is not necessary to match group members by some external judgment about whether their abuse experiences were equally traumatic (Briere, 1995). As I have indicated, similar external events can have very different internal effects on different abused individuals. What is crucial is to match what Briere calls "therapeutic windows" (see Chapter 7) to be sure that group members will be able to deal with approximately the same level of psychic stress. Otherwise, there is a risk, for example, of retraumatizing a man who is not ready to hear another group member express himself with an intense level of affect, or, on the other hand, of making the second man feel he has to monitor what he says in order to not disturb the first man. In this second situation, the second man would be forced to become the first man's emotional caretaker, a position he may have had in his family of origin.

In Horsley's (1997) interviews with clinicians leading group therapies for sexually abused men, additional criteria identified for entering groups included stability and commitment, being sober for an extended period (two years was often mentioned), and having been stable for a sustained period of time if there was a history of suicide attempts or hospitalizations. The additional factor of a man's tendency to project blame onto others emerges when Horsley quotes a clinician about the screening process:

"What I'm looking at in terms of whether they are appropriate for the group is their ability to relate to me, their anger level. If they are very angry at the person who abused them, that is one thing. But if it's somebody who has a whole series of people they are angry at, therapists, bosses, so on and so forth, that's something I'm going to look at. It shows a lot of displacement going on and they haven't really come to terms yet and haven't been able to put it in the right place yet. And that's for sure going to happen in the group." (p. 48)

Exclusion criteria identified in Horsley's interviews included psychosis, multiple personality disorder (unless fairly well integrated), and severe personality disorder. The feeling expressed was that such patients cannot remain reality-based. Some of her respondents excluded people who have not addressed the abuse in therapy previously, unless the screening is for a psychoeducational group or another type of beginning group. A few therapists said the groups were inappropriate for young men whose abuse had ended only a short time earlier. Others excluded men who had been ritually abused, saying that other group members could not tolerate listening to such stories.

Horsley also notes that some of her respondents used the screening process to tell group members what to expect in the group, to describe themes that may emerge, and to see how the member may be affected by them. One clinician noted that, if anything, during the screening process the group leader should overarticulate the issues that are necessary to make group members feel safe. These include discussing guidelines for behavior in the group, a topic I will discuss later in this chapter.

Dimock (n. d.) believes groups for sexually abused men work best with a relatively small number of group members (he recommends five to seven; I limit my groups to eight members). He notes that the high intensity of the group experience and the need for a sense of safety and adequate time make small groups more manageable. He believes it is helpful, but not essential, that group members be concurrently in individual treatment. My own belief, however, is that, because of the emotionally laden material likely to emerge in psychodynamic groups centered around abuse, it is essential that a man have a place to go to process what the group has elicited in him. I therefore require that group members be in concurrent individual treatment (two-thirds of Horsley's respondents also stipulate that men be seen in individual therapy). For some men, this represents a financial burden that may stop them from entering a group. Yet I feel that to work otherwise will not provide every group member with the safety net he needs when facing his history of abuse. The only exceptions I have made have been for men who have had long-term individual treatment about abuse issues in the past or who, while still in the group, decide in consultation with their individual therapist that termination is appropriate. In either of these cases, I would want to monitor the man's reactions to the group in the individual sessions we have every three months, and perhaps recommend further individual treatment if over time he feels overwhelmed by the group process.

The most important factor in assessing a man's readiness for a group is his openness to participation. When actually in the group situation, however, some men who believe they are highly motivated to participate find it intolerable. In evaluating whether a man is ready for a group, Dimock (n. d.) recommends considering these factors: a positive experience in other group settings; a sense of how a group might be helpful to him; an ability to engage in supportive relationships; a recognition that such groups can be frightening; some knowledge of his sexual abuse history and a belief that it has had an impact on his life (whether or not he can articulate that impact); a willingness to learn about himself and his history; and, if he is prone to severe compulsive behaviors, a sense that he is addressing them or they are in remission. Noting many men's tendencies to be able to talk about sexual abuse histories dissociatively, as if describing someone else's experience, Dimock further recommends evaluating such a man's ability to acknowledge this tendency and his desire to explore his feelings.

Dimock also discusses mixing gay and straight men in a group. He believes that in a mixed group it is more likely that conflicts about sexuality and sexual orientation will be evoked and addressed in a safe environment. Commenting on the difficulty of arranging and then maintaining such a mixture in an ongoing group, however, he cautions against having only a single gay or straight member in a group. About the issue of mixing gay and straight men in a group, Lew (1988) originally wrote that it is preferable to run separate groups for gay and straight men because of the highly charged nature of feelings about sexual orientation for many men with sexual abuse histories. By the time he published the second edition of his book (1990), however, he had changed his mind, and wrote that "the advantages of heterosexual and gay men working together far outweigh any difficulties. . . . [W]e are dealing with issues of sexual child abuse, not sexual orientation" (p. xvii).

Addressing the thorny question of whether to include victimized men who have also been sexual abusers in groups for sexually abused men, Dimock (n. d.) divides men with this history into two subgroups. One includes men whose abusive behavior occurred in childhood or adolescence, and who are in treatment for help in acknowledging this behavior and working toward self-forgiveness. Men in this subgroup may be appropriate for a group that includes men who have never been abusive (see my discussion of Victor later in this chapter). Indeed, one member's disclosure of such abusiveness often elicits confessions of similar behavior from other group members.

The second subgroup of sexual abusers includes men with a more extensive history of victimizing behavior, often as adults. Here, the issues are more complicated. Even if it has been many years since the last abusive incident, the current task may be for him to take responsibility for his actions and understand his behavior. In such a situation, when the focus of an individual's therapy will be perpetration rather than victimization, Dimock recommends excluding him from a group of nonabusing sexual abuse survivors and referring him to an offender group (see M. Russell, 1995, for a discussion of abuser groups).

On the other hand, some men in this second subgroup have gone through offender treatment programs but have never had the opportunity to address their own victimization. Dimock says these men may benefit from a group for sexually abused men. They may, however, need additional support because working on the original victimization may trigger old feelings associated with prior offending behavior. Dimock recommends having a plan in place for addressing the possibility that such a man could relapse and become abusive. He does not say whether men in this category can be successfully integrated into a group with nonabusing men. While I have not treated men with extensive histories of being abusive, my own belief is that this would be difficult because of the strong antipathy most nonabusing men have toward habitual victimizers. If possible, I believe such men should be in groups with men having similar histories or in carefully constructed groups openly designed to mix men who have and have not been abusive.

In my own practice, I never knowingly include in a group a man who has been an abuser as an adult, but I have included some men who have sexually victimized others as children or adolescents if I feel that abusiveness is not a fundamental part of their adult behavior and/or psychology. Roughly, my other criteria for inclusion are a history of being able to address the abuse without severe decompensation or dissociation; a lack of psychosis, suicidality, and substance abuse in approximately the past two years; some ability to listen to other people's stories with empathy; some curiosity about his inner life and relationships with others; and a capacity to tolerate more or less the same levels of psychic stress as the other group members.

COMPOSITION OF THE GROUPS

In 1991, I started a group for men who had been sexually abused after I tried in vain to find one in New York City for my patient Patrick. I started a second, similar group in 1997. My discussion in this chapter is based on these two groups as well as others I have supervised or about which I have been consulted by other therapists. My groups meet weekly, with a long-term treatment emphasis and a slow evolution in group membership. All group members are seen concurrently in individual treatment. The exceptions, as noted above, are men already in the group for some time who decided in consultation with me and their individual therapists to stop that treatment, and the occasional man who has previously been in long-term therapy for abuse issues. A few group members are my individual patients; most, however, continue to see other therapists while consulting with me in individual sessions once every three months. I noted the transference implications of mixing these two kinds of patients earlier in this chapter.

The groups have ranged in size from four to eight men. As of this writing, there have been twenty-six men in my two groups combined. They have ranged in age from twenty-six to fifty-five. This is about the age range reported by Horsley's (1997) respondents' in their groups. Thirteen of my group members have been predominantly gay, eleven have been predominantly straight, and two used the group in part to sort out their sexual orientation confusion. Most group members have had problems in the area of personal relationships, work, or both. They have commonly had one or multiple addiction problems in the past, usually involving alcohol, drugs, sex, money, and/or food. The groups have included both men who were overtly abused and men who suffered covert abuse; men who were abused by male abusers and men whose abusers were female; men who were molested once and men whose abuse was chronic; and men who were incestuously abused and men whose victimization was extrafamilial. Somewhat to my surprise, none of these factors has seemed important to the group functioning. What has been crucial, as elucidated earlier in this chapter, has been grouping together men with similar "therapeutic windows." In other words, it has been important that men have similar ranges of psychological distur-bance and abilities to tolerate hearing painful material.

Each potential group member sees me in consultation at least three times before entering the group. In these consultations, I assess whether the man is committed to working on abuse issues. In addition, I explore his ability to form interpersonal connections and the degree to which he has already evolved psychologically as a result of facing his childhood abuse. I further assess each man in terms of the criteria described in the previous section of this chapter. These consultations also help prepare and orient him to the group experience, a process likely to minimize pre-mature withdrawal from the group (Yalom, 1975). I do not recommend group for some men. Such a man may need first to connect more deeply to his individual therapist or he may be too unstable in terms of job, family, living situation, or psychological state. For other men, I may recommend a short-term group as an initial experience. I am likely to do this if a man has had little time to reflect on his abuse, or if his feelings about being in a group make it impossible for him to make an initial commitment to a long-term group experience.

As I have indicated, the groups have had a mixture of gay and straight men, and, as Lew (1990) ultimately believed, in most cases this has enriched the groups rather than impeded their functioning (see Parker, 1990, for another point of view). Gay men who needed to find or strengthen a positive feeling about their orientation and straight men with strong heterosexist and homophobic beliefs have occasionally elected not to join a group because of this mixture. In general, however, mixing sexual orientations has seemed to enhance the groups. Like Lisak (1995; Lisak, Hopper, and Song, 1996), I have found on the whole that nonoffending straight men who come to treatment for sexual abuse are less homophobic and more sympathetic to the experience of gay men as victims than nonabused heterosexual men.

GROUND RULES

During the course of the pregroup consultations, I discuss with each man the ground rules for the group, rules I have adapted from those of Lew (1988). I also give them a written copy of these rules, which I reproduce here:

1. Privacy and confidentiality must be respected. You may discuss anything about your own experiences with anyone you choose, but any discussions must completely protect the privacy and identity of other group members.
2. Attend each session on time, sober and drug-free. Give ample notice of unavoidable absences and call in case of emergencies.
3. Only touch a group member physically with permission. Never under any circumstances use physical force or violence with another group member.
4. No sex between group members.
5. Contact with other group members outside the group is fine, but any such contact should be mentioned in group. It is very important that there be no secrets from the group in these contacts. In addition, there must be respect for one another's limits and needs for privacy. Every group member has the right to decline extending his participation beyond the group meeting time.

6. Every group member agrees to attend the group for ten sessions before making a decision to leave the group, and to give at least two sessions' warning if he does decide to leave. Group members who have attended the group for six months or more agree to give at least four sessions' notice if they are leaving.
7. No smoking, eating, gum chewing, or drinking during group sessions.
8. Fees should be paid by the tenth of the month for the previous month. Sessions must be paid for even if you do not attend for any reason.

The purpose of these rules is to make clear exactly how the group is structured, exactly what is expected and what is *not* expected from each member. Many of these rules are at least implicit at the beginning of most treatments, but I feel it is especially important with this population to make them explicit. Furthermore, it is equally important for each man to know that other men have agreed to these ground rules as it is for him to agree to them himself. This establishes a relative sense of safety for a man whose boundaries have been violated and whose current expectations about interpersonal connections are often distorted. His anxieties about relationships will be addressed repeatedly in the group, but having these guidelines allows him to enter the group in the first place.

The rules about confidentiality; attendance; consumption of food, drink and cigarettes; and payment of fees do not need further explication here. I will, however, elaborate on the other rules.

The rule about touch is crucial because of these men's history of physical or psychological boundary violation. Many sexually abused men find being touched an aversive experience, especially if the touch is unexpected or the person touching them is a stranger. This aversion even holds for everyday, ordinary experiences. Several men, for example, have brought up how uncomfortable they feel getting haircuts or shaking hands with others. It is important, therefore, that they know they will not be subject to unwelcome touching in the group. Yet I also feel that it is important to teach that touch can be nurturing and compassionate as well as hungering or exploitative. For this reason, I do not rule out the possibility of touch altogether.

It may seem unnecessary to articulate the rule prohibiting sexual involvement, but I think it is essential to make explicit that sexual involvement will not take place within the intimate relationships in the group. This is important because the men have received confusing messages about sex and intimacy, and may still confuse friendship with sexuality.

The rule about allowing contact outside the group touches on an area of disagreement in relation to groups for sexually abused adults. While traditional psychodynamic groups usually do not allow such contact, some writers (for example, Lew, 1988) believe that the extreme social isolation of many sexually abused men argues in favor of permitting extragroup contact while trying to monitor its effects on the group. I choose to allow group members to socialize outside the group, but ask them to bring up these contacts in the group and under no circumstances to keep secrets. I feel that, for this population, the issue of social isolation is so crucial that I am willing to deal in the group with any complications from extragroup contact (see R. M. Friedman, 1995, for another viewpoint).

The rule about attending ten sessions before deciding against being in the group as well as giving adequate notice before terminating is, of course, unenforceable. Yet it is important to state the issue and ask each man to commit personally to this promise. This is a way to communicate the message that frightening experiences may lessen with time. In addition, the man hears that the relationship he is establishing with the group is important, that it carries interpersonal responsibilities, and that he has a relational impact on other people.

I want to emphasize the importance of planning terminations if possible. This allows the man leaving and the other group members to talk about feelings, process any sense of abandonment, and learn that there can be a positive leave-taking, an experience they may never have had before (Horsley, 1997). As one of Horsley's respondents said about planned terminations:

> "[This] gives them hope. They say, here's a guy and they'll tell the guy whether they think he's leaving for positive reasons or if they think he has more work to do. But when a couple of guys have left for positive reasons, they'll recognize . . . their changes and . . . it's very positive. . . . There's some hope. This isn't just a . . . cloistered group where people who are outcasts just come . . . and stay and can't hope for anything better. . . . " (p. 67)

Over the years only two men have left my groups without giving adequate notice. Both these men left without warning within five weeks of starting in the group. Interestingly, they were both HIV-positive, the only men I have had in my groups whom I knew to be infected with HIV. Neither had yet told the group of his health status when he left. This suggests that HIV infection and a man's history of having addressed it are further variables to be considered in screening group members.

Lew (1988), all of Horsley's (1997) respondents, and most of the therapists surveyed by Crowder (1995) all identified explicit rules for their groups. Three in Horsley's sample wrote the rules out and gave them to members before beginning the group, as I do. The guidelines these clinicians suggested as a group roughly correspond to mine, dealing with confidentiality, giving notice of leaving the group, agreeing that emotional discharge not include hurting oneself or others, prohibiting sexual contact, not coming to the group under the influence of any drugs or alcohol, and limiting touch. All of these therapists also felt it was important to address socializing outside the group. Like me, none made a rule against extragroup contact, but several also cautioned about the importance of talking about this contact in the group.

STRUCTURE OF GROUP SESSIONS

I frame group sessions as follows: Each meeting lasts an hour and a half and begins with a "check-in." In this process, each man speaks briefly about his current state of mind (several of Horsley's [1997] respondents begin their groups in a similar way). Sometimes a check-in is only a sentence or two, but usually it is longer. Group members do not interact verbally during check-in, holding any reactions to one another's comments till everyone has finished. Men are asked to talk about their emotional states as they check in, and often this involves relating events of the week or reactions to the previous group session. The check-in process is important because it breaks the ice for any man who has trouble speaking, ensuring that he talks at least once during the group. It also gives us all a gauge of who may need to talk in the group, and to track how the group process affects each group member. Check-in usually lasts fifteen or twenty minutes, but has occasionally continued as long as forty minutes. After some experimenting, I found that it worked best for me to check in also, mainly because it reminded people of my active presence in the group. In my check-ins, which are generally brief, I may address a leftover issue from the previous session or I may simply say something about being ready to work that night.

When check-in is over, the group has a more traditional, free-form interactive process. Often this starts with a group member picking up on someone else's check-in, asking about it or reacting to it. My own behavior during this middle part of the group varies considerably. If I feel, as I often do, that the group is able to work on its issues without my active intervention, I remain quiet. I intervene if I feel there is an impasse, or an issue is being ignored, or a member in distress is not speaking. Sometimes I make an overarching comment about the group, such as "The group seems to be dealing with problems about trust tonight" or "I don't know that [man's name] will be able to hear you if you all bombard him this way about this topic." Such interventions are intended to give the group some perspective on its process. Sometimes my comments are virtually ignored. At other times they seem to move the group along. On still other occasions they elicit some kind of emotional reaction or turmoil in one or more group members.

Fifteen minutes before the group is scheduled to end, I announce that it is time for "check-out." Similar to check-in but usually briefer, check-out gives each man a chance to begin to synthesize what that group session has meant to him, to tie up any loose ends, and to gradually detach from the group prior to its ending for the week. As with check-in, men are asked not to interact during check-out, and I also make a check-out comment. My statements are usually about the group process but occasionally I address further an issue that arose in the group. I am careful in my check-outs, however, to try to make observations that will help a man move toward a sense of closure for the evening rather than to open him up emotionally any further.

Group sessions thus include both individual statements and interactional processes. The individual statements were at one time dubbed the "moving monologue" by a group member, and sometimes the interactional part of the group has included similar solo expressions about a man's life. In general, however, the interactive part of the group is where interrelating skills and deepening identifications are fostered. Individual personal statements and interpersonal dialogues are both essential to the group's functioning, though I believe that it is in learning to tolerate and indeed thrive on interaction with others that the most important healing takes place in the groups. As Abe put it after seven years in a group, "The group has been tremendously important to me. Sitting with a group of peers—not just a therapist who gets paid—and seeing their willingness to get naked in front of you, go to their core in front of you, and not using it to manipulate or get something from you—I've never experienced that anywhere else in my life. Plus, their willingness to hear me—these men listen!—there is something enormously healing in that process. It makes revealing yourself less fearful, helps you get from behind the wall you've built up—this is what happens both for them and for me. It's miraculous—but only possible on a long-term basis. Short-term groups can't work that way. It requires a lot of time because the distrust has to be battered down over and over and over through time."

In the rest of this chapter, I will describe how themes identified and discussed throughout this book can be dealt with in a group situation. In addition, I will highlight how some themes are uniquely developed in a group.

PROBLEMS IN DIFFERENTIATING
AFFECTION AND ABUSE

As I discussed in Chapter 8, many sexually abused men have little real sense of the differences among sex, love, nurturance, affection, and abuse. They view these emotional states as basically similar. Thus, affectionate touch is highly suspect and may be experienced as both sexual and abusive, erotic and violating. This issue is highlighted in a group setting. Johanek (1988) comments:

> For many of the men, this is likely to be the first time they have allowed themselves to experience a close emotional relationship with other men, especially if they were abused in childhood by a male abuser. To avoid panic, the bonding process must be monitored closely by the therapists and discussed in the sessions. Otherwise, male group members may take flight from the group and friendship with other men becomes confused with sexual interest. Many of them have already had the life experience of confusing affectionate feelings, intimacy, and trust with sexual feelings. . . . (p. 112)

For example, when I began working with my first group, I reiterated the rule that only with permission could group members touch one another. The men laughed at my "uptightness" and grumbled about my "authoritarian" imposition of rules. In the elevator going down from an early group meeting, however, one of the men leaned over to straighten another's coat collar. The second man, Max, exploded, and for months afterward brought up the incident in the group as an example of a time he had been violated. Max had little sense of the possible difference between a friendly, partly affectionate though potentially seductive grooming behavior, and an abusive, probably sexual, violation of his personal space. The man who had straightened Max's collar likewise was not altogether certain whether he had intended affection, seduction, or abuse. The incident prompted other group members to consider their own problems differentiating these feelings.

TRANSFERENCE TO THE
ALL-MALE ENVIRONMENT

In Chapter 3, I discussed men's gender shame, and emphasized the inner struggles sexually abused men often go through about having been victimized. These conflicts may emerge as strong, sometimes overpowering feelings when a sexually victimized man thinks about being in an all-male group, especially one with a male leader. This is particularly true of men who had male victimizers, as they may be more prone to expect victimization from men. But recall also that even men abused by women may feel shamed discussing their victimization with a man.

One of the clinicians responding to Horsley's (1997) survey of therapists working with these groups addresses the problems men are likely to have in this area:

> "[M]en who go to men's groups are often . . . alienated from their own gender . . . and don't have the slightest idea what it means to be a man. They walk around like a lone wolf, walk around like a man trying to pretend. . . . [M]ost men don't have a sense of community or relatedness to other men except as a threat and one of the threats that another man poses is that you could be found out by them." (pp. 38–39)

In Chapter 10, we saw a prime example of a sexually abused man's terror of an all-male environment in the description of Greg. His shadowy recollections of abuse by his father and grandfather in childhood, as well as clear memories of abuse by his pastor in young adulthood, rendered him almost unable to step into a room full of men. Yet over time he became an active and valued member of the group, enjoyed his relationships with other group members, and for the first time developed a substantial love relationship with another man outside the group.

Some men abused by a man in boyhood may choose to work in group with a male therapist after an initial period of individual treatment with a woman. This has been true of many of the patients who have been referred to my groups. Of the twenty-one men not initially in my own practice who have entered my groups since 1991, fourteen (67 percent) were in treatment with female therapists, six (27 percent) were seeing male therapists, and one (5 percent) was not currently in treatment till I referred him to a colleague. Of those men seeing women therapists, eleven (79 percent) had been abused by men. By contrast, two-thirds of the men seeing male therapists were abused by women. Many of the female therapists commented to me that only after considerable work on abuse issues had their patients evolved to the point of feeling prepared to work with a man about the abuse, and at that point they were referred to my group.

CROSS-IDENTIFICATIONS
AND CROSS-VALIDATIONS

The group process allows members to identify with one another's strengths and creativity as varying modes of dealing with the original abuse are revealed. For example, Neal, a man in his late twenties who had been forced to fellate his father from ages six to ten, told the group in a matter-of-fact manner that as a seven-year-old he had run away from home and lived for several weeks in a gazebo in a public park. As he disclosed the remarkable ways in which he had taken care of himself during this period, the group began to help him see himself as a person with resources and courage, not a passive victim, a self-concept he shared with other group members. Neal was astonished that the men saw him in this light, and in the ensuing discussion, other men began tentatively to recast their views of their own childhood reactions. Neal then told the group that, when he finally returned home as winter set in, his parents seemed not to be curious about where he had been. The group mourned his lost childhood with him, and offered him enormous support and validation for his deep sense of parental neglect as well as abuse.

Similarly, the group allows men who blame themselves for their abuse to see the inappropriateness of this self-blame when it is expressed by others. For example, Teo once turned suddenly to another man who was saying he himself should have done more to set limits on his abuser, and said, "Have you ever seen a three-year-old? Do you realize how little and defenseless they are? You'd never blame that little kid for what some adult did to him!" This comment sent shock waves of self-recognition throughout the group, and even caused Teo to reconsider his own early experiences of abuse.

RAGE AND OTHER EMOTIONAL STATES

The man who was sexually abused as a boy may bring to his therapy a transference filled with rage about having been molested, along with a childlike wish to be refathered and protected from violation (see Chapters 8, 9, and 10). This volatile transferential mixture can overwhelm or derail the entire treatment. I learned this the hard way in my work with Max, the man who reacted explosively when another man straightened his collar. Max was the subject of seductive abuse by a possibly psychotic mother. Among other things, she habitually told him when he was nine years old to massage her legs and thighs as she sat naked on the toilet. Furious at her and at the father who had not protected him from her, Max as an adult confronted his mother shortly before her death about her seductiveness. Her taunting, derisive reply was that she was foreign-born and because of her cultural heritage was freer about her body than Max, whom she thought prudish and silly. (In fact, the culture she grew up in is not noted for its open acceptance of sexuality.) Max's father remained a bystander in this confrontation, as he had when Max was a boy.

Max entered my group while in individual treatment with a male therapist, having had several abortive earlier individual and group treatments with both male and female therapists. Although I had some doubts about his capacity for interpersonal connection, he was convinced that he was now ready for a group experience, and I allowed him to enter the group. Once there, however, he quickly exhibited arrogance and hostility, frightening other group members with his rage. He could not tolerate periods when he was not the focus of the group, and he alienated other group members by his naked, angry neediness. When group members confronted him, he turned his fury on me, derisively calling me weak, passive, and unprotecting. While he recognized the parallels with his feelings about his father, he found the situation too dangerous, left the group precipitously, and terminated with his individual therapist as well.

The group was deeply disturbed by Max's volatility. For a time, group members' trust in my ability and willingness to protect them wavered. I had, after all, permitted Max to join the group and was not able to stop his verbal assaults on them. They were relieved when he left, and his departure elicited important expressions of fear about their safety and about the difficulty they had had standing up to him. This particular group was newly formed when Max was in it. I believe that if it had been a more mature, cohesive group, with established norms of behavior and more connections among its members, it might have dealt more effectively with Max's behavior. Nevertheless, I think the outcome would have been the same and it was better for all concerned that he left.

Despite this experience with Max, rage may be more permissible in a men's group than a mixed group, particularly rage at women. Recall, for example, that when Beau erupted in a near-psychotic fury as he railed about abusive men and cruel women, the other members of his group were generally not frightened, but instead were supportive and even envious of his ability to express his rage. As their reactions indicate, these men often lack positive models for expressing their anger, and consequently are afraid of being angry. Like Beau, in a group they may feel safe experiencing their rage more fully, knowing it will be contained (Dimock, n. d.).

Other strong feelings besides rage are also frightening to sexually abused men. The emotions identified by Horsley's (1997) sample of group therapists as being problematic and important to address in groups include guilt, shame, hopelessness, hurt, pain, anger, depression, and disgust. In addition, men may be afraid of being perceived as fraudulent, different, abnormal, or likely to act out anger abusively. These emotions are not easily experienced by men. The therapist and other group members may be required to encourage a man to express and safely manage them in ways other than the self-blame, disgust, and distrust he has used in the past.

In the next section, we will see how therapeutic work on these emotions in a group setting informs men's abilities to relate to others.

RELATIONSHIPS WITHIN THE GROUP

By its nature, group therapy forces men to look at how they live in relationship to others. As Seth put it, "The edge of relating is always hidden—there are mirrors within mirrors so no one knows where my edge is. The group is a place where I can experiment with that edge safely."

While group members can get effective advice from one another on how to deal better with their relationships outside the group, the most potent relationship learning comes from their here-and-now relationships with one another and with the therapist. This learning comes through listening and being open with one another about their reactions. Especially important is attempting interpersonal confrontation, which frequently frightens men whose early relational experience has been exploitation, manipulation, and abuse.

When family relationships have been re-created and reworked transferentially, the relational learning can then be applied outside the group. Several men have noted, for example, how their experiences with one another affected their relationships with siblings, particularly brothers. Consider the dynamic between Harris and Abe:

Harris was the oldest of several brothers, and throughout his life he had related to his brothers in a manner reminiscent of their father's: autocratic, condescending, and controlling. Abe was the younger of two brothers, and had a highly conflictual relationship with his older brother, whom he experienced as demeaning and hateful. As children, Abe and his brother had been openly encouraged to compete for their mother's favors, and this competitiveness had lasted throughout their adult lives.

When the two men met in group, war was quickly declared between them. In one incident recounted in Chapter 9, Harris felt Abe was able to manipulate me into being less nurturing to Harris. In other incidents, Abe was sensitized to any sense of superiority emanating from Harris, while Harris was angered by Abe's rejection of what he felt were his attempts at friendship. Each became very wary of the other, feeling the other could not possibly empathize with his position. Eventually, the parallels to their respective sibling positions became unmistakeable. While this helped give them each a cognitive map for the transference in their relationship, it did not prevent their conflicts from reerupting. With time, however, each grudgingly acknowledged that he had learned to negotiate with the other and that this had been somewhat helpful to him. Nevertheless, when Harris left the group, there was a certain relief on both sides that they would not have to deal with one another any more.

When Harris returned to the group a year and a half later, there had been a sea change in the relationships each had with his real siblings. Abe had begun to have personal conversations with his brother in which they each acknowledged the abuse they had seen the other endure. They became hungry for emotional contact with one another and developed a mutually nurturant relationship that each valued. Harris found that in the contact he had with his brothers he was forcing himself not to try to control their behavior, despite his continuing feeling that he knew better than they how to resolve their problems. Instead, he tried to be emotionally supportive of each of them, and encouraged them to talk to him without problem-solving for them. This was a long and arduous process for Harris, but it made him feel more connected to his brothers and less responsible for them. I believe the sea changes in both men's sibling relationships were inspired by the work each had done with the other, work through which over time each learned to negotiate, listen, and modify his behavior. When they encountered one another in the group again, Abe and Harris realized and openly acknowledged how fond they were of one another, and how much each respected the other's struggles in life.

Intimate love and sexual relationships are also affected by group process. For many men, talking about a variety of sexual issues seems more permissible in an all-male group than elsewhere. In this setting, they are able to ask for sexual information and describe for the first time the details of their abuse, their sexual experiences, and their current sexual acting-out behavior.

An area of concern to many men regarding intimate relationships is their difficulty saying no, either about sex or about commitment. When Greg for example, began to date a man, he felt he either had to commit himself to a relationship he was unsure about or never talk to the other man again. He had begun to date men after eighteen months of group exploration of his difficulties with intimacy. Following a year of dating, he began a long-term relationship that, while problematic in many ways, greatly enhanced his life. He stayed with this man for a year and a half, sometimes feeling grateful that he was with someone at all, at other times feeling he had made a mistake trying to be in a relationship. Eventually he ended the affair because he felt his partner did not have the capacity or desire to deepen their relationship by talking frankly about some important and problematic areas of intimacy. At that point, Greg began to feel terribly guilty that he had chosen a superficial person to relate to, even briefly becoming paranoid that others who were voicing sympathy about the breakup really believed he was a fake, an inauthentic and superficial person himself. But by this time he had developed the self-confidence to question the other group members and state his own fears about his ability ever to be in an intimate relationship. The feedback he got was uniformly positive, as people told him they admired him for having tried so hard and for so long to create intimacy with this man.

A problematic relationship issue that must be dealt with carefully involves exploiting and abusing others. In the second meeting of a newly formed group, Victor described two occasions when at age sixteen he enticed prepubescent boys into sexual activity, in each case touching their genitals and ejaculating while remaining dressed. Having a history of extensive abuse by his father as well as sexual stimulation by his grandparents, he had not let himself think of the full consequences of his actions with these boys until he blurted the stories out in his group. Among the other group members was Ezra, a man who at age ten had been lured into the woods and masturbated upon by a seventeen-year-old boy. Startled, Ezra reacted by naming Victor's actions as abusive molestations similar to those Ezra had himself suffered. He said he felt squeamish being in a group with Victor but simultaneously he tried to find a way not to exclude Victor from the group through his repugnance.

In Victor's subsequent individual sessions with me, he declared defensively that he would not allow Ezra to "do a guilt trip" on him. As we considered together what his actions with the boys meant, however, he became troubled and anxious. He had not wanted to think about the boys he had molested, and now said in despair, "I don't know how to find them. I can't find out what happened to them. I don't want to be an abuser, but I was." This led us to explore how in his current life he was sometimes exploitative in his relationships with his lover and his employers without letting himself recognize the implications of what he was doing. I also pressed him about his not ever telling me about the abusive incidents with the young boys in the two years we had worked together before he entered the group, and then spilling out the story in his second group session. I suggested that on some level he had understood what his behavior meant, that being with other abused men had increased his anxiety about his own abusiveness, and that he was putting the group to a test of whether it could accept all of him.

Victor digested this and returned to the group, where he and Ezra tried valiantly to find a way to relate to one another. Victor acknowledged what he had done, expressed in a more authentic way his shame and guilt in relation to the boys he had abused, and grieved for the unhappy teenager he had been at the time. Ezra and the other group members made it clear they were not in a position to forgive Victor, since they were not the boys harmed by him. But they also indicated they were able to accept that an abuser could have positive qualities and could atone for his actions. This work deepened a few months later, in a group session where Ezra talked feelingly about his molestation and Victor wept as he understood at a more profound level the possible consequences of his own abusive behavior.

REFATHERING AND MALE IDENTITY

Participation in a men's group can dramatically change how a sexually abused man feels about being a man, about fathering, and about being with other men. Harris, for example, described the effects of the group on his self-concept as a man a year and a half after starting the group. Referring to societal views of masculine and feminine characteristics (see Chapter 3), Harris said he always had accepted the idea that women are "repositories for feelings" and men are out of touch with their emotions. "Then, about six months after starting this group, I suddenly realized I was sitting every week with men who were sensitive, feeling, and courageous about opening up. For the first time in my life, I was proud to be a man."

The father of a preschool boy named Ivan, Harris described in the group the beauty of Ivan's emerging eroticism, which he saw when the boy was naked in his bath, "pulling on his pud." His reactions as a father who wanted to be loving but was afraid he could inadvertently be abusive, as a son who had indeed been abused, and as a transferential son who worried that he could be abused again, all had a powerful impact on him, me, and the men in the group who identified both with Ivan as a boy who could be abused and Harris as a man trying to break an abusive familial pattern.

I described in Chapters 9 and 10 how Harris's lifelong difficulties with men were related to his history of sexual abuse by an alcoholic father who was at best neglectful and who sexually abused Harris for years during latency. I also discussed how these difficulties played themselves out in the transference and countertransference. I will focus here on how the group enhanced his individual treatment in the areas of fathering and expression of rage.

When Harris began group therapy, the group provided him with a network of men who could relate to his history, and he quickly began to focus and express the rage underneath his orderly surface. This rage was chiefly directed at his father, and he spent hours in the group venting the feelings he had previously only been able to describe in a contained, intellectualized manner. He shouted with glee that he would love to deface his father's tombstone with graffiti naming him as a child molester. (This adolescent-like fury and glee has also been noted by Isely, 1992.)

After a year in the group, Harris movingly thanked the other men for helping him finally become a man. As he put it, "Seeing your courage and sensitivity helped me find my own. You've helped me finally grow into my penis. I always had it attached to my body, but I never felt it was mine. Instead, I believed my father neutered me when he forced me to have sex with him."

In contrast to Greg, who could only function in the group by dissociating my presence and making believe I was not there, Harris monitored me closely. In the context of internal struggles about me as a fathering figure that are detailed in Chapter 9, he began to talk in the group about his relationship with his son. He described the "awesome responsibility" he felt to acknowledge Ivan's beauty without acting inappropriately. I recognized that Harris was also giving me a covert message about my own awesome responsibility not to act inappropriately toward *him*. When I said this to Harris in a follow-up individual session, he was moved to tears. He had not previously been able to articulate how afraid he had been of my failing him, given how much he wanted from me. We then entered into a discussion of what Winnicott (1960) might call "good enough fathering," both from Harris to Ivan and from me to Harris. We also talked about the abusive fathering Harris had received in his own family, the fathering that had led him to accept sexual molestation because it was as close to love as he ever got from his father. Harris hesitantly agreed with me that mistakes are possible in the context of a healthy, nurturing relationship. This helped him calm down about mistakes he could make with Ivan as well as about mistakes he recurrently felt I was making with him.

When Harris talked about his relationship with his son, it had an enormous effect on the other group members as well. Ivan was having severe impulse control problems in his preschool class, and an attention deficit disorder was diagnosed. Hearing Harris agonize over the decisions he had to make about Ivan, the group identified with both father and son. As they offered their advice or expressed their fears for Ivan, the other men in the group seemed to be healing themselves while trying to help Harris. Indeed, I felt that Ivan had five involved, sympathetic godfathers in the group in addition to his own father, each of them symbolically refathering himself while trying to work out Ivan's dilemmas.

Afterword

Writing this book has compelled me go deeper into the personal experience of trauma than I ever had before. It forced me to distill my patients' histories and crystallize the crucial themes we encountered in their therapies. I found it both exciting and moving to gain new insights into the conditions childhood sexual trauma imposes on men.

As time went on, however, I began to feel permeated by the traumatic experience. This was not because of the heightened empathy for the men I discuss in the book, although that was certainly one outcome of my focusing on our therapeutic experiences. Rather, I was reacting to a new and intensified understanding of how trauma affects people, pervading their existence, mediating their responses to everything and everyone. Trauma suffused my waking and dream life, and I felt surrounded by it, penetrated by it, weakened by it, imbued and steeped in it. Some early readers of the material I present in this book have told me of similar personal reactions, and I assume this will be true of other readers as well. We are vicariously enduring the traumas suffered by the boys I describe.

This is a positive outcome if it makes readers more attuned to the experience of boyhood sexual abuse. On the other hand, clinicians who treat large numbers of sexually abused patients need to ensure that they do not traumatize themselves, which would both hurt them and render them incapable of helping their patients. In this book, I have indicated some of the ways to accomplish this. Of these, I want particularly to emphasize the importance of having personal and professional support systems when doing this kind of work.

To highlight how significant and vital my own support systems have been for me, I will first return to the four individuals I described in the Introduction to this book. In my own mind, they became the readers I addressed as I wrote. They included a young scientist who had recently discovered the extent of his boyhood sexual abuse, a male therapist who worked with a number of sexually abused men but who had no professional and/or colleagial support for his work, another male therapist who had never told anyone about the boyhood sexual trauma he had personally experienced more than fifty years earlier, and a female therapist trying to better understand the men she had begun to treat in a rape intervention program.

The setting where I met these four was the biannual conference of the National Organization on Male Sexual Victimization (NOMSV), a body founded formally in Columbus, Ohio, in the fall of 1994. NOMSV's Founding Congress was a group consisting of sexually abused men, therapists treating sexually abused men, and therapists who were themselves men with sexual abuse histories. The Columbus gathering was the outcome of a series of national conferences on male sexual victimization held since 1988 by an informal federation of people interested in the topic. These people came from all over the United States and Canada, with some traveling from overseas as well. They had in common a feeling of being isolated personally and/or professionally, and had found that at these periodic national meetings they felt connected, educated, and supported in ways they had not imagined were possible.

I was privileged to be a member of the Congress that founded NOMSV, and have since valued tremendously the personal and professional network I gained along with my affiliation with this group. This network has buttressed the personal and professional networks I have relied on throughout my years of practice. As of this writing, I am serving on the board of directors of the still-fledgling organization. The fact that such a group exists, and that web sites have been developed (www.malesurvivor.org) to reach out to sexually abused men and therapists who work with them, says that we have come a long way in the last two decades.

When people hear me speak about male sexual victimization or learn that I work with sexually abused men, they often still voice expressions of disbelief that boys can be sexually abused. Or they may ask misinformed questions. They may assume that all these men have themselves been abusive, or that they are all gay, or that their abusers were always strangers and always male. Yet, more and more frequently, people who hear me speak have considered the problem before, and are eager to learn about the effects of boyhood sexual victimization and the vicissitudes of psychotherapeutic work with men having such histories. I have directed this book to the people in these audiences, and to people like those I met at the NOMSV conference. I have tried to communicate to them a psychoanalytically informed understanding of men who were sexually abused as children. Emphasizing the relational impact of these experiences, I have illustrated diverse aftereffects of early sexual betrayal on men, focusing especially on how these sequelae emerge in psychotherapy.

My final communication to therapists is this: The crucial initial task in working with a sexually abused adult is to bear witness. This is fundamental both for men and for women. It is essential to allow them to say what has been unsayable. For men, this means not only articulating previously undescribable experiences. It is also vital to understand internalized cultural ideas that have interfered with a man's capacity to process what happened, as well as the effect abuse experiences have had on his internal and relational worlds. Equally important is that we not retreat emotionally because of the countertransferential horror we do indeed inevitably feel. Once a man feels his trauma has been recognized, once he feels heard and knows his therapist can stay with him emotionally, then the tasks of constructing interpersonal boundaries, understanding symptoms in terms of intrusion and abuse, critiquing internalized masculine gender ideals, differentiating loving from abusive relationships, and helping him create a life for himself—all these become possible.

My messages to sexually abused men are simpler: You are not alone. You do not have to become an abuser yourself. Your sexual orientation was not dictated by premature sexual experiences. It is better to put appalling experiences into words and find someone who can hear them than to suffer in miserable, unarticulated silence. You will never change the fact that you were abused, but you can get to a point where you no longer spend your time dwelling in that part of your memory.

I end with a metaphoric tale. A patient of mine once recalled the story of Pandora's box. In this story, the Furies come flying out when Pandora opens the forbidden box. All manner of woes, tribulations, and sorrows are unleashed on humankind. My patient told the story to explain his motivation for not wanting to investigate any further the interior world created by his abuse. He was terrified of the personal furies that might fly out of his own darkness if he opened the box they dwelt in. But he changed his mind after he was reminded by another man in his therapy group that at the bottom of Pandora's box, after the Furies leave, is Hope.

APPENDIX

———————

Cross-References
to Personal Histories

References

Abelin, E. (1980). Triangulation, the role of the father, and the origins of core gender identity during the rapprochement subphase. In R. Lax, S. Bach, and J. Burland (Eds.), *Rapprochement* (pp. 151–170). Northvale, NJ: Aronson.

Adams, K. (1991). *Silently seduced.* Deerfield Beach, FL: Health Communications.

Alexander, F. (1948). *Fundamentals of psychoanalysis.* New York: Norton.

Alexander, F., and French, T. M. (1946). *Psychoanalytic therapy: Principles and application.* New York: Ronald Press.

Alpert, J. L., Brown, L. S., Ceci, S., Courtois, C., Loftus, E., and Ornstein, P. (1994). *Interim report of the APA working group on investigation of memories of childhood abuse.* Washington, DC: American Psychological Association.

Andronico, M. (Ed.). (1995). *Men in groups: Realities and insights.* Washington: American Psychological Association.

Aponte, H., and Hoffman, L. (1973). The open door: A structural approach to a family with an anorectic child. *Family Process, 12,* 1–44.

Bachmann, K. M., Moggi, F., and Stirnemann-Lewis, F. (1994). Mother–son incest and its long-term consequences: A neglected phenomenon in psychiatric practice. *Journal of Nervous and Mental Disease, 182,* 723–725.

Balint, M. (1968). *The basic fault: Therapeutic aspects of regression.* London: Tavistock.

Banning, A. (1989). Mother–son incest: Confronting a prejudice. *Child Abuse and Neglect, 13,* 563–570.

Baraff, A. (1991). *Men talk.* New York: Penguin.

Baron, R., Burgess, M., and Kao, C. (1991). Detecting and labeling prejudice: Do female perpetrators go undetected? *Personality and Social Psychology Bulletin, 17,* 115–123.

Bauserman, R., and Rind, B. (1997). Psychological correlates of male child and adolescent sexual experiences with adults: A review of the nonclinical literature. *Journal of Sexual Behavior, 16,* 213–223.

Bear, E., and Dimock, P. (1988). *Adults molested as children: A survivor's manual for women and men.* Orwell, VT: Safer Society Press.

Benjamin, J. (1988). *The bonds of love.* New York: Pantheon Books.

Benjamin, J. (1996). In defense of gender ambiguity. *Gender and Psychoanalysis, 1,* 27–43.

Berendzen, R., and Palmer, L. (1993). *Come here: A man overcomes the tragic aftermath of childhood sexual abuse.* New York: Villard Books.

Bergler, E. (1956). *Homosexuality: Disease or way of life?* New York: Hill and Wang.

Bergler, E. (1959). *One thousand homosexuals: Conspiracy of silence, or curing and deglamorizing homosexuals?* Paterson, NJ: Pageant Books.

Bieber, I., Dain, H., Dince, P., Drellich, M., Grand, H., Gundlach, R., Kremer, M., Rifkin, A., Wilbur, C., and Bieber, T. (1962). *Homosexuality: A psychoanalytic study of male homosexuals.* New York: Basic Books.

Black, C., and DeBlassie, R. (1993). Sexual abuse in male children and adolescents: Indicators, effects, and treatments. *Adolescence, 28,* 123–133.

Blanchard, G. (1986). Male victims of child sexual abuse: A portent of things to come. *Journal of Independent Social Work, 1,* 19–27.

Blechner, M. J. (1993). Homophobia in psychoanalytic writing and practice. *Psychoanalytic Dialogues, 3,* 627–637.

Blechner, M. J. (1995a). The shaping of psychoanalytic theory and practice by cultural and personal biases about sexuality. In T. Domenici and R. Lesser (Eds.), *Disorienting sexuality* (pp. 265–288). New York: Routledge.

Blechner, M. J. (1995b, September). Societal prejudice, psychodiagnosis, and treatment aims. *Round Robin,* pp. 9–12.

Blechner, M. J. (1996, January). Values, bigotry, and the aims of psychoanalysis. *Round Robin,* pp. 7–9.

Blechner, M. J. (1998). Maleness and masculinity. *Contemporary Psychoanalysis, 34,* 597–613.

Bloom, S. (1997). *Creating sanctuary: Toward the evolution of sane societies.* New York: Routledge.

Bly, R. (1992). *Iron John: A book about men.* New York: Vintage.

Bolton, F., Morris, L., and MacEachron, A. (1989). *Males at risk: The other side of child sexual abuse.* Newbury Park, CA: Sage.

Boyle, P. (1994). *Scout's honor: Sexual abuse in America's most trusted institution.* Rocklin, CA: Prima.

Brandt, R., and Tisza, V. (1977). The sexually misused child. *American Journal of Orthopsychiatry, 47,* 80–90.

Breuer, J., and Freud, S. (1893–1895). Studies on hysteria. *Standard Edition, 2,* 1–306. London: Hogarth Press, 1962.

Briere, J. (1988). The long-term clinical correlates of child sexual victimization. *Annals of the New York Academy of Sciences, 528,* 327–334.

Briere, J. (1989). *Therapy for adults molested as children: Beyond survival.* New York: Springer.

Briere, J. (1991). *Treating victims of child sexual abuse.* San Francisco: Jossey-Bass.

Briere, J. (1992). *Child abuse trauma: Theory and treatment of the lasting effects.* Newbury Park, CA: Sage.

Briere, J. (1995, October 5). *Treating male survivors of sexual abuse.* Workshop presented at the Sixth World Interdisciplinary Conference on Male Sexual Victimization, sponsored by the National Organization on Male Sexual Victimization, Columbus, OH.

Briere, J., and Conte, J. (1993). Self-reported amnesia for abuse in adults molested as children. *Journal of Traumatic Stress, 6,* 21–31.

Briere, J., Evans, D., Runtz, M., and Wall, T. (1988). Symptomatology in men who were molested as children: A comparison study. *American Journal of Orthopsychiatry, 58,* 457–451.

Briere, J., and Runtz, M. (1987). Post sexual abuse trauma: Data and implications for clinical practice. *Journal of Interpersonal Violence, 2,* 367–379.

Briere, J., and Runtz, M. (1988). Symptomatology associated with childhood sexual victimization in a non-clinical population. *Child Abuse and Neglect, 12,* 51–59.

Briggs, F., and Hawkins, R. (1996). A comparison of the childhood experiences of convicted male child molesters and men who were sexually abused in childhood and claimed to be nonoffenders. *Child Abuse and Neglect, 20,* 221–233.

Brod, H., and Kaufman, M. (Eds.). (1994). *Theorizing masculinities.* Thousand Oaks, CA: Sage.

Bromberg, P. M. (1991). On knowing one's patient inside out: The aesthetics of unconscious communication. *Psychoanalytic Dialogues, 1,* 399–422.

Bromberg, P. M. (1993). Shadow and substance: A relational perspective on clinical process. *Psychoanalytic Psychology, 10,* 147–168.

Bromberg, P. M. (1994). "Speak! That I may see you": Some reflections on dissociation, reality, and psychoanalytic listening. *Psychoanalytic Dialogues, 4,* 517–547.

Bromberg, P. M. (1995a). Psychoanalysis, dissociation, and personality organization. *Psychoanalytic Dialogues, 5,* 511–528.

Bromberg, P. M. (1995b). A rose by any other name: Commentary on Lerner's "Treatment issues in a case of possible multiple personality disorder." *Psychoanalytic Psychology, 12,* 143–149.

Bromberg, P. M. (1995c). Resistance, object-usage, and human relatedness. *Contemporary Psychoanalysis, 31,* 173–192.

Bromberg, P. M. (1996a). Hysteria, dissociation, and cure: Emmy von N revisited. *Psychoanalytic Dialogues, 6,* 55–71.

Bromberg, P. M. (1996b). Standing in the spaces: The multiplicity of self and the psychoanalytic relationship. *Contemporary Psychoanalysis, 32,* 509–535.

Bromberg, P. M. (1998). *Standing in the spaces: Essays on clinical process, trauma, and dissociation.* Hillsdale, NJ: Analytic Press.

Brooks, G. R. (1995). *The centerfold syndrome: How men can overcome objectification and achieve intimacy with women.* San Francisco: Jossey-Bass.

Brooks, G. R., and Silverstein, L. B. (1995). Understanding the dark side of masculinity. In R. F. Levant and W. S. Pollack (Eds.), *A new psychology of men* (pp. 280–333). New York: Basic Books.

Brown, J. (1990). The treatment of male victims with mixed-gender, short-term group psychotherapy. In M. Hunter (Ed.), *The sexually abused male* (Vol. 2, pp. 137–169). Lexington, MA: Lexington Books.

Brownmiller, S. (1975). *Against our will: Men, women, and rape.* New York: Simon and Schuster.

Bruckner, D. F., and Johnson, P. E. (1987, February). Treatment for adult male victims of childhood sexual abuse. *Social Casework,* pp. 81–87.

Burgess, A., and Holstrom, L. (1979). *Rape: Crisis and recovery.* Bowie, MD: Robert J. Brady.

Butler, J. (1990). *Gender trouble: Feminism and the subversion of identity.* London: Routledge.

Butler, J. (1992). Gender. In E. Wright (Ed.), *Feminism and psychoanalysis* (pp. 140–145). Oxford, UK: Blackwell.

Byne, W., Hamer, D., Isay, R., and Stein, T. (1995). *Sexual orientation is primarily a biological phenomenon: A debate.* Paper presented at the meeting of the American Psychiatric Association,

Caruth, C. (Ed.). (1995). *Trauma: Explorations in memory.* Baltimore: Johns Hopkins University Press.

Cassese, J. (Ed.). (In press). *Integrating the shattered self: Gay men and childhood sexual trauma.* New York: Haworth.

Chandy, J., Blum, R., and Resnick, M. (1997). Sexually abused male adolescents: How vulnerable are they? *Journal of Child Sexual Abuse, 6,* 1–16.

Charcot, J. M. (1887). *Lessons on the illnesses of the nervous system held at the Salpêtrière* (Vol. 3). Paris: Progrès Médical en A. Delahaye and E. Lecrosnie.

Chauncey, G. (1994). *Gay New York.* New York: Basic Books.

Cheselka, O. (1996). *Betrayal: Common and extraordinary.* Paper presented at the William Alanson White Institute Clinical Services Case Conference, New York, NY.

Chodorow, N. (1978). *The reproduction of mothering.* Berkeley and Los Angeles: University of California Press.

Chodorow, N. (1989). *Feminism and psychoanalytic theory.* New Haven, CT: Yale University Press.

Coates, S. (1990). Ontogenesis of boyhood gender identity disorder. *Journal of the American Academy of Psychoanalysis, 18,* 414–438.

Coates, S. (1992). The etiology of boyhood gender identity disorder: An integrative model. In J. Barron, M. Eagle, and D. Wolitzky (Eds.), *Interface of psychoanalysis and psychology* (pp. 245–265). Washington, DC: American Psychological Association.

Coates, S., Friedman, R. C., and Wolfe, S. (1991). The etiology of boyhood gender identity disorder: A model for integrating temperament, development, and psychodynamics. *Psychoanalytic Dialogues, 1,* 481–523.

Collings, S. J. (1995). The long-term effects of contact and noncontact forms of child sexual abuse in a sample of university men. *Child Abuse and Neglect, 19,* 1–6.

Condy, S. R., Templer, D. I., Brown, R., and Veaco, L. (1987). Parameters of sexual contact of boys with women. *Archives of Sexual Behavior, 16,* 379–394.

Conte, J. R. (1985). The effects of sexual abuse on children: A critique and suggestions for future research. *Victimology, 10,* 110–130.

Corbett, K. (1993). The mystery of homosexuality. *Psychoanalytic Psychology, 10,* 345–357.

Corbett, K. (1996). Homosexual boyhood: Notes on girlyboys. *Gender and Psychoanalysis, 1,* 429–461.

Courtois, C. (1988). *Healing the incest wound.* New York: Norton.

Courtois, C. (1992). The memory retrieval process in incest survivor therapy. *Journal of Child Sexual Abuse, 1,* 15–31.

Crewdson, J. (1988). *By silence betrayed: Sexual abuse of children in America.* Boston: Little, Brown.

Crowder, A. (1995). *Opening the door: A treatment model for therapy with male survivors of sexual abuse.* New York: Brunner/Mazel.

Daskovsky, D. (1998). The abuser and the abused: Sources of resistance to resolving splits in the countertransference in the treatment of adults who were sexually abused as children. *Psychoanalytic Psychology, 15,* 3–13.

Davies, J. M. (1994). Love in the afternoon: A relational reconsideration of desire and dread in the countertransference. *Psychoanalytic Dialogues, 4,* 153–170.

Davies, J. M. (1996a, April). *The multiple aspects of multiplicity.* Paper presented at the Spring meeting of Division 39 (Psychoanalysis) of the American Psychological Association, NY.

Davies, J. M. (1996b). Linking the "pre-analytic" with the postclassical: Integration, dissociation, and the multiplicity of unconscious process. *Contemporary Psychoanalysis, 32,* 553–576.

Davies, J. M. (1997). Dissociation, repression, and reality testing in the countertransference. In R. B. Gartner (Ed.), *Memories of sexual betrayal: Truth, fantasy, repression, and dissociation* (pp. 45–75). Northvale, NJ: Aronson.

Davies, J. M., and Frawley, M. G. (1992). Dissociative processes and transference–countertransference paradigms in the psychoanalytically-oriented treatment of adult survivors of childhood sexual abuse. *Psychoanalytic Dialogues, 2,* 5–36.

Davies, J. M., and Frawley, M. G. (1994). *Treating the adult survivor of childhood sexual abuse: A psychoanalytic perspective.* New York: Basic Books.

Dhaliwal, G., Gauzas, L., Antonowicz, D., and Ross, R. (1996). Adult male survivors of childhood sexual abuse: Prevalence, sexual abuse characteristics, and long-term effects. *Clinical Psychology Review, 16,* 619–639.

Diamond, M. (1997a). The unbearable agony of being: Interpreting tormented states of mind in psychoanalysis of adult sexually traumatized patients. *Bulletin of the Menninger Clinic, 61,* 495–519.

Diamond, M. (1997b, February). *Becoming a man: The consolidation of masculinity in adulthood.* Paper presented at the spring meeting of Division 39 (Psychoanalysis) of the American Psychological Association, Denver, CO.

Dimen, M. (1991). Deconstructing difference: Gender, splitting, and transitional space. *Psychoanalytic Dialogues, 1,* 335–352.

Dimen, M. (1995a). The third step: Freud, the feminists, and postmodernism. *American Journal of Psychoanalysis, 55,* 303–321.

Dimen, M. (1995b). On "our nature": Prolegomenon to a relational theory of sexuality. In T. Domenici and R. Lesser (Eds.), *Disorienting sexuality* (pp. 129–152). New York: Routledge.

Dimen, M. (1997). The engagement between psychoanalysis and feminism: A report from the front. *Contemporary Psychoanalysis, 33,* 527–548.

Dimock, P. (1988). Adult males sexually abused as children. *Journal of Interpersonal Violence, 3,* 203–221.

Dimock, P. (1989a). Factors in underreporting. National Organization on Male Sexual Victimization Web Page (www.malesurvivor.org).

Dimock, P. (1989b). Differences between adult male and adult female victims of childhood sexual abuse. National Organization on Male Sexual Victimization Web Page (www.malesurvivor.org).

Dimock, P. (1996). Recovery for the male sexual abuse survivor: Critical steps in the healing process. National Organization on Male Sexual Victimization Web Page (www.malesurvivor.org).

Dimock, P. (n. d.). Group work with adult male sexual abuse survivors. National Organization on Male Sexual Victimization Web Page (www.malesurvivor.org).

Dolan, Y. M. (1991). *Resolving sexual abuse.* New York: Norton.

Domenici, T., and Lesser, R. (Eds.). (1995). *Disorienting sexuality.* New York: Routledge.

Drescher, J. (1996). A discussion across sexual orientation and gender boundaries: Reflections of a gay male analyst to a heterosexual female analyst. *Gender and Psychoanalysis, 1,* 223–237.

Drescher, J. (1998). *Psychoanalytic therapy and the gay man.* Hillsdale, NJ: Analytic Press.

Duberman, M. (1991). *Cures.* New York: Dutton.

Duberman, M., Vicinus, M., and Chauncey, G. (Eds.). (1989). *Hidden from history: Reclaiming the gay and lesbian past.* New York: Penguin.

Ehrenberg, D. (1992). Abuse and desire. In D. Ehrenberg, *The intimate edge* (pp. 159–191). New York: Norton.

Elise, D. (1997, February). *Unlawful entry: Male fears of psychic penetration.* Paper presented at the spring meeting of Division 39 (Psychoanalysis) of the American Psychological Association, Denver, CO.

Elliott, M. (Ed.). (1994). *Female sexual abuse of children.* New York: Guilford Press.

Estrada, H. (1990). *Recovery for male victims of child sexual abuse.* Santa Fe, NM: Red Rabbit Press.

Etherington, K. (1995). Adult male survivors of childhood sexual abuse. *Counseling Psychology Quarterly, 8,* 233–241.

Evans, M. (1990). Brother to brother: Integrating concepts of healing regarding male sexual assault survivors and Vietnam veterans. In M. Hunter (Ed.), *The sexually abused male* (Vol. 2, pp. 57–78). Lexington, MA: Lexington Books.

Everstine, D., and Everstine, L. (1989). *Sexual trauma in children and adolescents: Dynamics and treatment.* New York: Bruner/Mazel.

Fast, I. (1984). *Gender identity: A differentiation model.* Hillsdale, NJ: Analytic Press.

Fausto-Sterling, A. (1985). *Myths of gender: Biological theories about men and women.* New York: Basic Books.

Ferenczi, S. (1930). The principles of relaxation and neo-catharsis. In M. Balint (Ed.), *Final contributions to the problems and methods of psychoanalysis* (pp. 108–125). New York: Brunner/Mazel.

Ferenczi, S. (1933). Confusion of tongues between adults and the child. Reprinted in *Contemporary Psychoanalysis* (1988), *24,* 196–206.

Fields, E. (1994). Countertransference issues in the treatment of victims of abuse. In A. Sugarman (Ed.), *Victims of abuse: The emotional impact of child and adult trauma* (pp. 187–212). Madison, CT: International Universities Press.

Figley, C. (Ed.). (1985). *Trauma and its wake, Vol. 1: The study and treatment of post-traumatic stress disorder.* New York: Brunner/Mazel.

Figley, C. (Ed.). (1986). *Trauma and its wake, Vol. 2: Traumatic stress theory, research, and intervention.* New York: Brunner/Mazel.

Fine, C. G. (1991). Treatment stabilization and crisis intervention: Pacing the therapy of the multiple personality disorder patient. *Psychiatric Clinics of North America, 14,* 661–675.

Finkelhor, D. (1981). The sexual abuse of boys. *Victimology, 6,* 76–84.

Finkelhor, D. (1984). *Child sexual abuse: New theory and research.* New York: Free Press.

Finkelhor, D., and Associates. (1986). *A sourcebook on child sexual abuse.* Newbury Park, CA: Sage.

Fiscalini, J. (1995). Transference and countertransference as interpersonal phenomena. In M. Lionells, J. Fiscalini, C. Mann, and D. Stern (Eds.), *Handbook of interpersonal psychoanalysis* (pp. 603–616). Hillsdale, NJ: Analytic Press.

Fischer, R. (1991). The unresolved rapprochement crisis: An important constitu-
ent of the incest experience. In S. Kramer and S. Akhtar (Eds.), *The trauma
of transgression* (pp. 41–56). Northvale, NJ: Aronson.

Freedman, A. M., Kaplan, H. I., and Sadock B. J. (1976). *Comprehensive textbook of psychiatry.* Baltimore: Williams and Wilkins.

Freeman-Longo, R. E. (1986). The impact of sexual victimization on males.
Child Abuse and Neglect, 10, 411–414.

Freud, S. (1896). The aetiology of hysteria. *Standard Edition, 3,* 189–221. London: Hogarth Press, 1962.

Freud, S. (1900). The interpretation of dreams. *Standard Edition, 4,* entire; *5,* 1–
630. London: Hogarth Press, 1962.

Freud, S. (1905). Three essays on the theory of sexuality. *Standard Edition, 7,*
130–245. London: Hogarth Press, 1962.

Freyd, J. (1996). *Betrayal trauma.* Cambridge, MA: Harvard University Press.

Friday, N. (1981). *Men in love: Men's sexual fantasies: The triumph of love over
rage.* New York: Dell.

Friday, N. (1998). *My secret garden: Women's sexual fantasies* (rev. ed.). New
York: Pocket Books.

Friday, N., and Rubenstein, J. (Eds.). (1993). *Women on top: How real life has
changed women's sexual fantasies.* New York: Pocket Books.

Friedman, R. C. (1988). *Male homosexuality: A contemporary psychoanalytic
perspective.* New Haven, CT: Yale University Press.

Friedman, R. M. (1995). Psychodynamic group therapy for male survivors of
sexual abuse. *GROUP, 18,* 225–234.

Friedrich, W. (1995). *Psychotherapy with sexually abused boys: An integrated
approach.* Thousand Oaks, CA: Sage.

Friedrich, W., Beilke, R., and Urquiza, A. (1987). Children from sexually abusive
families: A behavioral comparison. *Journal of Interpersonal Violence, 2,*
391–402.

Friedrich, W., Beilke, R., and Urquiza, A. (1988). Behavior problems in young
sexually abused boys. *Journal of Interpersonal Violence, 3,* 21–28.

Friedrich, W., Berliner, A., Urquiza, A., and Beilke, R. (1986). Brief diagnostic
group treatment of sexually abused boys: A comparison study. *Journal of
Interpersonal Violence, 3,* 331–343.

Friedrich, W., and Luecke, W. (1988). Young school-age sexually aggressive children. *Professional Psychology: Research and Practice, 19,* 155–164.

Friedrich, W., Urquiza, A., and Beilke, R. (1986). Behavior problems in sexually
abused young children. *Journal of Pediatric Psychology, 11,* 47–57.

Fromuth, M. E., and Burkhart, B. R. (1987). Childhood sexual victimization
among college men: Definitional and methodological issues. *Violence and
Victims, 2,* 241–253.

Fromuth, M. E., and Burkhart, B. R. (1989). Long-term psychological correlates
of childhood sexual abuse in two samples of college men. *Child Abuse and
Neglect, 13,* 533–542.

Fuentes, L. A. (Ed.). (1995). *Sexual abuse in nine North American cultures.*
Thousand Oaks, CA: Sage.

Gabbard, G. O. (Ed.). (1989). *Sexual exploitation in professional relationships.*
Washington, DC: American Psychiatric Press.

Gabbard, G. O. (1992). Commentary on "Dissociative processes and transference–countertransference paradigms . . . " by Jody Messler Davies and
Mary Gail Frawley. *Psychoanalytic Dialogues, 2,* 37–47.

Gabbard, G. O., and Twemlow, S. W. (1994). Mother–son incest in the pathogenesis of narcissistic personality organization. *Journal of the American Psychoanalytic Association, 42,* 171–190.

Galperin, L. (1998, March 20). *Integration and trauma resolution.* Presentation at "Trauma and Intimacy: Self/Other Adaptations," a conference sponsored by the Masters and Johnson Treatment Programs at River Oaks Hospital, New York, NY.

Ganzarain, R., and Buchele, B. (1990). Incest perpetrators in group therapy: A psychodynamic perspective. *Bulletin of the Menninger Clinic, 54,* 295–310.

Gartner, R. B. (1994, April). *When the analyst and the sexually abused patient are both men.* Paper presented at the spring meeting of Division 39 (Psychoanalysis) of the American Psychological Association, Washington, DC.

Gartner, R. B. (1996a). Incestuous boundary violations in families of borderline patients. *Contemporary Psychoanalysis, 32,* 73–80.

Gartner, R. B. (1996b, April). *The de-masculinization of sexually abused men: Crises about gender identity and sexual orientation.* Paper presented at the spring meeting of Division 39 (Psychoanalysis) of the American Psychological Association, New York, NY.

Gartner, R. B. (1997a). Considerations in the psychoanalytic treatment of men who were sexually abused as children. *Psychoanalytic Psychology, 14,* 13–41.

Gartner, R. B. (1997b). An analytic group for sexually abused men. *International Journal of Group Psychotherapy, 47,* 373–383.

Gartner, R. B. (Ed.). (1997c). *Memories of sexual betrayal: Truth, fantasy, repression, and dissociation.* Northvale, NJ: Aronson.

Gartner, R. B. (1997d). The controversy in context. In R. B. Gartner (Ed.), *Memories of sexual betrayal: Truth, fantasy, repression, and dissociation* (pp. 13–27). Northvale, NJ: Aronson.

Gartner, R. B., Bass, A., and Wolbert, S. (1979). The use of the one-way mirror in restructuring family boundaries. *Family Therapy, 6,* 27–37.

Gelinas, D. (1983). The persisting negative effects of incest. *Psychiatry, 46,* 313–332.

Gerber, P. (1990). Victims becoming offenders: A study in ambiguities. In M. Hunter (Ed.), *The sexually abused male* (Vol. 1, pp. 153–176). Lexington, MA: Lexington Books.

Gilgun, J. (1990). Factors mediating the effects of childhood maltreatment. In M. Hunter (Ed.), *The sexually abused male* (Vol. 1, pp. 177–190). Lexington, MA: Lexington Books.

Gilgun, J. (1991). Resilience and the intergenerational transmission of child sexual abuse. In M. Q. Patton (Ed.), *Family sexual abuse* (pp. 93–105). Newbury Park, CA: Sage.

Gilgun, J., and Reiser, E. (1990). The development of sexual identity among men sexually abused as children. *Journal of Contemporary Human Services, 71,* 515–523.

Gill, M., and Tutty, L. (1997). Sexual identity issues for male survivors of childhood sexual abuse: A qualitative study. *Journal of Child Sexual Abuse, 6,* 31–47.

Gilligan, C. (1982). *In a different voice.* Cambridge, MA: Harvard University Press.

Gillman, R. (1986). Physical trauma and actual seduction. In A. Rothstein (Ed.), *The reconstruction of trauma: Its significance in clinical work* (pp. 73–94). Madison, CT: International Universities Press.

Glaser, D. (1998, March 21). *Unfinished business: Erotophobia vs. erotophilia.* Presentation at "Trauma and Intimacy: Self/Other Adaptations," a conference sponsored by the Masters and Johnson Treatment Programs at River Oaks Hospital, New York, NY.

Goldberg, P. (1995). "Successful" dissociation, pseudovitality, and inauthentic use of the senses. *Psychoanalytic Dialogues, 5,* 493–509.

Goldner, V. (1991). Toward a critical relational theory of gender. *Psychoanalytic Dialogues, 1,* 249–272.

Gonsiorek, J., Bera, W., and LeTourneau, D. (1994). *Male sexual abuse: A trilogy of intervention strategies.* Thousand Oaks, CA: Sage.

Gonsiorek, J., and Weinrich, J. (1991). The definition and scope of sexual orientation. In J. Gonsiorek and J. Weinrich (Eds.), *Homosexuality: Research implications for public policy* (pp. 1–12). Newbury Park, CA: Sage.

Gornick, L. (1986). Developing a new narrative: The woman therapist and the male patient. *Psychoanalytic Psychology, 3,* 299–325.

Grame, C. J. (1993). Internal containment in the treatment of patients with dissociative disorders. *Bulletin of the Menninger Clinic, 57,* 355–361.

Grand, S. (1997). The paradox of innocence: Dissociative "adhesive" states in perpetrators of incest. *Psychoanalytic Dialogues, 7,* 465–490.

Green, R. (1987). *The "sissy boy" syndrome and the development of homosexuality.* New Haven, CT: Yale University Press.

Greenberg, J., and Mitchell, S. (1983). *Object relations in psychoanalytic theory.* Cambridge, MA: Harvard University Press.

Greenson, R. (1966). A transsexual boy and a hypothesis. In *Explorations in psychoanalysis* (pp. 289–305). New York: International Universities Press.

Greenson, R. (1968). Dis-identifying from mother: Its special importance for the boy. *International Journal of Psycho-Analysis, 49,* 370–374.

Groth, A. N. (1979). *Men who rape: The psychology of the offender.* New York: Plenum.

Groth, A. N. (1982). The incest offender. In S. Sgroi (Ed.), *Handbook of clinical intervention in child sexual abuse* (pp. 215–218). Lexington, MA: Lexington Books.

Groth, A. N., and Oliveri, F. (1989). Understanding sexual abuse behavior and differentiating among sexual abusers. In S. Sgroi (Ed.), *Vulnerable populations* (Vol. 2, pp. 309–327). Lexington, MA: Lexington Books.

Grubman-Black, S. (1990). *Broken boys/mending men.* Blue Ridge Summit, PA: TAB Books.

Haley, J. (1973). *Uncommon therapy: The psychiatric techniques of Milton H. Erickson.* New York: Norton.

Haley, J. (1976). *Problem-solving therapy: New strategies for effective family therapy.* San Francisco: Jossey-Bass.

Halperin, D. (1989). Sex before sexuality: Pederasty, politics, and power in classical Athens. In M. Duberman, M. Vicinus, and G. Chauncey (Eds.), *Hidden from history: Reclaiming the gay and lesbian past* (pp. 37–53). New York: Penguin (Meridian).

Hamer, D., Hu, S., Magnuson, V., Hu, N., and Pattatucci, A. (1993). A linkage between DNA markers on the X chromosome and male sexual orientation. *Science, 261,* 321–327.

Harper, J. F. (1993). Prepuberal male victims of incest: A clinical study. *Child Abuse and Neglect, 17,* 419–421.

Harris, A. (1991). Gender as contradiction. *Psychoanalytic Dialogues, 1,* 197–224.

Harris, A. (1994, April). *Gender practices and speech practices: Towards a model of dialogical and relational selves.* Paper presented at the spring meeting of Division 39 (Psychoanalysis) of the American Psychological Association. Washington, DC.

Harrison, J., and Morris, L. (1995). Group therapy treatment for adult male survivors of sexual child abuse. In M. Andronico (Ed.), *Men in groups: Realities and insights* (pp. 339–356). Washington, DC: American Psychological Association.

Hastings, A. S. (1998). *Treating sexual shame: A new map for overcoming dysfunctions, abuse, and addiction.* Northvale, NJ: Aronson.

Hedges, L. (1994). *Remembering and working through childhood trauma.* Northvale, NJ: Aronson.

Hegeman, E. (1995a). Transferential issues in the psychoanalytic treatment of incest survivors. In J. Alpert (Ed.), *Sexual abuse recalled: Treating trauma in the era of the recovered memory debate* (pp. 185–213). Northvale, NJ: Aronson.

Hegeman, E. (1995b). Resolution of traumatic transference: Two cases. *Contemporary Psychoanalysis, 31,* 409–422.

Hegeman, E. (1997, November 8). *Discussion: Dissociated states, possession, and shamanism.* Discussion of a panel presented at "Building New Bridges," a conference sponsored by the William Alanson White Institute, New York, NY.

Heim, S. (1995). *Mysterious skin.* New York: HarperCollins.

Henton, D., and McCann, D. (1995). *Boys don't cry: The struggle for justice and healing in Canada's biggest sex abuse scandal.* Toronto: McClelland and Stewart.

Hepburn, J. (1994). The implications of contemporary feminist theories of development for the treatment of male victims of sexual abuse. *Journal of Child Sexual Abuse, 3,* 1–18.

Herdt, G. (1981). *Guardians of the flutes.* New York: McGraw-Hill.

Herek, G. (1991). Stigma, prejudice, and violence against lesbians and gay men. In J. Gonsiorek and J. Weinrich (Eds.), *Homosexuality: Research implications for public policy* (pp. 60–80). Newbury Park, CA: Sage.

Herek, G. (Ed.). (1998). *Stigma and sexual orientation: Understanding predjudice against lesbians, gay men, and bisexuals.* Newbury Park, CA: Sage.

Herman, J. L. (1981). *Father–daughter incest.* Cambridge, MA: Harvard University Press.

Herman, J. L. (1992). *Trauma and recovery.* New York: Basic Books.

Hirsch, I. (1993). Countertransference enactments and some issues related to external factors in the analyst's life. *Psychoanalytic Dialogues, 3,* 343–366.

Hirsch, I. (1995). Therapeutic uses of countertransference. In M. Lionells, J. Fiscalini, C. Mann, and D. Stern (Eds.), *Handbook of interpersonal psychoanalysis* (pp. 643–660). Hillsdale, NJ: Analytic Press.

Hirsch, I. (1997, February). *Reflections on the concepts of dissociation and repression.* Paper presented at the spring meeting of Division 39 (Psychoanalysis) of the American Psychological Association, Denver, CO.

Holmes, W., and Slap, G. (1998). Sexual abuse of boys: Definition, prevalence, correlates, sequelae, and management. *Journal of the American Medical Association, 280,* 1855–1862.

Hooker, E. (1957). The adjustment of the overt male homosexual. *Journal of Projective Techniques, 21,* 18–31.

Hopenwasser, K. (1998a). Dissociative disorders in women: Long-term consequences of violence against children. *Journal of the American Medical Women's Association, 53,* 179–184.

Hopenwasser, K. (1998b). Listening to the body: Somatic representations of dissociated memory. In L. Aron and F. S. Anderson (Eds.), *Relational perspectives on the body* (pp. 215–236). Hillsdale, NJ: Analytic Press.

Hopkins, B. (1993, Fall). A question of child abuse. *Raritan*, pp. 33–55.

Hopper, J. (1997). Sexual abuse of males: Prevalence, lasting effects, and resources. Jim Hopper Web Page (www.jimhopper.com/male-ab).

Horsley, K. C. (1997). *A place for healing: Group leaders' perspectives on groups for men sexually abused as children.* Unpublished master's thesis, Smith College School for Social Work, Northampton, MA.

Huizenga, J. (1990). Incest as trauma: A psychoanalytic case. In H. Levine (Ed.), *Adult analysis and childhood sexual abuse* (pp. 117–135). Hillsdale, NJ: Analytic Press.

Hunter, M. (1990a). *Abused boys: The neglected victims of sexual abuse.* Lexington, MA: Lexington Books.

Hunter, M. (Ed.). (1990b). *The sexually abused male, Vol. 1: Prevalence, impact, and treatment.* Lexington, MA: Lexington Books.

Hunter, M. (Ed.). (1990c). *The sexually abused male, Vol. 2: Application of treatment strategies.* Lexington, MA: Lexington Books.

Hunter, M., and Gerber, P. (1990). Use of the terms "victim" and "survivor" in the grief stages commonly seen during recovery from sexual abuse. In M. Hunter (Ed.), *The sexually abused male* (Vol. 2, pp. 79–89). Lexington, MA: Lexington Books.

Isay, R. (1989). *Being homosexual.* New York: Farrar, Straus, and Giroux.

Isay, R. (1991). The homosexual analyst: Clinical considerations. *Psychoanalytic Study of the Child, 46,* 199–216.

Isay, R. (1998). Heterosexually married homosexual men: Clinical and developmental issues. *American Journal of Orthopsychiatry, 68,* 424–432.

Isely, P. J. (1992). A time-limited group therapy model for men sexually abused as children. *GROUP, 16,* 233–246.

Janet, P. (1887). L'anesthésie systemisée et la dissociation des phénomènes psychologiques. *Revue Philosophique, 23,* 449–472.

Janet, P. (1889). *L'automatisme psychologique.* Paris: Alcan.

Janet, P. (1898). *Nevroses et idées fixes.* Paris: Alcan.

Janet, P. (1907). *The major symptoms of hysteria.* New York: Macmillan.

Jenny, C., Roesler, T., and Poyer, K. (1994). Are children at risk for sexual abuse by homosexuals? *Pediatrics, 94,* 41–44.

Johanek, M. (1988). Treatment of male victims of child sexual abuse in military service. In S. Sgroi (Ed.), *Vulnerable populations* (Vol. 1, pp. 103–114). Lexington, MA: Lexington Books.

Johnson, R., and Shrier, D. (1985). Sexual victimization of boys: Experience at an adolescent medicine clinic. *Journal of Adolescent Health Care, 6,* 372–376.

Johnson, R., and Shrier, D. (1987). Past sexual victimization by females of male patients in an adolescent medicine clinic population. *American Journal of Psychiatry, 144,* 650–652.

Jones, E. (1957). *The life and work of Sigmund Freud* (Vol. 3). New York: Basic Books.

Jung, C. (1933). *Modern man in search of a soul.* New York: Harvest Books.

Kaftal, E. (1991). On intimacy between men. *Psychoanalytic Dialogues, 1,* 305–328.

Kasl, C. D. (1990). Female perpetrators of sexual abuse: A feminist perspective. In M. Hunter (Ed.), *The sexually abused male* (Vol. 1, pp. 259–274). Lexington, MA: Lexington Books.

Katz, J. N. (1995). *The invention of heterosexuality.* New York: Dutton.

Kendall-Tackett, K., and Simon, A. (1992). A comparison of the abuse experiences of male and female adults molested as children. *Journal of Family Violence, 7,* 57–62.

Khairallah, T. (1995). Traditional male socialization and propensity for addiction. *SPSMM Bulletin* (Division 51, American Psychological Association), *1, 5.*

King, N. (1995). *Speaking our truth.* New York: Harper Perennial.

Kinsey, A. C., Pomeroy, W. B., and Martin, C. E. (1948). *Sexual behavior in the human male.* Philadelphia: Saunders.

Kirschner, S., Kirschner, D. A., and Rappaport, R. L. (1993). *Working with adult incest survivors: The healing journey.* New York: Brunner/Mazel.

Kite, M., and Whitley, B. (1998). Do heterosexual women and men differ in their attitudes toward homophobia?: A conceptual and methodological analysis. In G. Herek (Ed.), *Stigma and sexual orientation: Understanding prejudice against lesbians, gay men, and bisexuals* (pp. 39–61). Thousand Oaks, CA: Sage.

Kluft, R. (Ed.). (1989a). Treatment of victims of sexual abuse. *Psychiatric Clinics of North America, 12,* 237–503.

Kluft, R. (1989b). Playing for time: Temporizing techniques in the treatment of multiple personality disorder. *American Journal of Clinical Hypnosis, 32,* 90–98.

Kluft, R. (1990a). On the apparent invisibility of incest: A personal reflection on things known and forgotten. In R. Kluft (Ed.), *Incest-related syndromes of adult psychopathology* (pp. 11–34). Washington, DC: American Psychiatric Press.

Kluft, R. (1990b). Incest and subsequent revictimization: The case of therapist–patient sexual exploitation, with a description of the sitting duck syndrome. In R. Kluft (Ed.), *Incest-related syndromes of adult psychopathology* (pp. 263–287). Washington, DC: American Psychiatric Press.

Knight, C. (1993). The use of a therapy group for adult men and women sexually abused as children. *Social Work with Groups, 16,* 81–94.

Knoblauch, S. (1993, April). *Forms and transformations of aggression in a male patient who was sexually abused.* Paper presented at the spring meeting of Division 39 (Psychoanalysis) of the American Psychological Association, New York, NY.

Kramer, S. (1974). Episodes of severe ego regression in the course of adolescent analysis. In M. Harley (Ed.), *The analyst and the adolescent at work* (pp. 190–231). New York: Quadrangle Press.

Kramer, S. (1990). Residues of incest. In H. Levine (Ed.), *Adult analysis and childhood sexual abuse* (pp. 149–170). Hillsdale, NJ: Analytic Press.

Krug, R. (1989). Adult male report of childhood sexual abuse by mothers. *Child Abuse and Neglect, 13,* 111–119.

Krystal, H. (1975). Affect tolerance. *Annual of Psychoanalysis, 3,* 179–217.

Kupers, T. A. (1993). *Revisioning men's lives: Gender, intimacy, and power.* New York: Guilford Press.

Kwawer, J. (1980). Transference and countertransference in homosexuality: Changing psychoanalytic views. *American Journal of Psychotherapy, 34,* 72–80.

Lachmann, F. (1996). How many selves make a person? *Contemporary Psychoanalysis, 32,* 595–614.

Laing, R. D., and Esterson, A. (1964). *Sanity, madness, and the family.* New York: Basic Books.

Lesser, R. (1993). A reconsideration of homosexual themes. *Psychoanalytic Dialogues, 3,* 639–641.

Levant, R. F. (1990). Psychological services designed for men: A psychoeducational approach. *Psychotherapy, 27,* 309–315.

Levant, R. F. (1995). Toward the reconstruction of masculinity. In R. F. Levant and W. S. Pollack (Eds.), *A new psychology of men* (pp. 229–251). New York: Basic Books.

Levant, R. F., and Brooks, G. (Eds.). (1997). *Men and sex: New psychological perspectives.* New York: Wiley.

Levant, R. F., and Kopecky, G. (1995). *Masculinity reconstructed: Changing the rules of manhood—at work, in relationships, and in family life.* New York: Dutton.

Levant, R. F., and Pollack, W. S. (Eds.). (1995). *A new psychology of men.* New York: Basic Books.

LeVay, S. (1993). *The sexual brain.* Cambridge, MA: MIT Press.

Levesque, R. (1994). Sex differences in the experience of child sexual victimization. *Journal of Family Violence, 9,* 357–369.

Lew, M. (1988; 2nd ed., 1990). *Victims no longer.* New York: Harper and Row.

Lew, M. (1993, November 19). *Men recovering from childhood sexual abuse: Sexual abuse and chemical dependency.* Workshop jointly sponsored by the Learning Alliance and People Against Sexual Abuse, New York, NY.

Lewes, K. (1988). *The psychoanalytic theory of male homosexuality.* New York: Simon and Schuster.

Lichtenberger, B., and Buttenheim, M. (1998). Sexual orientation and family development: Introduction. *American Journal of Orthopsychiatry, 68,* 344–351.

Lindsay, D. S., and Read, J. D. (1994). Psychotherapy and memories of child sexual abuse: A cognitive perspective. *Applied Cognitive Psychology, 8,* 281–338.

Lionells, M. (1998, February). *What happens matters, and what really happened really matters.* Paper presented at "The Seduction Hypothesis One Hundred Years Later: Trauma, Fantasy, and Reality Today," a conference sponsored by the Symposium of the Journals of the PEP CD-ROM, New York, NY.

Lisak, D. (1993). Men as victims: Challenging cultural myths. *Journal of Traumatic Stress, 6,* 577–580.

Lisak, D. (1994, April 30). *Sexual abuse, gender, and male socialization: Research findings from the UMass study.* Presentation at "Men and Traumatic Life Experience: The Impact of Gender Identity and Socialization on How Males Cope with Psychological Trauma," a conference sponsored by the Trauma Clinic of The Erich Lindemann Mental Health Center, Boston, MA.

Lisak, D. (1995). Integrating a critique of gender in the treatment of male survivors of childhood abuse. *Psychotherapy, 32,* 258–269.

Lisak, D. (1998). Confronting and treating empathic disconnection in violent men. In W. S. Pollack and R. F. Levant (Eds.), *New psychotherapy for men* (pp. 215–236). New York: Wiley.

Lisak, D., Hopper, J., and Song, P. (1996). Factors in the cycle of violence: Gender rigidity and emotional constriction. *Journal of Traumatic Stress, 9,* 721–743.

Lisak, D., and Luster, L. (1994). Educational, occupational, and relationship histories of men who were sexually and/or physically abused as children. *Journal of Traumatic Stress, 7,* 507–523.

Lisman-Pieczanski, N. (1990). Countertransference in the analysis of an adult who was sexually abused as a child. In H. Levine (Ed.), *Adult analysis and childhood sexual abuse* (pp. 137–147). Hillsdale, NJ: Analytic Press.

Love, P. (1990). *The emotional incest syndrome.* New York: Bantam.

Lymberis, M. (1994). Boundary violations in psychotherapy: Sexual and nonsexual. In A. Sugarman (Ed.), *Victims of abuse: The emotional impact of child and adult trauma* (pp. 165–186). Madison, CT: International Universities Press.

MacIntosh, H. (1994). Attitudes and experiences of psychoanalysts in analyzing homosexual patients. *Journal of the American Psychoanalytic Association, 42,* 1183–1207.

Maddock, J. W., Larson, P. R., and Lally, C. F. (1991). An evaluation protocol for incest family functioning. In M. Q. Patton (Ed.), *Family sexual abuse* (pp. 162–177). Newbury Park, CA: Sage.

Madison, M. (1995, October 7). *The fragmented self: Understanding and working with the dissociative process in male survivors.* Workshop presented at the Sixth World Interdisciplinary Conference on Male Sexual Victimization, sponsored by the National Organization on Male Sexual Victimization, Columbus, OH.

Maletzky, B. M. (1991). *Treating the sexual offender.* Newbury Park, CA: Sage.

Maloney, B. (1995, October 7). *When the perpetrator is Mom.* Workshop presented at the Sixth World Interdisciplinary Conference on Male Sexual Victimization, sponsored by the National Organization on Male Sexual Victimization, Columbus, OH.

Maltz, W. (1991). *The sexual healing journey: A guide for survivors of sexual abuse.* New York: HarperCollins.

Marcuse, J. J. (1994, February). *Dissociation and enactment: Countertransference considerations in work with adult survivors of abuse.* Paper presented at the William Alanson White Institute Clinical Services Case Conference, New York, NY.

Margolis, M. (1977). A preliminary report of a case of consummated mother–son incest. *Annual of Psychoanalysis, 5,* 267–293.

Margolis, M. (1984). A case of mother–adolescent son incest. *Psychoanalytic Quarterly, 53,* 355–385.

Maroda, K (1991). *The power of countertransference.* New York: Wiley.

Martin, H. (1991). The coming-out process for homosexuals. *Hospital and Community Psychiatry, 42,* 158–162.

Marvesti, J. (1986). Incestuous mothers. *American Journal of Forensic Psychiatry, 7,* 63–69.

Mathews, R., Matthews, J., and Speltz, K. (1990). Female sexual offenders. In M. Hunter (Ed.), *The sexually abused male* (Vol. 1, pp. 275–293). Lexington, MA: Lexington Books.

May, R. (1995). Re-reading Freud on homosexuality. In T. Domenici and R. Lesser (Eds.), *Disorienting sexuality* (pp. 153–166). New York: Routledge.

McCann, I. L., and Pearlman, L. A. (1990). Vicarious traumatization: A framework for understanding the psychological effects of working with victims. *Journal of Traumatic Stress, 3,* 131–150.

Mendel, M. P. (1995). *The male survivor.* Thousand Oaks, CA: Sage.

Mennon, F., and Meadow, D. (1993). Process to recovery: In support of long-term groups for sexual abuse survivors. *International Journal of Group Psychotherapy, 42,* 29–44.

Mezey, G., and King, M. (Eds.). (1992). *Male victims of sexual assault.* Oxford, UK: Oxford University Press.

Miletski, H. (1997). *Mother–son incest: The unthinkable broken taboo.* Brandon, VT: Safer Society Press.

Minuchin, S., Montalvo, B., Guerney, B. G., Rosman, B. L., and Schumer, F. (1967). *Families of the slums.* New York: Basic Books.

Minuchin, S., Rosman, B., and Baker, L. (1978). *Psychosomatic families: Anorexia nervosa in context.* Cambridge, MA: Harvard University Press.

Mitchell, S. (1978). Psychodynamics, homosexuality, and the question of pathology. *Psychiatry, 41,* 254–263.

Mitchell, S. (1981). The psychoanalytic treatment of homosexuality: Some technical considerations. *International Review of Psycho-Analysis, 8,* 63–80.

Mitchell, S. (1992). True selves, false selves, and the ambiguity of authenticity. In N. J. Skolnick and S. C. Warshaw (Eds.), *Relational perspectives in psychoanalysis* (pp. 1–20). New York: Analytic Press.

Mitchell, S. (1993). *Hope and dread in psychoanalysis.* New York: Basic Books.

Mitchell, S. (1996). Gender and sexual orientation in the age of postmodernism: The plight of the perplexed clinician. *Gender and Psychoanalysis, 1,* 45–73.

Mitchell, S. (1998). Emergence of features of the analyst's life. *Psychoanalytic Dialogues, 8,* 187–194.

Monette, P. (1992). *Becoming a man.* New York: Harcourt Brace Jovanovich.

Money, J. (1988). *Gay, straight, and in-between: The sexology of erotic orientation.* New York: Oxford University Press.

Money, J., and Ehrhardt, A. A. (1972). *Man and woman, boy and girl.* Baltimore: Johns Hopkins University Press.

Morris, L. (1997). *The male heterosexual.* Thousand Oaks, CA: Sage.

Morris, L., Hunter, M., Struve, J., and Fitzgerald, R. (1997, September 18). *Everything you ever wanted to know about male survivors but were afraid to ask: Ask.* Workshop presented at the Seventh World Interdisciplinary Conference on Male Sexual Victimization, sponsored by the National Organization on Male Sexual Victimization, Orinda, CA.

Moss, D. (1992). Introductory thoughts: Hating in the first person plural: The example of homophobia. *American Imago, 49,* 277–291.

Mura, D. (1987). *A male grief: Notes on pornography and addiction.* Minneapolis, MN: Milkweed Editions.

Myers, M. (1989). Men sexually assaulted as adults and sexually abused as boys. *Archives of Sexual Behavior, 18,* 203–215.

Nasjleti, M. (1980). Suffering in silence: The male incest victim. *Child Welfare, 49,* 269–275.

Neilsen, T. (1983, November). Sexual abuse of boys: Current perspectives. *Personnel and Guidance Journal,* pp. 139–142.

Nelson, D., Higginson, G., and Grant-Worley, J. (1994). Using the risk behavior survey to estimate prevalence of sexual abuse among Oregon high school students. *Journal of School Health, 64,* 413–416.

Nicolosi, J. (1991). *Reparative therapy of male homosexuality: A new clinical approach.* Northvale, NJ: Aronson.

Olson, P. (1990). The sexual abuse of boys: A study of the long-term psychological effects. In M. Hunter (Ed.), *The sexually abused male* (Vol. 1, pp. 137–152). Lexington, MA: Lexington Books.

Parker, S. (1990). Healing abuse in gay men: The group component. In M. Hunter (Ed.), *The sexually abused male* (Vol. 2, pp. 177–198). Lexington, MA: Lexington Books.

Paul, D. (1994, August). *The psychoanalysis of dissociative states and self blame in victims of childhood sexual abuse.* Paper presented at the annual convention of the American Psychological Association, Los Angeles, CA.

Peake, A. (1989). Issues of under-reporting: The sexual abuse of boys. *Educational and Child Psychology, 6,* 42–50.

Pearlman, L. A., and Saakvitne, K. (1995). *Trauma and the therapist: Countertransference and vicarious traumatization in psychotherapy with incest survivors.* New York: Norton.

Perchuk, A., and Posner, H. (1995). *The masculine masquerade: Masculinity and representation.* Cambridge, MA: MIT Press.

Pescosolido, F. (1989). Sexual abuse of boys by males: Theoretical and treatment implications. In S. Sgroi (Ed.), *Vulnerable populations* (Vol. 2, pp. 85–109). Lexington, MA: Lexington Books.

Pierce, L. (1987). Father–son incest: Using the literature to guide practice. *Social Casework, 68,* 67–74.

Pierce, R., and Pierce, L. (1985). The sexually abused child: A comparison of male and female victims. *Child Abuse and Neglect, 9,* 191–199.

Piers, C. (1998). Contemporary trauma theory and its relation to character. *Psychoanalytic Psychology, 15,* 14–33.

Pizer, S. (1996a). The distributed self: Introduction to symposium on "The multiplicity of self and analytic technique." *Contemporary Psychoanalysis, 32,* 499–507.

Pizer, S. (1996b, October 16). *The capacity to tolerate paradox: Bridging multiplicity within the self.* Paper presented at the William Alanson White Psychoanalytic Society Scientific Program, New York, NY.

Pizer, S. (1998). *Building bridges: The negotiation of paradox in psychoanalysis.* Hillsdale, NJ: Analytic Press.

Pleck, J. H. (1981). *The myth of masculinity.* Cambridge, MA: MIT Press.

Pleck, J. H. (1995). The gender role strain paradigm: An update. In R. F. Levant and W. S. Pollack (Eds.), *A new psychology of men* (pp. 11–32). New York: Basic Books.

Pollack, W. S. (1990). Men's development and psychotherapy: A psychoanalytic perspective. *Psychotherapy, 27,* 316–321.

Pollack, W. S. (1995). No man is an island: Toward a new psychoanalytic psychology of men. In R. F. Levant and W. Pollack (Eds.), *A new psychology of men* (pp. 33–67). New York: Basic Books.

Pollack, W. S. (1998). *Real boys: Rescuing our sons from the myths of boyhood.* New York: Random House.

Porter, E. (1986). *Treating the young male victim of sexual assault.* Syracuse, NY: Safer Society Press.

Price, M. (1994). Incest: Transference and countertransference implications. *Journal of the American Academy of Psychoanalysis, 22,* 211–229.

Price, M. (1997). Knowing and not knowing: Paradox in the construction of historical narratives. In R. B. Gartner (Ed.), *Memories of sexual betrayal: Truth, fantasy, repression, and dissociation* (pp. 129–148). Northvale, NJ: Aronson.

Prince, M. (1890). Some of the revelations of hypnotism. Reprinted in N. G. Hale (Ed.), *Morton Prince: Psychotherapy and multiple personality: Selected essays.* Cambridge, MA: Harvard University Press, 1975.

Prince, M. (1905). *The dissociation of a personality.* New York: Longmans Green.

Putnam, F. (1989). *The diagnosis and treatment of multiple personality disorder.* New York: Guilford Press.

Putnam, F. (1992). Dissociative phenomena. *Review of Psychiatry, 10,* 145–160.

Real, T. (1994, April 30). *Wounded and wounding: Empathy and accountability in working with men.* Presentation at "Men and Traumatic Life Experience: The Impact of Gender Identity and Socialization on How Males Cope with Psychological Trauma," a conference sponsored by the Trauma Clinic of the Erich Lindemann Mental Health Center, Boston, MA.

Reinhart, M. (1987). Sexually abused boys. *Child Abuse and Neglect, 11,* 229–235.

Risin, L. I., and Koss, M. P. (1987). The sexual abuse of boys: Prevalence and descriptive characteristics of childhood victimizations. *Journal of Interpersonal Violence, 2,* 309–323.

Rivera, M. (1989). Linking the psychological and the social: Feminism, poststructuralism, and multiple personality. *Dissociation, 2,* 24–31.

Robertshaw, K. (1997, December 2). *Addictions in survivors of childhood trauma.* Presentation at the Eating Disorders and Substance Abuse Program Clinical Seminar, William Alanson White Institute, New York, NY.

Rosenberg, L. (1995, August). *Trauma with a difference: Abuse of gay and bisexual men.* Paper presented at the annual convention of the American Psychological Association, New York, NY.

Ross, C. (1989). *Multiple personality disorder: Diagnosis, clinical features, and treatment.* New York: Wiley.

Rothstein, A. (1979). Oedipal conflicts in narcissistic personality disorders. *International Journal of Psychoanalysis, 60,* 189–199.

Rusinoff, J., and Gerber, P. (1990). Crossing typological boundaries in treating the shame cycle. In M. Hunter (Ed.), *The sexually abused male* (Vol. 2, pp. 99–115). Lexington, MA: Lexington Books.

Russell, D. (1983). The incidence and prevalence of intrafamilial and extrafamilial sexual abuse of female children. *Child Abuse and Neglect, 7,* 133–146.

Russell, D. (1984). *Sexual exploitation: Rape, child sexual abuse, and workplace harassment.* Beverly Hills, CA: Sage.

Russell, D. (1986). *The secret trauma: Incest in the lives of girls and women.* New York: Basic Books.

Russell, M. (1995). *Confronting abusive beliefs: Group treatment for abusive men.* Thousand Oaks, CA: Sage.

Ryan, M. (1995). *Secret life.* New York: Vintage.

Saigh, P. (Ed.). (1992). *Posttraumatic stress disorder: A behavioral approach to assessment and treatment.* Needham Heights, MA: Allyn and Bacon.

Salter, A. (1995). *Transforming trauma.* Thousand Oaks, CA: Sage.

Sanders, T. (1991). *Male survivors: Twelve-step recovery program for survivors of childhood sexual abuse.* Freedom, CA: Crossing Press.

Sanderson, C. (1990). *Counselling adult survivors of child sexual abuse.* London: Jessica Kingsley.

Sands, S. (1994). What is dissociated? *Dissociation, 7,* 145–152.

Sarrel, P. M., and Masters, W. H. (1982). The sexual molestation of men by women. *Archives of Sexual Behavior, 2,* 117–131.

Scarce, M. (1997). *Male on male rape: The hidden toll of stigma and shame.* New York: Insight Books (Plenum Press).

Schafer, R. (1995). The evolution of my views on nonnormative sexual practices. In T. Domenici and R. Lesser (Eds.), *Disorienting sexuality* (pp. 187–202). New York: Routledge.

Schwartz, D. (1993). Heterophilia—The love that dare not speak its aim. *Psychoanalytic Dialogues, 3,* 643–652.

Schwartz, D. (1995). Current psychoanalytic discourses about sexuality: Tripping over the body. In T. Domenici and R. Lesser (Eds.), *Disorienting sexuality* (pp. 115–126). New York: Routledge.

Schwartz, D. (1996). Questioning the social construction of gender and sexual orientation. *Gender and Psychoanalysis, 1,* 249–260.

Schwartz, H. L. (1994). From dissociation to negotiation: A relational psychoanalytic perspective on multiple personality disorder. *Psychoanalytic Psychology, 11,* 189–231.

Schwartz, M. (1998, March 20). *Development of the capacity for intimacy and bonding.* Presentation at "Trauma and Intimacy: Self/Other Adaptations," a conference sponsored by the Masters and Johnson Treatment Programs at River Oaks Hospital, New York, NY.

Schwartz, M., Galperin, L., and Masters, W. (1995a). Sexual trauma within the context of traumatic and inesapable stress, neglect, and poisonous pedagogy. In M. Hunter (Ed.), *Adult survivors of sexual abuse: Treatment innovations* (pp. 1–17). Thousand Oaks, CA: Sage.

Schwartz, M., Galperin, L., and Masters, W. (1995b). Dissociation and treatment of compulsive reenactment of trauma: Sexual compulsivity. In M. Hunter (Ed.), *Adult survivors of sexual abuse: Treatment innovations* (pp. 42–55). Thousand Oaks, CA: Sage.

Sebold, J. (1987). Indicators of child sexual abuse in males. *Social Casework, 68,* 75–80.

Sedgwick, E. K. (1990). *Epistemology of the closet.* Berkeley and Los Angeles: University of California Press.

Selvini Palozzoli, M., Boscolo, L., Cecchin, G., and Prata, G. (1978). *Paradox and counterparadox.* New York: Aronson.

Sepler, F. (1990). Victim advocacy and young male victims of sexual abuse: An evolutionary model. In M. Hunter (Ed.), *The sexually abused male* (Vol. 1, pp. 73–85). Lexington, MA: Lexington Books.

Sgroi, S. (1989). Stages of recovery for adult survivors of child sexual abuse. In S. Sgroi (Ed.), *Vulnerable populations* (Vol. 2, pp. 111–130). Lexington, MA: Lexington Books.

Shapiro, S. (1993). Gender role stereotypes and two person psychology. *Psychoanalytic Dialogues, 3,* 371–388.

Shapiro, S. (1994, April). *Discussion: Issues for male analysts working with survivors of sexual abuse.* Discussion of a panel presented at the spring meeting of Division 39 (Psychoanalysis) of the American Psychological Association, Washington, DC.

Shapiro, S. (1997). Makes me want to shout. In R. B. Gartner (Ed.), *Memories of sexual betrayal: Truth, fantasy, repression, and dissociation* (pp. 95–110). Northvale, NJ: Aronson.

Shengold, L. (1980). Some reflections on a case of mother–adolescent son incest. *International Journal of Psycho-Analysis, 61,* 461–475.

Shengold, L. (1989). *Soul murder.* New York: Fawcett Columbine.

Siegel, E. V. (1996). *Transformations: Countertransference during the psychoanalytic treatment of incest, real and imagined.* Hillsdale, NJ: Analytic Press.

Silber, A. (1979). Childhood seduction, parental pathology and hysterical symptomatology: The genesis of altered states of consciousness. *International Journal of Psycho-Analysis, 60,* 109–116.

Silverstein, O., and Rashbaum, B. (1994). *The courage to raise good men.* New York: Penguin.

Simari, C. G., and Baskin, D. (1982). Incestuous experiences within homosexual populations: A preliminary study. *Archives of Sexual Behavior, 11,* 329–344.

Simon, B. (1992). "Incest—see under Oedipus complex": The history of an error in psychoanalysis. *Journal of the American Psychoanalytic Association, 40,* 955–988.

Singer, E. (1968). The reluctance to interpret. In E. Hammer (Ed.), *Use of interpretation in treatment* (pp. 364–371). New York: Grune and Stratton.

Singer, J. (Ed.). (1990). *Repression and dissociation: Implications for personality, psychopathology, and health.* Chicago: University of Chicago Press.

Singer, K. (1989). Group work with men who experienced incest in childhood. *American Journal of Orthopsychiatry, 59,* 468–472.

Singer, K. (n. d.). Characteristics observed in male sexual abuse victims. National Organization on Male Sexual Victimization Web Page (www.malesurvivor.org).

Slavin, J. (1997). Memory, dissociation, and agency in sexual abuse. In R. B. Gartner (Ed.), *Memories of sexual betrayal: Truth, fantasy, repression, and dissociation* (pp. 221–236). Northvale, NJ: Aronson.

Slavin, J., and Pollock, L. (1997). The poisoning of desire: The destruction of agency and the recovery of psychic integrity in sexual abuse. *Contemporary Psychoanalysis, 33,* 573–593.

Smith, S. (1984). The sexually abused patient and the abusing therapist: A study in sadomasochistic relationships. *Psychoanalytic Psychology, 1,* 89–98.

Socarides, C. (1968). *The overt homosexual.* New York: Grune and Stratton.

Socarides, C. (1978). *Homosexuality.* New York: Aronson.

Socarides, C. (1995). *Homosexuality: A freedom too far.* Phoenix, AZ: Adam Margrave Books.

Spiegel, D. (1990). Trauma, dissociation, and hypnosis. In R. Kluft (Ed.), *Incest-related syndromes of adult psychopathology* (pp. 247–261). Washington, DC: American Psychiatric Press.

Sprei, J. E. (1987). Group treatment of adult women incest survivors. In C. M. Brody (Ed.), *Women's therapy groups: Paradigms of feminist treatment* (pp. 198–216). New York: Springer.

Stanton, A. (1973, September). *Orientation talk for psychology interns.* McLean Hospital, Belmont, MA.

Steele, B. (1981). Long-term effects of sexual abuse in childhood. In P. Mrazek and C. Kempe (Eds.), *Sexually abused children and their families* (pp. 223–234). New York: Pergamon Press.

Steele, B. (1990). Some sequelae of the sexual maltreatment of children. In H. Levine (Ed.), *Adult analysis and childhood sexual abuse* (pp. 21–34). Hillsdale, NJ: Analytic Press.

Steele, B. (1991). The psychopathology of incest participants. In S. Kramer and S. Akhtar (Eds.), *The trauma of transgression* (pp. 13–37). Northvale, NJ: Aronson.

Steele, K., and Colrain, J. (1990). Abreactive work with sexual abuse survivors: Concepts and techniques. In M. Hunter (Ed.), *The sexually abused male* (Vol. 2, pp. 1–55). Lexington, MA: Lexington Books.

Stern, D. (1983). Unformulated experience. *Contemporary Psychoanalysis, 19,* 71–99.

Stern, D. (1987). Unformulated experience and transference. *Contemporary Psychoanalysis, 23,* 484–491.

Stern, D. (1989). The analyst's unformulated experience of the patient. *Contemporary Psychoanalysis, 25,* 1–33.

Stern, D. (1997). *Unformulated experience: From dissociation to imagination in psychoanalysis.* Mahwah, NJ: Analytic Press.

Stoller, R. J. (1968). *Sex and gender.* New York: Aronson.

Stoller, R. J. (1973). Facts and fancies: An examination of Freud's concept of bisexuality. In J. Strouse (Ed.), *Women and analysis* (pp. 343–364). Boston: Hall, 1985.

Stoller, R. J. (1985). *Presentations of gender.* New Haven, CT: Yale University Press.

Stoltenberg, J. (1993). *The end of manhood.* New York: Plume.

Sugarman, A. (1994). Trauma and abuse: An overview. In A. Sugarman (Ed.), *Victims of abuse* (pp. 1–21). Madison, CT: International Universities Press.

Sullivan, H. S. (1953). *The interpersonal theory of psychiatry.* New York: Norton.

Sullivan, H. S. (1956). *Clinical studies in psychiatry.* New York: Norton.

Tauber, E. S. (1954). Exploring the therapeutic use of countertransference data. *Psychiatry, 17,* 331–336.

Thomas, T. (1989). *Men surviving incest.* Walnut Creek, CA: Launch Press.

Thompson, S. (1988). Child sexual abuse redefined: Impact of modern culture on the sexual mores of the Yuit Eskimo. In S. Sgroi (Ed.), *Vulnerable populations* (Vol. 1, pp. 299–308). Lexington, MA: Lexington Books.

Urquiza, A., and Capra, M. (1990). The impact of sexual abuse: Initial and longterm effects. In M. Hunter (Ed.), *The sexually abused male* (Vol. 1, p. 105–136). Lexington, MA: Lexington Books.

Urquiza, A., and Keating, L. M. (1990). The prevalence of sexual victimization in males. In M. Hunter (Ed.), *The sexually abused male* (Vol. 1, pp. 89–104). Lexington, MA: Lexington Books.

van der Kolk, B. (Ed.). (1987). *Psychological trauma.* Washington: American Psychiatric Press.

van der Kolk, B. (1995). The body, memory, and the psychobiology of trauma. In J. Alpert (Ed.), *Sexual abuse recalled* (pp. 29–60). Northvale, NJ: Aronson.

van der Kolk, B. (1996). The body keeps the score: Approaches to the psychobiology of posttraumatic stress disorder. In B. van der Kolk, A. McFarlane, and L. Weisaeth (Eds.), *Traumatic stress: The effects of overwhelming experience on mind, body, and society* (pp. 217–241). New York: Guilford Press.

van der Kolk, B., and Greenberg, M. (1987). The psychobiology of the trauma response: Hyperarousal, constriction, and addiction to traumatic reexposure. In B. van der Kolk (Ed.), *Psychological trauma* (pp. 63–87). Washington: American Psychiatric Press.

van der Kolk, B., McFarlane, A., and Weisaeth, L. (Eds.). (1996). *Traumatic stress: The effects of overwhelming experience on mind, body, and society.* New York: Guilford Press.

Vander Mey, B. (1988). The sexual victimization of male children: A review of previous research. *Child Abuse and Neglect, 12,* 61–72.

Vasington, M. (1989). Sexual offenders as victims: Implications for treatment and the therapeutic relationship. In S. Sgroi (Ed.), *Vulnerable populations* (Vol. 2, pp. 329–350). Lexington, MA: Lexington Books.

Violato, C., and Genuis, M. (1993). Problems in research in male child sexual abuse: A review. *Journal of Child Sexual Abuse, 2,* 33–54.

Watkins, B., and Bentovin, A. (1992). Male children and adolescents as victims: A review of current knowledge. In G. Mezey and M. King (Eds.), *Male victims of sexual assault* (pp. 27–66). Oxford, UK: Oxford University Press.

Watzlawick P., Weakland, J., and Fisch, R. (1974). *Change: Principles of problem formation and problem resolution.* New York: Norton.

Weeks, J. (1985). *Sexuality and its discontents: Meanings, myths, and modern sexualities.* London: Routledge and Kegan Paul.

Welldon, E. V. (1988). *Mother, madonna, whore: The idealization and denigration of motherhood.* New York: Columbia University Press.

Wiedemann, G. (1962). Survey of psychoanalytic literature on overt male homosexuality. *Journal of the American Psychoanalytic Association, 10,* 386–409.

Wiehe, V. (1996). *The brother–sister hurt: Recognizing the effects of sibling abuse.* Brandon, VT: Safer Society Press.

Williams, L. M. (1994). Recall of childhood trauma: A prospective study of women's memories of child sexual abuse. *Journal of Consulting and Clinical Psychology, 62,* 1167–1176.

Winnicott, D. W. (1949). Hate in the countertransference. *International Journal of Psychoanalysis, 30,* 69–74.

Winnicott, D. W. (1960). Ego distortion in terms of the true and false self. In D. W. Winnicott, *Maturational processes and the facilitating environment* (pp. 179–192). Madison, CT: International Universities Press, 1965.

Wolstein, B. (1954). *Transference.* New York: Grune and Stratton.

Wolstein, B. (1959). *Countertransference* New York: Grune and Stratton.

Wolstein, B. (Ed.). (1988). *Essential papers on countertransference.* New York: New York University Press.

Wright, D. (1995). Acknowledging the continuum from childhood abuse to male prostitution. *British Columbia Institute on Family Violence Journal, 4,* 7–8.

Wright, D. (1997a, September 19). *Homophobia: The socially embedded barrier to recovery.* Workshop presented at the Seventh World Interdisciplinary Conference on Male Sexual Victimization, sponsored by the National Organization on Male Sexual Victimization, Orinda, CA.

Wright, D. (1997b, September 20). *Socialized denial of male sexual victimization and its impact on disclosure and recovery.* Workshop presented at the Seventh World Interdisciplinary Conference on Male Sexual Victimization, sponsored by the National Organization on Male Sexual Victimization, Orinda, CA.

Wyatt, G. (1985). The sexual abuse of Afro-American and white women in childhood. *Child Abuse and Neglect, 9,* 507–519.

Yalom, I. (1975). *The theory and practice of group psychotherapy.* New York: Basic Books.

Zhang, S.-D., and Odenwald, W. F. (1995). Misexpression of the white (w) gene triggers male–male courtship in *Drosophilia. Proceedings of the National Academy of Sciences, USA, 92,* 5525–5529.

Index